ANNUAL REVIEW OF NURSING RESEARCH

Volume 16, 1998

ANNUAL REVIEW OF NURSING RESEARCH

Volume 16, 1998

Focus on
Heath Issues in Pediatric Nursing

Joyce J. Fitzpatrick, PhD

Editor

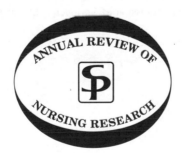

 SPRINGER PUBLISHING COMPANY

New York

Order ANNUAL REVIEW OF NURSING RESEARCH, Volume 17, 1999, prior to publication and receive a 10% discount. An order coupon can be found at the back of this volume.

Copyright © 1998 by Springer Publishing Company, Inc.

Springer Publishing Company, Inc.
536 Broadway
New York, NY 10012

98 99 00 01 02 / 5 4 3 2 1

ISBN-0-8261-8235-6
ISSN-0739-6686

ANNUAL REVIEW OF NURSING RESEARCH is indexed in *Cumulative Index to Nursing and Allied Health Literature* and *Index Medicus*.

Printed in the United States of America.

Contents

Preface

The *Annual Review of Nursing Research* (ARNR) series is now in its sixteenth volume. As the series has progressed, so has nursing research. Thus, we are now in a position to more specifically target each volume, particularly in relation to the clinical nursing research section. With each volume we have witnessed the narrowing of research topics, just as the field of nursing research has become more precise.

Volume 16 includes eight chapters in the area of nursing practice and three chapters in the area of nursing care delivery. The theme of the volume is health promotion and disease prevention, particularly among the vulnerable populations of children/adolescents and the elderly. In keeping with this focus, the majority of chapters are targeted toward nursing research related to health promotion.

In chapter 1, Christine Kennedy explores the research on childhood nutrition. Next, Kathleen Long and David Williams review the research on health care for the school-aged child, and Patricia Brandt discusses behavioral research on childhood diabetes. In chapter 4, Susan Kools describes research focused on prevention of mental health problems in adolescence. Then, in chapter 5, Rosemary Jadack and Mary Keller discuss sexual risk taking and development in adolescence. In chapter 6, Nola Pender reviews research related to motivations for health behaviors. In chapter 7, Susan Heidrich reviews research on health promotion in old age. Barbara and Charles Given describe research on promoting health for family caregivers, In the nursing care delivery section, Paulette Hoyer describes research on programs for adolescent mothers.

In addition to the above chapters on health-promotion programs, there are two chapters in the Other Research section. Janet Larson and Nancy Kline Leidy review research on chronic obstructive pulmonary disease and Jeanne Fox and Catherine Kane describe research on schizophrenia.

As we approach the second half of the second decade of the ARNR series, we welcome topic suggestions from readers, and invite submissions by authors who are expert researchers in their content area.

As with any major publication of this magnitude, producing this volume requires a team effort. In particular, I would like to acknowledge the work of Laree Moser Schoolmeesters, PhD student at Case Western Reserve University, for her monumental efforts on this project. In addition, the Advisory Board members, chapter reviewers, and authors are thanked for their continuing contributions to the discipline.

Joyce J. Fitzpatrick
Editor

Contributors

Patricia Brandt, PhD
School of Nursing
University of Washington
Seattle, Washington

Jeanne C. Fox, PhD
SE Rural Mental Health Research
    Center
School of Nursing
University of Virginia
Charlottesville, Virginia

Barbara A. Given, PhD
College of Nursing
Michigan State University
East Lansing, Michigan

Charles W. Given, PhD
College of Human Medicine
Michigan State University
East Lansing, Michigan

Susan M. Heidrich, PhD
School of Nursing
University of Wisconsin—
    Milwaukee
Milwaukee, Wisconsin

Paulette J. Perrone Hoyer, PhD
College of Nursing
Wayne State University
Detroit, Michigan

Rosemary A. Jadack, PhD
College of Nursing
The Ohio State University
Columbus, Ohio

Catherine F. Kane, PhD
SE Rural Mental Health Research
    Center
School of Nursing
University of Virginia
Charlottesville, Virginia

Mary L. Keller, PhD
School of Nursing
University of
    Wisconsin—Madison
Madison, Wisconsin

Christine M. Kennedy, PhD
School of Nursing
University of California—
    San Francisco
San Francisco, California

Susan Kools, PhD
School of Nursing
University of California—
    San Francisco
San Francisco, California

Janet L. Larson, PhD
College of Nursing
University of Illinois at Chicago
Chicago, Illinois

Nancy Kline Leidy, PhD
Health Outcomes Research
MEDTAP International, Inc.
Bethesda, Maryland

Kathleen Ann Long, PhD
College of Nursing
University of Florida
Gainesville, Florida

Nola J. Pender, PhD
School of Nursing
University of Michigan
Ann Arbor, Michigan

David Williams, PhD
College of Nursing
University of Florida
Gainesville, Florida

Forthcoming

ANNUAL REVIEW OF
NURSING RESEARCH, Volume 17

Tentative Contents

PART I

Health Promotion Across the Life Span

Chapter 1

Childhood Nutrition

CHRISTINE M. KENNEDY
SCHOOL OF NURSING
UNIVERSITY OF CALIFORNIA—SAN FRANCISCO

ABSTRACT

This review focuses on the research in normative nutrition for children aged 2 to 12, published from 1985 to 1996. The chapter uses a primary prevention framework and the *Healthy People 2000* (Public Health Service, 1990) objectives to identify and review those areas relevant for childhood health promotion and nursing practice. Current research demonstrates that food intake in early childhood is causally linked to health-related problems later in life, therefore obesity and cardiovascular research are highlighted in this review. Environmental and societal factors affect the nutritional health of children, thus the contribution of the media, poverty, cultural, and family practices are also reviewed. The chapter concludes with a summary of strengths and weaknesses of the body of research and suggestions for a nursing agenda in the area of childhood nutrition.

Keywords: Cardiovascular Health, Diet, Eating Behavior, Family Intervention, Food Attitudes, Health-Promotion Models, *Healthy People 2000*, Hispanic, Homelessness, Malnutrition, Nutritional Status, Obesity, Poverty, Television

This review is focused on the research on normative nutrition in children aged 2 to 12, published from 1985 to 1996. Normative nutrition was defined here on the basis of a review of the nutritional status of children in the United States today and on current governmental and policy recommendations, such as *Healthy People 2000* (Public Health Service, 1990). Unfortunately, approximately a fourth of the children in the United States are living in poverty, which translates into a normative risk for malnutrition among many children.

Diet is a known risk factor for the development of the nation's three leading causes of death by disease: coronary heart disease, cancer, and stroke; diet is also a factor in diabetes, high blood pressure, overweight, and osteoporosis (Centers for Disease Control [CDC], 1996). Better control of a limited number of risk factors, diet, exercise, and the use of tobacco, alcohol, and other drugs, could prevent at least 40% of all premature deaths, a third of all short-term disability cases, and two thirds of all chronic disability cases (National Commission on Children, 1991). Current research demonstrates that food intake in early childhood is causally linked to health-related problems later in life. Concern about dietary intake therefore is not limited to adults, and diet is being targeted by pediatric health care providers for early intervention.

Research was sought on the environmental and social factors affecting the nutritional health of children, including the media, which influence food attitudes, eating behavior, and body image. The research reviewed also included investigations of the role of parents and other family members in forming dietary habits and changing the eating behaviors of children.

The best age at which to lay the groundwork and to intervene in children's eating behavior patterns was also considered using Bloom's (1996) primary prevention framework. Research has demonstrated that children develop life-long habits and attitudes during the period of dependence, and by late childhood (9 to 11 years of age) many of these learned behaviors and attitudes are already formed, suggesting that interventions would be best timed for the 3- to 8-year-old age range (Bush & Iannotti, 1988; Farrand & Cox, 1993; Gochman, 1985; K. E. Green & Bird, 1986; Mechanic, 1979; Radius, Dillman, & Becker, 1980).

The literature search for the review was conducted using a variety of data collection techniques. Online computer searches of the MEDLINE, Psychological Abstracts Information Services, and the Cumulative Index to Nursing and Allied Health Literature (CINAHL) databases yielded most of the studies reviewed. These databases provided some unique and overlapping references. Relevant citations were pulled from certain articles using the ancestry approach, and some citations were obtained through informal sharing among faculty and student colleagues. The search was limited to U.S.-authored literature with a few Canadian and British sources. In reviewing the research, we originally scanned all author credentials for a nursing affiliation. Then, because of the relative lack of nursing-authored research in this area, the review was expanded to include child nutrition research of other disciplines relevant to nursing practice in primary care. In total over 943 citations were obtained and 93 research articles reviewed. Studies were reviewed for prevention area, subject source, intervention characteristics, and use of theoretical models. Eighty studies met criteria for relevance and scientific acceptability.

Because of the health promotion framework used for this review, research on the nutritional needs of children with chronic illnesses or those coping with life-threatening conditions was not included. Recognizing the special nutritional needs of children in the ages of dependence and interdependence, adolescence was not reviewed unless specific links were made to earlier childhood issues. Also not addressed were the needs of premature or full-term infants. The author recognizes that there is a wealth of nursing-authored research on infancy, especially in areas such as breast-feeding, neonatal sucking behaviors (Gill, Behnke, Conlon, & Anderson, 1992; C. Kennedy & Lipsitt, 1993; Kinneer & Beachy, 1994; McCain, 1995; Medoff-Cooper, 1991; Medoff-Cooper & Gennaro, 1996; Medoff-Cooper, Weininger, & Zukowsky, 1989; Meier & Anderson, 1987; H. D. Miller & Anderson, 1993; Siddell & Froman, 1994; Swartz, Moody, Yarandi, & Anderson, 1987; Weaver & Anderson, 1988), and the area of nutritional delivery and nursing techniques such as parenteral and enteral feeding (for reviews see Bodkin & Hansen, 1991; Moore, Guenter, & Bender, 1986).

STATUS OF NUTRITION IN AMERICAN CHILDREN

U.S. children, like their parents, consume large amounts of dietary fat, cholesterol, sodium, and sugar. Surveys suggested that children rarely consume vegetables and fruits, have low fiber intake, consume large amounts of refined carbohydrates, and drink soft drinks or whole milk (high in saturated fat); favorite "junk" foods account for various nutritional problems (Saltz et al., 1983; Tell, 1982). Fewer than 20% of children consume the recommended number of servings of grains, vegetables and fruits, and less than one third eat the suggested number of servings from the milk or meat group (E. Kennedy, 1996).

In developing this review, the *Healthy Children 2000: National Health Promotion and Disease Prevention Objectives* (U.S. Department of Health and Human Services [USDHHS], 1990) was consulted. This included 21 nutrition objectives, 8 of which contain specific provisions for children and adolescents (USDHHS, 1990). Mid-decade data were derived from *Healthy People 2000 Review, 1994* (National Center for Health Statistics, 1995). Some of these objectives address ongoing concerns about adequate nutrient intakes of children. Objective 2.4 proposes a reduction in growth retardation among low-income children (5 years and younger) caused by inadequate nutrient/

caloric intake to less than 10%. Baseline in 1987 was 16% and 1992 middecade data showed an overall decrease to 8%. With the dismantling of federal health and nutrition programs during the mid 1990s, however, it is not clear whether this positive trend will continue; this will need monitoring by child advocates. Calcium intake has still not reached adequate levels; Objective 28 (revised in 1995) recommends an increase in calcium intake so that youth aged 11 to 24 years would have 1,200 mg of calcium for the recommended dietary allowance. From 1989 to 1991, only about half of children aged 2 to 10 met the average daily goal of two or more servings of milk and milk products. The National Health and Nutrition Examination Survey (NHANES II, 1976–1980) baseline found a 10% to 21% iron deficiency among low-income children, but no interim report has been published (Yip, Binkin, Fleshood, & Trowbridge, 1987). Objective 2.10 proposes a reduction in iron deficiency to less than 3% among children aged 1 to 4 years.

There is a growing focus on other dietary components, especially saturated fat, sodium, and cholesterol and a related health outcome: adolescent obesity. Objective 2.3 aims to keep obesity among adolescents (12 to 19 years) at no more than 15%. NHANES II estimates were 15%; 1988 to 1991 data showed that adolescent obesity actually increased to 21%. Objective 2.5 calls for a reduction in total dietary fat to 30% of calories among people aged 2 years and over. In 1992, 34% of caloric intake for the population as a whole was from total fat, which is a slight decrease from the 1987 baseline of 36%.

A few of the objectives address the fact that children from all socioeconomic levels are spending a greater part of their day away from home, as do parents, and they are eating away from home at day care centers, (pre)schools, and restaurants. Nutritional interventions, guidelines, and research sites are therefore expanding to include new providers. Objective 2.17 proposes that the proportion of school lunches and breakfasts serve menus consistent with nutrition principles in the "Dietary Guidelines for Americans" (DGA) should increase to at least 90% (U.S. Department of Agriculture & USDHHS, 1990). Only 1% of school lunches and 44% of school breakfasts were consistent with the Dietary Guidelines for total fat in 1992. Objective 2.19 calls for the proportion of the nation's schools that provide nutrition education from preschool through grade 12, preferably as part of school health education, to increase to at least 75%. Data from 1991 show that 60% of schools provided nutrition education.

Objective 2.16 calls for an increase to 90% in the proportion of restaurants and institutional food service operations that offer identifiable low-fat, low-calorie food choices consistent with the DGA. The proportion of restaurants offering at least one low-fat, low-calorie food choice increased from 70% in 1989 to 75% in 1990 according to a National Restaurant Association Survey

(USDHHS, 1996). More processed foods with reduced fat are available in supermarkets; the number of such products increased from 2,500 in 1986 to 5,600 in 1991 (USDHHS, 1996).

Healthy People 2000 Objective 2.21 calls for an increase to at least 75% in the proportion of primary care providers who provide nutrition assessment, counseling, and/or referral to qualified nutritionists or dietitians. In 1988 physicians reported providing diet counseling to approximately 40% to 50% of patients (C. E. Lewis, 1988). Studies of pediatricians range from those who report giving relatively little dietary advice to patients who reported giving such advice (Nader, Taras, Sallis, & Patterson, 1987) to over 53% (Office of Disease Prevention and Health Promotion, 1992). The 1992 Primary Care Provider Survey also reported that 46% of nurse practitioners inquired about their patients' diet/nutrition and 31% formulated a diet/nutrition plan with patients.

THEORETICAL MODELS USED IN CHILDHOOD NUTRITION RESEARCH

Primary prevention, as framed by Bloom (1996), is "coordinated actions seeking to prevent predictable problems, to protect existing states of health and healthy functioning, and to promote desired potentialities in individuals and groups in their physical and sociocultural settings over time" (p. 2). Other theories and models used in primary prevention include the health belief model (Rosenstock, Strecher, & Becker, 1990), the health promotion model (Ponder, 1982), the theory of reasoned action (Fishbein & Ajzan, 1975), the social stress approach (Bloom, 1996), social learning theory (Bandura, 1986), and Caplan's recurrent themes model of primary prevention (Caplan, 1989). Nutrition research typically has emanated from either the public health domain (e.g., supplementation programs) or the biomedical model of disease treatment (e.g., diagnosis and treatment of specific nutrient deficiencies), however. The first of these approaches has led to national education efforts targeted primarily to food labeling and development of dietary guidelines and their public usage (e.g., Food Guide Pyramid). The second approach has contributed to viewing nutrition from the perspective of pathology and has led to the overmedicalization of contemporary nutrition issues.

In the studies reviewed for this chapter, many researchers used a biomedical model, though this was often implicit rather than articulated. More interesting theoretical models were used by those studying nutrition and health-promoting interventions. Such interventions are sometimes directed toward the individual but are most effective when they also address the influences of family and other factors on a child's eating behavior. In the research reviewed, these factors were addressed using a variety of models, most commonly social learning theory or a variation of it, to guide the intervention and inquiry. According to social learning theory (Bandura, 1986), behaviors are acquired through transactions between the child and social models and eating is influenced by three types of factors: individual, environmental, and behavioral. Social learning theory and theories of organizational change have been used to create programs directed toward improving nutrition in schools (Parcel et al., 1987, 1995; Stone, Perry, & Luepker, 1989). School-based intervention studies based on social learning theory have been supported by the National Heart, Lung, and Blood Institute (NHLBI). The health belief model has also guided nutrition interventions in combination with social learning theory (Walter, Hofman, Vaughan, & Wynder, 1988).

A few of the studies reviewed used an implicit, undefined family-based theory as the rationale for involving both parents and children in interventions. Social cognitive theory identified self-efficacy as the pivotal construct in understanding and modifying human behaviors such as dietary intake (Nader, 1993). Reciprocal determinism derived from social cognitive theory was used to frame an understanding of the interaction of the environment, caregivers' personal factors, and behavior and their combined influence on a child's eating behavior (Crockett, Mullis, & Perry, 1988; Domel et al., 1993). Drawing on nursing theory, Orem's (1980) self-care model has been used to construct research into a mother's knowledge, practices, and values and their effects on her child's eating and weight (Blank & Alexander, 1988). The American Cancer Society's "Changing the Course" nutrition curriculum used the PRECEDE model (predisposing, reinforcing, and enabling constructs in educational diagnosis and evaluation), derived from public health, using behavioral-change processes to identify predisposing factors (knowledge, beliefs, attitudes), enabling factors (e.g., skills), and reinforcing factors (rewards, support from family and peers) to evaluate nutrition education programs (L. W. Green, Kreuter, Deeds, & Partridge, 1980).

PROMOTION OF CARDIOVASCULAR HEALTH

Cardiovascular health has received the most attention by researchers in the past several years. Coronary heart disease is the leading cause of death by disease in the United States. Dietary risk factors such as high cholesterol, high blood pressure, and obesity can all be reduced by consuming less (saturated) fat and cholesterol and by increasing physical activity. Thirty to 60% of school-age youth are now estimated to have one or more risk factors associated with heart disease: obesity, high blood pressure, high cholesterol, sedentary lifestyle, cigarette smoking, or diabetes (Department of Health, Education, and Welfare, 1979; Lauer, Connor, Leaverton, Reiter, & Clarke, 1975; Oganov, Tubol, Zhukovskii, Perova, & Ilchenko, 1988; Rabbia et al., 1994; Wheeler, Marcus, Cullen, & Konugres, 1983; Wilmore & McNamara, 1974). This overall prevalence rate is similar to estimates from other industrialized countries, where these risk factors range from 25% to 65%.

Studies of cardiovascular-related health questions have ranged from the role of specific nutrients to the relationships between variables such as exercise and personality profiles. In nursing, Hayman's (Hayman, 1988; Hayman, Meininger, Coates, & Gallagher, 1995; Hayman, Meininger, Gallagher, & Chandler, 1992; Hayman, Meininger, Stashinko, Gallagher, & Coates, 1988; Hayman & Ryan, 1991, 1994; Hayman, Weill, Tobias, Stashinko, & Meininger, 1988a, 1988b; Meininger, Hayman, Coates, & Gallagher, 1988; Meininger, Hayman, Gallagher, & Coates, 1992; Meininger, Stashinko, & Hayman, 1991; Shamir et al., 1996) program of research has been focused on biobehavioral risk factors for cardiovascular disease in childhood and adolescence and the promotion of cardiovascular health in early childhood. Her research team at the University of Pennsylvania identified both physiologic and behavioral nongenetic influences through rigorous longitudinal twin cohort studies using sophisticated methods and analyses. The investigators identified factors in two age groups (school age and adolescence) that are essential groups for primary prevention of cardiovascular disease (CVD). In particular the Hayman group delineated the role that obesity–lipid associations play in CVD risk profiles and the implications for primary care. Further, they contributed some controversial developmental findings with their study of Type A behavior in school-age twin children. They suggest that a global Type A personality may not be indicative of cardiovascular risk, but rather suppression of impatient-aggressive emotions may selectively contribute to activation of neuroendocrine processes. A limitation acknowledged by this group is that their samples have consisted only of White middle-class children.

Obesity in childhood continues to increase yearly, despite a national obsession with thinness. Conservative estimates now suggest that approximately 20% to 30% of children are overweight and sedentary. Ten years ago Gortmaker, Dietz, Sobol, and Wehler (1987), using triceps skinfold data from the NHANES II, documented that the prevalence of obesity and superobesity had increased over the previous 2 decades between 17% and 306% depending on age, sex, and race. Their landmark study also revealed that not only were children getting fatter, but the fatter ones were becoming more obese. Data from the NHANES III (1988 to 1994) clearly indicates a dramatic increase again during the past decade (CDC, 1994, 1997). The increased prevalence is evident among all sex and age groups regardless of whether overweight was defined as a body mass index (BMI) exceeding the 85th or 95th percentile. Using the 85 percentile for all race–ethnic groups combined, the prevalence is now 22% (Troiano et al., 1995).

Research has generally pursued issues of obesity and cholesterol as singular variables amenable to prevention or intervention. Yet over 10 years ago the National Children and Youth Fitness Studies, which included 8,800 students, revealed that half of the students did not engage in sufficient physical activity to maintain effective cardiovascular functioning (Ross & Gilbert, 1985; Ross & Pate, 1987). Given the limitations of self-report measures, these statistics are believed to be underestimates. Data from the Bogalusa Heart Study (Nicklas, Rarris, Srinivasan, Webber, & Berenson, 1989) indicated that increased weight is not accompanied by an increase in height or energy (calorie) intake, but rather a major contributor to increasing overweight is decreased physical activity (E. Kennedy, 1996). Recent studies have documented significant decreases in school-age and adolescent physical education leading to increased sedentary lifestyles for children, though extensive secular trend data does not exist (Heath, Pratt, Warren, & Kann, 1994). Missing from the research literature are studies that address changes in safety, parental work habits, and other changes in the social and cultural aspects of the environment that further decrease opportunities and motivation for exercise and physical play. The role of the media and its powerful effect in transmission of culture via television as a mediator of health behavior is just beginning to be addressed. Though outside of the scope of this review, there also appears to be a lack of activity prevention and intervention research, which could guide health care providers to ensure successful approaches to individual and community behavior changes in physical activity level.

Schools, from day care to high school, have served as a focus of many recently funded intervention studies, particularly in the cardiovascular health area. Nearly 55 million children (5 to 18 years of age) or approximately 95% of all youth in the United States are enrolled in school; 22.3 million of these children have working mothers and many of them require care outside of school hours (Bureau of the Census, 1995; National Center for Education Statistics, 1984). Over 50% of preschool children have mothers employed outside the home and an estimated 9.9 million children under 5 need child care. At least 9.1 million are enrolled in either child-care centers or family homes offering day care, with 70% of those in family day care attending full time. Thus these settings have become a significant source of American children's daily dietary intake with estimates running from one third to two thirds of the total food intake for any given day.

Nursing has contributed in this area of school-based intervention. Harrell and colleagues in the Cardiovascular Health in Children study (CHIC) tested a classroom-based intervention of 1,274 third and fourth graders targeting exercise, nutrition, and smoking (Harrell & Frauman, 1994; Harrell et al., 1996; McMurray et al., 1993). These researchers, using a randomized controlled field trial in 12 schools, were able to demonstrate an increase in knowledge, physical activity, aerobic power, and a drop in total cholesterol level (though not statistically significant), body fat, and a smaller rise in diastolic blood pressure in the intervention group compared to controls.

Limitations were imposed by the use of only a posttest measure of health knowledge instead of any direct assessment of changes in nutritional behavior. But the CHIC study was also able to demonstrate similar changes in the intervention groups in a shorter time frame and less resource intensive model than the 3-year Child and Adolescent Trial for Cardiovascular Health (CATCH) study (Luepker et al., 1996). It will be important to note whether these investigators report sustained effects on diets longitudinally as other follow-up studies that demonstrated an initial postintervention significance found that the effects fade after 1 year (Perry et al., 1989).

Though the CHIC and CATCH studies report no significant changes in serum cholesterol in children with levels within the acceptable range, other studies have been successful in at-risk populations. The Dietary Intervention Study in Children (DISC I) was a multicenter, randomized clinical trial of 663 children that studied the feasibility and long-term efficacy, safety, and acceptability of a fat-modified diet in 8- to 10-year-old children with moderately elevated plasma low-density lipoprotein cholesterol levels (Obarzanek et al., 1997; Van Horn et al., 1993; The Writing Group for the DISC Collaborative Research Group, 1995). A behaviorally based, personalized family intervention was designed to have children consume a diet reduced in total fat, saturated fat, and cholesterol. The study achieved modest lowering of low-density lipoprotein (LDL) cholesterol levels over 3 years with significant differences in total dietary fat, saturated fat, and cholesterol in the intervention group while supporting growth.

Four generations of school-based health-promotion research laid the groundwork for National Heart, Lung, and Blood Institute funding of 10 studies in the past decade on cardiovascular health promotion for youth and families. These studies provided substantial information to inform nursing practice in primary prevention. Over 19,000 students and, in some studies, their families and teachers from over 127 public and 2 private schools in 10 states participated. Stone et al. (1989) and Ernst and Obarzanek (1994) provided in-depth presentations of these cardiovascular risk-reduction demonstration-and-education studies.

The findings from the Minnesota Heart Health Program, a community-intervention education-and-demonstration trial, illustrated the contributions these studies can make to nursing practice. The emphasis for the Minnesota Heart Health Program was adult behavior and risk-factor change, yet youth education and prevention were seen as major components and were given more emphasis in Minnesota than in the other three major community-wide CVD prevention programs at Stanford, CA, Rhode Island, and Pennsylvania. Targeted behaviors included eating, activity, and smoking. Four of the eight youth programs tested interventions aimed at nutritional behavioral goals in elementary and high-school populations. For an extensive review of 10 years of findings, see Perry, Hearn, Kelder, and Klepp (1991).

The largest and most rigorous of the pediatric studies is the Child and Adolescent Trial for Cardiovascular Health. The CATCH intervention involved four field centers made up of 5,000 third-grade students and was aimed at changing eating, activity, and smoking behaviors. The interventions consisted of school- and family-based components with a school-only versus school-plus-family treatment arm. Interventions were able to modify the fat content in school lunches, increase physical activity at school, and modify food-related behaviors for intake of cholesterol, total and saturated fat, but not sodium. In comparison to the school-only arm, the addition of the family program did not significantly improve the child's physiological or behavioral measures. Results supported changes in knowledge and attitudinal effects only. Secondary analysis revealed significant dose effects (as adult participation increased, children's scores improved) for knowledge and attitudes related to diet and physical activity. These effects were greater for the minority and male subjects. This finding supports the need to develop and evaluate new approaches that are responsive to the cultural differences and individual needs of racially and ethnically diverse minority populations.

The use of multiple sites and teams of investigators to increase the power of the sample size and diversity of subjects greatly enhances the use of these results. Consideration should be given by nursing scientists and clinicians to developing large, consortium-based, multicenter trials of child and family health promotion in order to maximize statistical power, combine resources, and enhance grant and funding possibilities. These school-based intervention studies have approached cardiovascular health and the concomitant issues of nutrition, obesity, and activity from a multidisciplinary and multifactorial perspective and have used sophisticated designs with interventions targeted at child, family, and community levels. As a group, these studies are relevant to nursing science not just for their practice application but as forerunners of social ecological interventions aimed at community-level interventions that affect individual and populations' health.

Notwithstanding these successes, many studies continue to approach individual behavior change through health-education interventions and suffer from important methodological and theoretical limitations. For example, despite health care providers' almost exclusive reliance on a didactic teaching model with parents and children (anticipatory guidance approaches), lack of knowledge or information about health-compromising behaviors does not appear to be the main problem. Several investigators have found both children and parents to be very knowledgeable about practices that promote health in nutritional areas (Goldman, Withney-Saltiel, Granger, & Rodin, 1991; S. R. Johnson et al., 1994), but knowing the "right thing" has not translated into "doing the right thing," (i.e., positive health behaviors). As Cataldo et al. (1985) pointed out, educationally based programs have assumed that knowledge automatically alters behavior! To design more efficacious interventions, the field needs to develop a fuller and more systematic understanding of the complex range of behaviors involved in establishing, adopting, and sustaining behavioral strategies for health. Approaches that continue to emphasize only personal factors and strategies, however, are inadequate to address determinants of health-related behaviors. In the next section, research addressing changing environmental influences on behavior is addressed.

SOCIETAL ISSUES AND THE INFLUENCE OF MEDIA

Outside of sleeping, American children spend more hours watching television and other forms of media than going to school (Dietz & Strasburger, 1991). Television, which is influential in both cognitive and emotional domains, has been the most studied of the media experiences. Over the years several studies have been published on the effects of television, particularly in the areas of aggression and violence. The studies reviewed here focus on nutritional effects relevant for nursing practice (Dietz & Gortmaker, 1985; Signorielli & Lears, 1992; Taras, Sallis, Patterson, Nader, & Nelson, 1989; Wallack & Dorfman, 1992).

In 1982 the National Institute of Mental Health concluded that television advertising and programs were doing a poor job educating people about health and nutrition (Pearl, 1982). Studies since then have been criticized for being atheoretical and lacking generalizability primarily because of the use of experimental laboratory settings rather than natural settings and studying short-term stimuli instead of the long-term effects of exposure. To address this, Dietz and Gortmaker (1985), using data collected during Cycles II and III of the National Health Examination Survey, examined over 9,000 children (6–17 years of age) in two cross-sectional and one prospective study. The prevalence of obesity and the time spent watching television were significantly correlated and the correlation persisted even when several independent variables were controlled (prior obesity, region, season, population density, race, socioeconomic class, and several family variables). A dose–response effect for time spent watching television was also established in adolescence (2% prevalence increase in obesity for every hourly increment of viewing). Robinson et al. (1993) were unable to replicate this finding, but their study used a smaller sample and did not use national data. Other studies have established amount of time spent watching television as indicators of high cholesterol (Wong et al., 1992) and overall poor eating habits and notions about food (Signorielli & Lears, 1992).

Signorielli and Lears (1992) surveyed 209 fourth- and fifth-grade children (21.3% minorities, race not stated) from different socioeconomic groups. They tested two hypotheses: (a) the relation between watching television and having poor eating habits would be positive and (b) the relation between watching television and having "unhealthy conceptions" about food and the principles of nutrition would also be positive. Support was obtained for both hypotheses, though it was stronger for the former than the latter. Boys had significantly poorer eating habits than girls, and minority children had significantly poorer eating habits than White children. A regression analysis controlling for sex, race, reading level, occupational status, and parents' educational level revealed that television viewing was the only significant predictor of poor eating habits. Half (105) of the children could not answer questions regarding their parents' education or occupation, however, thereby limiting the sample size for this analysis.

Though it has been documented that obesity occurs among televised characters far less frequently than in the general population, the literature has not determined whether the implicit message that it is possible to eat frequently and remain thin, is operating (Kaufman, 1980). What role the absence of obese characters on television may play in the obsession with thinness now seen in even young children is unclear. Although a relatively large body of research has explored the prevalence and indicators of eating disorders among adolescent and young adult women, similar investigations are just beginning with children. By third grade nearly one third of boys and girls have already tried to lose weight (Maloney, McGuire, Daniels, & Specker, 1989). In a study of children in second-, fourth-, and sixth-grade classes at a Midwestern elementary school, fourth- and sixth-grade girls indicated more concern than second graders for being or becoming overweight and a preference to be thinner than their current weight. Among fourth and sixth graders, girls had more concern than boys about being or becoming overweight, more concern about the effects of eating food, a greater desire to be thinner than their perceived body image, and a history of more dieting behavior. This indicates that pressures leading girls to become dissatisfied with their weight and body image begin by middle to late childhood (Thelan, Powell, Lawrence, & Kuhnert, 1992). None of the studies have included enough non-White subjects to analyze differences between White children and other racial or ethnic groups, however, such as Black, Latino, or Asian children's eating and body-image concerns.

An average child sees an estimated 20,000 advertisements per year (an increase from 11,000 documented in 1982), more than half of which are for food; yet only about 3% are for healthy foods (Brown & Walsh-Childers, 1994; Kunkel & Gantz, 1991; Strasburger, 1992). The contribution of television commercials to unhealthy eating patterns is rarely addressed in the applied health science literature (for a notable exception, see the review by Dietz & Strasburger, 1991); yet multiple studies have documented a relationship between viewing or television exposure, expressed preference, purchase-influencing attempts, and overconsumption of food (Galst & White, 1976; Goldberg, Gorn, & Gibson, 1978; Gorn & Goldberg, 1982; Jeffrey, McLellan, & Fox, 1982; Sallis et al., 1995; Taras et al., 1989).

For example, in a study of 80 first-grade children, Goldberg et al. (1978) tested the effect of exposure to an ad for sugared foods versus a nutritional snack embedded in a television program. Those who saw the sugar-snack commercial chose a sugared food choice at a significantly higher rate than those in the healthy snack group. Galst and White (1976) observed 40 3- to 5-year-olds and their mothers grocery shopping and found prior amount of television viewing positively associated with number of requests; the kinds of products requested were those more often advertised on children's programming. In an experimental study using a direct measure of actual food consumption, Jeffrey et al. (1982) found that low-nutrition advertisements were responsible for increasing total calorie consumption, the advertisements affected boys more than girls, and they were not mediated by cognitive development. In the same year Gorn and Goldberg (1982) tested 288 children ranging from 5 to 8 years of age, who for 14 Saturdays watched morning programs with fruit and fruit-juice commercials, candy, Kool-Aid™ commercials, pronutritional public service announcements, or no commercials. They found the commercial viewed made a significant difference in the child's choice of snack immediately after viewing.

In an attempt to capture mothers' beliefs about television's influence on children's diets and physical activity, Taras et al. (1989) interviewed 66 mothers of children aged 3 to 8, 63% of whom were Hispanic. They found that regardless of ethnicity, the foods that children requested were the foods frequently advertised on television. Children were successful in getting what they requested: parents reported purchasing 22% to 58% of the high salt, fat, or sugar items advertised. Requests and purchases for high-fat foods were significantly correlated with intake in all three categories (sugar, fat, salt); high sugar requests and purchases were correlated only with high sugar intake by the child and the relationship did not hold for the salt category.

Sallis et al. (1995) in a more recent study involving both Mexican and Anglo American mothers of preschool children found that mothers' BMI and skinfold measures were positively associated with purchasing a higher percentage of food items the child requested after seeing them on television. Mothers reported that they purchase on average 61% of the food children request because of television. These results are similar to several older studies that, though imprecise, range from 45% to 87% for parents' self-report of yielding to purchase requests for food items (Adler et al., 1980). The findings of these studies support the need to design interventions. Mothers reported being well aware of the associations, however, and thus mere educational interventions may prove pointless. Further work needs to address what strategies would help parents modify television's influence on the family's purchasing behavior. Limitations to note in this study were the low test–retest reliability on some items on the questionnaire and the lack of acculturation data on this primarily Spanish-speaking, low-income, bordertown population sample.

The Wallack and Dorfman (1992) content analysis of commercial time during a composite day sought to explore the nature of health messages on television. Because a substantial portion of children's viewing is of adult fare, the study did not distinguish between adult and children's programming times. Seventy-six percent of the 654 commercial spots were advertisements, and over a third contained "health" messages, 40% of which were for food and beverages. Nutritional adequacy or veracity was not assessed, though the authors said that most messages did not provide useful information for consumers but claimed "good nutrition" as a characteristic of the product. The notion of a child or viewer "acquiring health" by using certain products needs to be investigated. In addition, this study points to the need for a content analysis method that captures the child's perspective and analysis, in contrast to the adult investigators' interpretation of what the child audience may perceive.

In the meantime, a guiding principle for looking at the effects of television can be gained from the research done at the Center for the Study of Language and Information at Stanford, notably from the investigations of Reeves and Nass (1996). Their work documented that all people (children included) automatically and unconsciously respond socially and naturally to media; viewers assume that what they perceive is real and assume it is the truth.

Primary care interventions for childhood nutrition continue to take an assumptive model that "correct" knowledge will lead to behavioral change, devoid of an understanding of the powerful influence of consumptive advertising. No studies have documented that nurse practitioners include a careful television history during patient visits despite the epidemic proportions of obesity now; nor have any interventions based on this body of work been tested, despite the pervasive role that television plays in the lives of children and their families. The American Academy of Pediatrics Committee on Communications (1990) has gone on record that obesity represents one of the two areas in which research has demonstrated a causal effect rather than a merely contributory one, yet intervention research has not followed or reflected this level of concern. Some researchers are beginning to explore nutrition in relation to the cultural and ethnic beliefs of the diverse population of the United States today. Yet there is a general paucity of television research using diverse populations, and nutrition studies are no exception, limiting their generalizability.

FAMILY AND CULTURE

Traditionally, research in nutrition has taken a quantitative perspective, for example, with codifying of growth and development by growth charts. These analytical tools have become part of the practice perspective of many health care providers in Western populations (Pelto, 1987). A contextual approach, however, could shed more light on food practices within both subcultures and the dominant culture. Nutrition occurs within the context of family life for most children, and families exist within a community, embedded in cultural, religious, and social niches. Nowhere is this more evident than in those nutritional vestiges of culture called cuisine. Families' food habits often mirror their cultural beliefs and values, and these are transmitted through traditional family foods, for example, during holidays (Mennella & Beauchamp, 1996).

Research has used the household as the unit of data collection, and given its central role in food management and child rearing, variations would be expected to be associated with nutrition and health outcomes. The types of variables that have been investigated, however, are limited to maternal–child health dyads and infant feeding practices; and much remains to be learned using true family research methods. Findings that family-based nutrition interventions are more effective than those focused on an individual provide support for this approach (Brownell, Heckerman, Westlake, Hayes, & Monti, 1978; Dubbert & Wilson, 1984; Epstein, Wing, Koeske, Andrasik, & Ossip, 1981; Patterson, Rupp, Sallis, Atkins, & Nader, 1988).

Nutrition researchers have recognized the important role of families in childhood nutrient provision; but despite this recognition, empirical investigations of the ways in which food knowledge, behaviors, and practice are transmitted in families are still limited. Parental attitudes and interaction patterns in families with preschool and elementary-school-aged children were examined in 1989 by Gillespie and Achterberg using an ecosystems model. The authors found that positive nutrition attitudes and interaction behaviors increased with increasing education for both parents, even after the effects of income and mother's employment status were removed. Interestingly, mothers employed part time had higher scores on both attitudes and interaction behaviors than mothers employed full time or unemployed mothers. This raises questions about time compression and stress-interaction variables experienced by the other mothers.

In the 1990s over 50% of households with preschool children use alternative care during the daytime, and more than two thirds of all infants receive nonparental child care during their first year of life, with most enrolled for 30 hours a week (National Institute of Child Health and Human Development, 1995). Seventy-five percent of women with school-aged children are in the work force compared with 40% in 1970 (U.S. Bureau of Labor Statistics, 1987). These significant shifts in parental responsibility heighten the need for research to address the relationship of parents' work patterns to child nutrition. Mackenzie (1995), who has reviewed dining practices across cultures, argued that shared family meals in the United States are an endangered cultural tradition as a result of pressures faced by adults and changing definitions of family. A 1995 survey by Gerber Products revealed that only 43% of households with children under 6 years reported eating dinner together an average of five times a week, and only 26% of families with teens reported eating dinner together an average of 4.2 meals a week (cited in Mackenzie, 1995).

Food preferences are the major determinants of children's food intake, and correlations between preferences and intake are very strong, ranging from 0.60 to 0.80 (Birch, 1979a, 1979b). During the formative years of infancy through preschool, establishment of food intake via familial influence appears to be linked to sensory-affective factors, anticipated consequences, and ideational factors. Birch attempted to delineate parental behavior contributions and the role of food composition on food-preference behavior in these three realms. Birch's work indicated the power of the social milieu in establishing food preferences in young children (for a complete review, see Birch & Fisher, 1995). She demonstrated that preschool children increased their preference for foods that are presented as preferred by elders, heroes, or peers; preference is enhanced if used as a reward (but not a bribe, which reduces its value), and repeated exposure helps youngsters overcome initial rejection of foods (Birch, 1979a, 1979b, 1980; Sullivan & Birch, 1994). This work has obvious implications for the formation of food habits in families and day-care centers. It also offers an explanation of the influence of commercialized culture via television and the present poor food intake of American children. Familiarity is a powerful influence on food preferences.

Families' choices of food are determined far more by attitudes than by health knowledge; and these attitudes are susceptible to cultural and social influences. The role of the mother's belief system was highlighted in the Contento et al. (1993) study, which found that Latino families of Caribbean heritage could be predictably segmented into six typologies ranging from "high health" to "high taste." Three of the groups (42% of the sample) selected foods based on their health-related perceptions and the other 36% selected food based on how it tasted. The typology of families was based on mothers' beliefs about the healthfulness of food and predicted dietary intake of their children, an association that held even when knowledge was controlled. The findings were consistent with expectancy value theory (Deci & Ryan, 1985) of motivation in that children of mothers who were knowledgeable about the health consequences of food and valued healthfulness in choosing foods for their children had diets that were more health enhancing and disease-risk reducing. The authors suggested timely implications that are relevant for primary care.

In an attempt to examine the familial aggregation of dietary habits and cultural factors, Patterson et al. (1988) studied family influences on dietary habits in 206 families (95 Anglo and 111 Mexican American). Most families shared only the evening meal, though within families dietary similarities were evident at other meals, suggesting that families' habits and preferences operate outside the household. Parents' dietary habits were significantly correlated with those of younger children in Anglo and Mexican American families. This correlation held with older children only in Mexican American families. The role of families in a primarily Hispanic population is reviewed in the extensive publications from the University of California: San Diego's Family Health Project funded by the NHLBI as one of the 10 Cardiovascular School-Based Health Promotion studies in project CATCH, as discussed earlier in the Promotion of Cardiovascular health section (Nader, Sallis, & Patterson, 1989; Nader et al., 1986; Patterson et al., 1988; Sallis, Patterson, Buona, & Nader, 1988).

Understanding of the determinants of food habits (food beliefs, preferences and choices, and how they affect each other) is very incomplete. Determinants of food choice have been investigated in five realms: biological mechanisms, availability, cultural factors, personal food systems, and miscellaneous (such as advertising). The finding that food habits appear to be among the last practices of a family or group that are assimilated (if at all) into a new culture (Rozin, 1984) is important for nursing practices. This would appear to affect the exposure, attitudes, and values that are conveyed. However, work on childhood preferences and correlations with adult family member practices demonstrates that there are enormous differences within a culture, and children may be the first to initiate change toward the dominant culture's food patterns. Few studies have examined this issue. Further, most of the research on ethnic food diversity in the United States and childhood nutrition is about Hispanic families. Few studies have been done for other ethnic groups, except for singular work on Vietnamese children (Thuy, Tam, Craig, & Zimmerman, 1983) and Hmong families (Ikeda, Ceja, Glass, & Hardwood, 1991).

One area of cultural variation that has begun to be addressed by nursing research is obesity development in children. A high prevalence of obesity has been reported among children in several minority groups, though rates vary by age and ethnic group and do not necessarily correspond to prevalence in the adult population (Kumanyika, 1993). Factors that may account for this variation include birthweight, infant feeding, and childhood eating and activity patterns. Sherman, Alexander, and colleagues have focused on primary prevention of obesity in Mexican American children (Alexander & Blank, 1988; Blank & Alexander, 1988; Sherman, Alexander, Clark, Dean, & Welter, 1992). They examined the role that mothers' knowledge, feeding practices, and values play in relation to preschool children's weight. Their findings indicated that if a Mexican American mother prefers a chubby baby, is overweight herself, and is from a lower socioeconomic stratum, then her child is at higher risk of being overweight during the preschool years.

A series of studies from the family-based Cuidando El Corazon (Taking Care of Your Heart) prevention program also substantiate parenting differences for Mexican American children that are consistent with attribution theory (i.e., highly directive techniques, threats, and bribes are negatively associated with children's intake) and are consistent with Birch's work on the negative effects of adult bribes on children's food preferences (Contento et al., 1993; Cousins, Power, & Olvera-Ezzell, 1993; Olvera-Ezzell, Power, & Cousins, 1990). Obese mothers of nonobese children used context-specific parenting techniques: permissive when encouraging the child to eat a new food, authoritarian when the child did not want to eat, and authoritative when discouraging eating. Both cultures report significant differences depending on the child's gender, with boys being encouraged to eat more than girls. Level of acculturation and of formal education influence parents' behavior; associations between nutrition and types of parenting strategies changed when these are factored in. Health locus-of-control beliefs were covariates, however: Only modest effects were seen for education when locus of control was held constant (Cousins et al., 1993).

There are strong indications that family influences on diet vary by developmental level and ethnicity and warrant further investigation. For example, nationally no significant differences in obesity occur between Black and White girls ages 6 to 11; however, in the teen years Black girls have a significantly greater prevalence of obesity (NHANES II, reported in Gartside, Khoury, & Glueck, 1984). Dietary intake and activity levels have been documented as responsible for this difference (Falkner, 1993). Because of the implications of obesity for hypertension and cardiovascular disorders in Black women, this has obvious health implications. However, Black girls also report fewer eating disorders and less extreme preoccupation with body image; less dissatisfaction with body size; and less attendant low self-esteem, which is associated with overweight in White teen girls (Falkner, 1993; Kumanyika, 1993). These findings suggest protective factors associated with race and gender.

It is instructive to review the research explicating children's health beliefs and practices relative to diet, especially when they move out of the period of parental control, because children's attitudes and health behaviors significantly affect their health in childhood and in later life. From a health-promotion perspective, it is easier both to establish healthful habits and to prevent the formation of unhealthful habits early in life. It would appear that some children are quite knowledgeable about diet though this is not true of all ethnic groups or socioeconomic levels.

Olvera-Ezzell, Power, Cousins, Guerra, and Trujillo (1994) found that 4- to 8-year-old Mexican American children scored higher on safety and hygiene than on nutrition. They were less likely to provide reasons for eating healthy foods than to know the rationale for engaging in hygiene or safety behaviors, and their nutrition knowledge tended to be global or undifferentiated. The authors suggested that children do not understand the long-term effect of nutrition, and this hindered the development of sound nutritional concepts. S. R. Johnson et al. (1994) found that minority, predominantly Black, elementary students (first to fifth grade), became more knowledgeable about obesity as they grew older, though many lacked basic knowledge about the types of foods that promote obesity. Few children (7%) cited lack of exercise as a cause of obesity. These results paralleled those for 4- to 6-year-olds who had difficulty understanding how certain food components, such as sugar, make foods unhealthy (Goldman et al., 1991).

Results of other studies are contrary to the above findings. For instance, Singleton, Achterberg, and Shannon (1992) using a sophisticated analysis of concept maps found that 4- to 7-year-old children perceived nutrition as a meaningful concept in relation to health, and the experimental group demonstrated a significant increase in knowledge about food and nutrition postintervention. By using the content mapping analysis method, the investigators were able to detect changes in perception that were not detected by standard closed-ended questions in objective tests.

Murphy, Youatt, Hoerr, Sawyer, and Andrews (1995) found that kindergarten students understood the general relationship among food choices, exercise, body fat, and health. They were able to name foods high in salt, fat, and sugar. Nevertheless, their food preferences were poor compared to national dietary guidelines. The authors concluded that the students knew what to eat, but their practices were inconsistent with their knowledge. Taken together, these studies suggested that young children possess the ability to comprehend abstract concepts in nutrition and that greater efforts should be made to work with them.

According to several surveys, older children show deterioration in eating habits; older children (grades 3 to 12) snack more, and consume more fast food, salt, and red meat than younger children (Adeyanju, 1990; Cohen, Brownell, & Felix, 1990; Groër, Thomas, & Droppleman, 1991). At the same time, 95% of students in this age range report that school is their primary source of nutritional information ("Who Decides," 1991). Yet in 1985 only 12 states required nutrition education from preschool through Grade 12 (USDHHS, 1992).

Research related to interventions to influence, modify, or change children's food choices and habits generally falls into two categories: behavioral (contingencies/correspondence training) and cognitive (educational/informational). Studies in the behavioral realm have been focused on changing food choices in children and have attempted to include parents so as to extrapolate to the home setting (Contento, Balch, & Bronner, 1995; Contento, Manning, & Shannon, 1992; Friedman, Greene, & Stokes, 1990; Horne, Lowe, Fleming, & Dowey, 1995; Lytle & Achterberg, 1995; Pelchat & Pliner, 1995; Stark, Collins, Osnes, & Stokes, 1986). Cognitive approaches have more frequently been in the school setting with less involvement of family or home (for review see Weiss & Kien, 1987). Education has proven to be important in the adoption of healthy eating, but cognitive-focused studies have typically resulted in gains in knowledge with little effect on behavior (Byrd-Bredbenner, O'Connell, & Shannon, 1982; Byrd-Bredbenner, O'Connell, Shannon, & Eddy, 1984; Byrd-Bredbenner, Shannon, Hsu, & Smith, 1988; Domel et al., 1993; German, Pearce, Wyse, & Hansen, 1981; Lewis, Brun, Talmage, & Rasher, 1988; Shannon & Chen, 1988). Educational programs that encourage or incorporate parent participation have also reported low or no effects (Petchers, Hirsch, & Bloch, 1987). Those programs that incorporate both behavioral and cognitive approaches across both home and school settings have reported more consistent positive program evaluation outcomes (Crockett, Mullis, Perry, & Luepker, 1989; Crockett et al., 1988; Perry et al., 1988). In 1996 the CDC issued "Guidelines for School Health Programs to Promote Lifelong Healthy Eating" in which a multidisciplinary expert panel concluded that "knowledge alone does not enable young persons to adopt healthy eating behaviors" thus "current scientific knowledge indicates that a focus on behavior is a key determinant in the success of nutrition education programs" (p. 17).

It appears that children do not find nutritional health a potent motive; other motives, however, may be more potent in generating healthy food behaviors. These might include the child's wish to experience pleasure on eating, be physically strong and active, socially acceptable or attractive in appearance, to advance academically, and so forth. Health or wellness motivation has classically been elaborated within the psychological sciences and has not been systematically examined (Gochman, 1985). Once these motivators are identified, it would be useful to examine how family factors enter into this changing equation. Interventions that tap children's everyday activities and intrinsic motivations, such as play and its attendant pleasures, are called for and have just begun to surface in the literature (Bartfay & Bartfay, 1994; Rickard, Gallahue, Bewley, & Tridle, 1996). Certainly there are sufficient data to show that family-based interventions, such as behavior modification, are superior to nutrition education alone (Epstein, 1993). Given that substantially changing nutritional practices appear to be a problem that resist school-based nutrition education, more comprehensive interventions based on joint cognitive and behavioral frameworks are required. Inclusion of the child and the family's total environment (individuals, household, school, and community) may be necessary to sustain significant lifelong changes.

ECONOMIC MALNUTRITION

The major source of malnourishment in American children is no longer malnutrition secondary to protein-calorie deficits or grossly reduced caloric intake. Instead, obesity secondary to imbalanced diets (high fat and/or sucrose intake along with gross deficits of fruits and vegetables) coupled with early sedentary lifestyle are culpable. Poverty and homelessness, however, increasingly create multiple risk factors for poor nutritional status and its sequelae in childhood. Although there is debate over the prevalence of hunger in American children, there is no doubt that the problem has increased over the past decade with the increase in childhood poverty (Kotelchuck, 1990). Recent estimates indicate that 2 to 5.5 million children within the United States are hungry (Community Childhood Hunger Identification Project, 1991; U.S. Congress, House of Representatives, Committee on Agriculture, 1990).

With the 1996 change in federal sources of nutritional support (Women, Infants, and Children [WIC], food stamps, Head Start, etc.), nutrition-related health issues are reemerging among impoverished and working-poor children and their families. Under the new welfare law, funding for nutrition programs over the next 6 years is to be cut by $30 billion, including deep cuts in the food stamp program and the elimination of some funding for programs providing breakfasts for schoolchildren. Several studies have documented the effectiveness of early intervention for the amelioration of individual and community nutritional deficits (e.g., iron fortification and supplements in infancy via the WIC program). In order to note outcome differences across at-risk populations, nurses may well need to reframe their research and move to a public policy and advocacy research agenda to provide effective interventions on the societal level rather than maintaining the traditional individualistic primary care provider stance.

Homeless families with children are the fastest growing group needing emergency food and shelter (Wiecha, Dwyer, & Dunn-Strohecker, 1991). Ten reports between 1983 and 1990 examined nutrition as a health service need among homeless children and their families (Acker, Fierman, & Dreyer, 1987; Alperstein & Arnstein, 1988; Alperstein, Rappaport, & Flanigan, 1988; Bass, Brennan, Mehta, & Kodzis, 1990; Bassuk, 1986; Hu, Covel, Morgan, & Arcia, 1989; Lewis & Meyers, 1989; Miller & Lin, 1988; Wood, Valdez, Hayashi, & Shen, 1990; Wright & Weber, 1987). Families with children comprised 20% to 34% of the samples in these studies; there was an average of three children per family, and 67% to 92% of the children were younger than 5 years of age. Sixty percent to 90% of the families studied were headed by unmarried or single women whose racial or ethnic affiliation reflected the local low-income population.

Nutrition-related health problems documented in most studies of homeless children included anemia, gastrointestinal difficulties (e.g., diarrhea and asymptomatic enteric infections), obesity, underweight and low height for age, lead poisoning, selected nutritional deficiencies, and dental problems. These problems are similar to those of housed but impoverished children. Prevalence rates varied between the two samples; however, many studies did not provide housed comparison groups. In three studies (Acker et al., 1987; Arnstein & Alperstein, 1987; Wright & Weber, 1987) anemia was twice as prevalent among the homeless as among other low-income children (rates varied from 2.2% to 50%). Overall rates of nutritional deficiencies, lead poisoning, gastrointestinal ailments, and dental problems were higher for homeless children. Coupled with their notably poor access to health care and transience, homeless children were also less likely to receive treatment for these problems, increasing the risks for subsequent sequelae.

Homeless families reported obtaining more meals from fast-food places and convenience stores than housed low-income families (Wood et al., 1990). Nationally only 50% of homeless families reported receiving food stamps (Burt & Cohen, 1988). However, none of the studies to date has addressed the issue of whether these children have access to healthy snacks or how many meals they consume daily. Given the young age of the children in shelters and the practice of many shelters to serve as sleeping quarters only, one can only conclude that the food practices may be poor. This needs to be addressed in future studies. Without regard to age, on average, only 1.4 meals are available per day per homeless person (Wiecha et al., 1991). Dietary intake data on homeless children have not been published and thus limit plans for systematic interventions.

The majority of studies of homeless children were descriptive surveys, some were supplemented by retrospective outpatient data obtained from clinic charts. Sampling strategies were primarily a census approach, though Acker et al. (1987) used consecutive records, Miller and Lin (1988) used probability sampling, and Hu et al. (1989) used a random sample. Generally samples were large enough to power the analysis and were obtained from multiple sites in one city or locale (Ns ranged from a low of 30 to over 2,100). Methodological problems in these and several adult-focused studies of the homeless reviewed by Wiecha et al. (1991) point to the need for consistent diagnostic criteria, inclusion of comparable control samples, and objective nutritional measures to complement self-reports and studies documenting the nature of the food-service component of homeless aid.

CONCLUSIONS AND RESEARCH DIRECTIONS

There is much that is meaningful and useful to health care providers in the childhood nutrition literature. Strengths identified are the theoretically sound, epidemiologically based prevalence and intervention work, particularly in the cardiovascular health prevention area and community-level interventions, which are based on well-designed, conceptually and methodologically sound approaches and sample sizes. Support is provided for continued theoretical development work, multidisciplinary approaches, and increased research in cultural variations of dietary practices and interventions. Weaknesses that need to be addressed are the lack of studies using family theory methodology, the paucity of longitudinal studies, and the absence of nutritional interventions in children's primary health care that show synthesis and integration of research findings generated from recent work.

Research design and analysis issues underlie all areas germane to intervention for nutrition and health promotion during childhood. Outside of the multisite collaborative studies sponsored by NHLBI, most research reports generally make no mention of addressing design sensitivity issues a priori. Early studies employed weak pre–postdesigns and used small convenience samples and weak measurement tools. Studies were often limited to survey and nonrandomized designs or used short-term self-report behavioral or knowledge instruments. Except for the D. W. Johnson and R. T. Johnson (1987) analysis of nutrition education in 1985, there were no reports using a meta-analysis technique. More recent studies used sophisticated design-and-analysis approaches, had theoretical models embedded to design interventions, generally addressed developmental factors, used better process measures, identified whether behavioral change was maintained, and carefully studied the multiple factors that operate in the child's larger environment.

A research agenda in nursing to foster healthy choices in meals and snacks and increase physical activity in children and their families would promote health in the American public. Increased understanding of singular intrinsic phenomena, such as motivation and complex multidimensional internal and external factors that support children's positive health behaviors, is clearly necessary from the results of this review. Nursing research using prescriptive nursing models in practice intervention would build on the theoretical work of nonnursing models of nutrition and health behaviors, but refocus nursing's attention toward a model of multidimensional health and away from the limitations imposed in single variable descriptive research. An example would be Cox's "Interaction Model of Client Health Behavior" (IMCHB). Using the IMCHB, Farrand and Cox (1993) in a study of middle-childhood health behaviors found that the model explained 53% of the variance in girls' behavior and 63% of variance in boys' behavior. The model, grounded in a multidisciplinary perspective, organized and elaborated the dynamic interplay between clients, elements of the health professionals' interaction with the child and family, and health outcomes (for review see Carter & Kulbok, 1995). The complexity of the model demonstrated the need to consider multiple influences on behavior.

The nursing literature on normative childhood nutrition is generally descriptive, informational, and nonresearch based. The advanced practice nursing literature does not reflect use of research findings for practice, nor reports of implementation on either an individual or community level of the rather substantial epidemiological findings that have been reported over the past 5 to 10 years. What is lacking are joint or collaborative efforts between nurses and nutritionists or other disciplines. Nursing science and clinical practice in child and family health would benefit from nurses conducting meaningful experiments based on recent nutritional science findings. Testing of interventions using a multidisciplinary and collaborative model is warranted given the present dismal status of the nutritional health of the American child.

ACKNOWLEDGMENT

Acknowledgment is given to Samantha Blackburn, R.N., whose assistance in preparing this chapter contributed at each phase of the process. This research was supported in part by the Division of Nursing, Department of Health and Human Services, USPHS, under Grant No. 1 D23 NU01161-01.

REFERENCES

Acker, P., Fierman, A. H., & Dreyer, B. P. (1987). An assessment of parameters of health care and nutrition in homeless children. *American Journal of Diseases of Children, 141,* 388.

Adeyanju, M. (1990). Adolescent health status, behaviors, and cardiovascular disease. *Adolescence, 25,* 155–169.

Adler, R. P., Lesser, G. S., Meringoff, L. K., Robertson, T. S., Rossiter, T. S., & Ward, S. (1980). *The effects of television advertising on children: Review and recommendations.* Lexington, MA: Lexington Books.

Alexander, M. A., & Blank, J. J. (1988). Factors related to obesity in Mexican-American preschool children. *IMAGE: The Journal of Nursing Scholarship, 20,* 79–82.

Alperstein, G., & Arnstein, E. (1988). Homeless children: A challenge for pediatricians. *Pediatric Clinics of North America, 35,* 1413–1425.

Alperstein, G., Rappaport, C., & Flanigan, J. M. (1988). Health problems of homeless children in New York City. *American Journal of Public Health, 78,* 1232–1233.

American Academy of Pediatrics, Committee on Communications. (1990). Children, adolescents, and television: Policy statement. *Pediatrics, 85,* 1019–1020.

Arnstein, E., & Alperstein, G. (1987). Healthcare for the homeless. *Public Health Currents, 27,* 29–34.

Bandura, A. (1986). *Social foundations of thought and action: A social cognitive theory.* Englewood Cliffs, NJ: Prentice Hall.

Barcus, F. E., & McLaughlin, L. (1978). *Food advertising on children's television. An analysis of appeals and nutritional content.* Newtonville, MA: Action for Children's Television.

Bartfay, W. J., & Bartfay, E. (1994). Promoting health in schools through a board game. *Western Journal of Nursing Research, 16,* 438–446.

Bass, J. L., Brennan, P., Mehta, K. A., & Kodzis, S. (1990). Pediatric problems in a suburban shelter for homeless families. *Pediatrics, 85,* 33–38.

Bassuk, E. L. (1986). Homeless families: Single mothers and their children in Boston shelters. In E. L. Bassuk (Ed.), *The mental health needs of homeless persons* (pp. 45–54). San Francisco: Jossey-Bass.

Birch, L. L. (1979a). Dimensions of preschool children's food preferences. *Journal of Nutrition Education, 11,* 189–192.

Birch, L. L. (1979b). Preschool children's food preferences and consumption patterns. *Journal of Nutrition Education, 11,* 77–80.

Birch, L. L. (1980). Effects of peer models' food choices and eating behaviors on preschoolers' food preferences. *Child Development, 51,* 489–496.

Birch, L. L., & Fisher, J. A. (1995). Appetite and eating behavior in children. *Pediatric Clinics of North America, 42,* 931–953.

Blank, J. J., & Alexander, M. A. (1988). Factors associated with obesity in Mexican-American preschool children—A cardiovascular risk. *Progress in Cardiovascular Nursing, 3,* 27–31.

Bloom, M. (1996). *Primary prevention practices: Issues in children's and families lives* (Vol. 5). Thousands Oaks, CA: Sage.

Bodkin, N. L., & Hansen, B. C. (1991). Nutritional studies in nursing. In J. J. Fitzpatrick, R. L. Tauton, & A. K. Jacox (Eds.), *Annual review of nursing research* (Vol. 9, pp. 203–220). New York: Springer Publishing Co.

Brown, J. D., & Walsh-Childers, K. (1994). Effects of media on personal and public health. In J. Bryant & D. Zillmann (Eds.), *Media effects: Advances in theory and research* (pp. 389–415). Hillsdale, NJ: Lawrence Erlbaum.

Brownell, K. D., Heckerman, C. L., Westlake, R. J., Hayes, S. C., & Monti, P. M. (1978). The effect of couples training and partner co-operativeness in the behavioral treatment of obesity. *Behavior Research and Therapy, 16,* 323–333.

Bureau of the Census. (1995). *What does it cost to mind our preschoolers?* Washington, DC: Population Division, Fertility Statistics Branch, U.S. Department of Commerce.

Burt, M. R., & Cohen, B. E. (1988). *Feeding the homeless: Does the prepared meals provision help?* (Report to the Congress on the prepared meal provision). Washington, DC: Urban Institute.

Bush, P. J., & Iannotti, R. J. (1988). Origins and stability of children's health beliefs relative to medicine use. *Social Science and Medicine, 27,* 342–352.

Byrd-Bredbenner, C., O'Connell, L. H., & Shannon, B. (1982). Junior high home economics curriculum: Its effect on students' knowledge, attitude, and behavior. *Home Economics Research Journal, 11,* 123–133.

Byrd-Bredbenner, C., O'Connell, L. H., Shannon, B., & Eddy, J. M. (1984). A nutrition curriculum for health education: Its effect on students' knowledge, attitude, and behavior. *Journal of School Health, 54,* 385–388.

Byrd-Bredbenner, C., Shannon, B., Hsu, L., & Smith, D. H. (1988). A nutrition education curriculum for senior high home economics students: Its effect on students' knowledge, attitudes, and behaviors. *Journal of Nutrition Education, 20,* 341–346.

Caplan, G. (1989). Recent developments in crisis intervention and the promotion of support services. *Journal of Primary Prevention, 10,* 3–25.

Carter, K. F., & Kulbok, P. A. (1995). Evaluation of the interaction model of client health behavior through the first decade of research. *Advances in Nursing Science, 18*(1), 62–73.

Cataldo, M. F., Dershewitz, R. A., Wilson, M., Christopherson, E. R., Finney, J. W., Fawcett, J. B., & Seekins, T. (1985). Childhood injury control. In N. A. Kasnegor, J. D. Arasten, & M. F. Cataldo (Eds.), *Child health behavior: A behavioral pediatrics perspective* (pp. 135–156). New York: Wiley-Interscience.

Centers for Disease Control. (1994). Health objectives for a nation: Prevalence of overweight among adolescents—United States, 1988–91. *Morbidity and Mortality Weekly Report (MMWR): Recommendations and Reports, 43*(44), 818–821.

Centers for Disease Control. (1996). Guidelines for school health programs to promote lifelong healthy eating. *Morbidity and Mortality Weekly Report (MMWR): Recommendations and Reports, 45*(RR-9), 1–41.

Centers for Disease Control. (1997). Update: Prevalence of overweight among children, adolescents, and adults—United States, 1988–1994. *Morbidity and Mortality Weekly Report (MMWR), 46*(29), 199–202.

Cohen, R., Brownell, K., & Felix, M. (1990). Age and sex differences in health habits and beliefs of school children. *Health Psychology, 9,* 208–224.

Community Childhood Hunger Identification Project. (1991). *A survey of childhood hunger in the United States* (p. 1). Washington, DC: Food Research and Action Center.

Contento, I., Balch, G. I., & Bronner, Y. L. (1995). Nutrition education for school-aged children. *Journal of Nutrition Education, 27,* 298–311.

Contento, I. R., Basch, C., Shea, S., Gutin, B., Zybert, P., Michela, J. L., & Rips, J. (1993). Relationship of mothers' food choice criteria to food intake of preschool children: Identification of family subgroups. *Health Education Quarterly, 20,* 243–259.

Contento, I. R., Manning, A. D., & Shannon, B. (1992). Research perspective on school-based nutrition education. *Journal of Nutrition Education, 24,* 247–260.

Cousins, J. H., Power, T. G., & Olvera-Ezzell, N. (1993). Mexican-American mothers' socialization strategies: Effects of education, acculturation, and health locus of control. *Journal of Experimental Child Psychology, 55,* 258–276.

Crockett, S. J., Mullis, R., & Perry, C. L. (1988). Parent nutrition education: A conceptual model. *Journal of School Health, 58,* 53–57.

Crockett, S. J., Mullis, R., Perry, C. L., & Luepker, R. V. (1989). Parent education in youth-directed nutrition interventions. *Preventive Medicine, 18,* 475–491.

Deci, E. L., & Ryan, R. M. (1985). *Intrinsic motivation and self-determination on human behavior.* New York: Plenum.

Department of Health, Education, and Welfare. (1979). *Healthy people: The surgeon general's report on health promotion and disease prevention* (PHS Publication No. 79-55071). Washington, DC: U.S. Government Printing Office.

Dietz, W. H., & Gortmaker, S. L. (1985). Do we fatten our children at the television set? Obesity and television viewing in children and adolescents. *Pediatrics, 75,* 807–812.

Dietz, W. H., & Strasburger, V. C. (1991). Children, adolescents, and television. *Current Problems in Pediatrics, 12,* 8–31.

Domel, S. B., Baranowski, T., Davis, H., Thompson, W. O., Leonard, S. B., Riley, P., Baranowski, J., Dudovitz, B., & Smyth, M. (1993). Development and evaluation of a school intervention to increase fruit and vegetable consumption among 4th and 5th grade students. *Journal of Nutrition Education, 25,* 345–349.

Dubbert, P., & Wilson, G. T. (1984). Goal-setting and spouse involvement in the treatment of obesity. *Behavior Research and Therapy, 22,* 227–242.

Epstein, L. H. (1993). Methodological issues and ten-year outcomes for obese children. *Annals of the New York Academy of Sciences, 699,* 237–249.

Epstein, L. H., Wing, R. R., Koeske, R., Andrasik, F., & Ossip, D. J. (1981). Child and parent weight loss in family-based behavior modification programs. *Journal of Consulting and Clinical Psychology, 49,* 674–685.

Ernst, N. D., & Obarzanek, E. (1994). Child health and nutrition: Obesity and high blood cholesterol. *Preventive Medicine, 23,* 427–436.

Falkner, F. (1993). Obesity and cardiovascular disease risk factors in prepubescent and pubescent black and white females. *Critical Reviews in Food Science and Nutrition, 33,* 397–402.

Farrand, L. L., & Cox, C. L. (1993). Determinants of positive health behavior in middle childhood. *Nursing Research, 42,* 208–213.

Fishbein, M., & Ajzan, I. (1975). *Belief, attitude, intention and behavior: An introduction to theory and research.* Reading, MA: Addison-Wesley.

Friedman, A. G., Greene, P. G., & Stokes, T. (1990). Improving dietary habits of children: Effects of nutrition education and correspondence training. *Journal of Behavior Therapy and Experimental Psychiatry, 21,* 263–268.

Galst, J. P., & White, M. A. (1976). The unhealthy persuader: The reinforcing value of television and children's purchase-influencing attempts at the supermarket. *Child Development, 47,* 1089–1096.

Gartside, P. S., Khoury, P., & Glueck, C. J. (1984). Determinants of high-density lipoprotein cholesterol in Blacks and Whites: The second National Health and Nutrition Examination Survey. *American Heart Journal, 108,* 641–653.

German, M. J., Pearce, J., Wyse, B. W., & Hansen, R. G. (1981). A nutrition component for high school health education curriculums. *Journal of School Health, 51,* 149–153.

Gill, N. E., Behnke, M., Conlon, M., & Anderson, G. C. (1992). Nonnutritive sucking modulates behavioral state for preterm infants before feeding. *Scandinavian Journal of Caring Sciences, 6*(1), 3–7.

Gillespie, A. H., & Achterberg, C. L. (1989). Comparison of family interaction patterns related to food and nutrition. *Journal of the American Dietetic Association, 89,* 509–512.

Gochman, D. S. (1985). Family determinants of children's concepts of health and illness. In D. C. Turk & R. D. Kerns (Eds.), *Health, illness, and families: A life-span perspective* (pp. 23–50). New York: Wiley.

Goldberg, M. E., Gorn, G. J., & Gibson, W. (1978). Some unintended consequences of TV advertising to children. *Journal of Consumer Research, 5,* 22–29.

Goldman, S. L., Withney-Saltiel, D., Granger, J., & Rodin, J. (1991). Children's representations of "everyday" aspects of health and illness. *Journal of Pediatric Psychology, 16,* 747–766.

Gorn, G. J., & Goldberg, M. E. (1982). Behavioral evidence of the effects of televised food messages on children. *Journal of Consumer Research, 9,* 200–205.

Gortmaker, S. L., Dietz, W. H., Sobol, A. M., & Wehler, C. A. (1987). Increasing pediatric obesity in the United States. *American Journal of Diseases of Children, 141,* 535–540.

Green, K. E., & Bird, J. E. (1986). The structure of children's beliefs about health and illness. *Journal of School Health, 56,* 325–328.

Green, L. W., Kreuter, M. W., Deeds, S. G., & Partridge, K. B. (1980). *Health education planning: A diagnostic approach.* Palo Alto, CA: Mayfield.

Groër, M., Thomas, S., & Droppleman, P. (1991, April). *A longitudinal study of adolescent blood pressure, lifestyle, stress and anger.* Paper presented at the Society of Behavioral Medicine, Washington, DC.

Harrell, J. S., & Frauman, A. C. (1994). Cardiovascular health promotion in children: Program and policy implications. *Public Health Nursing, 11,* 236–241.

Harrell, J. S., McMurray, R. G., Bangdiwala, S. I., Frauman, A. C., Gansky, S. A., & Bradley, C. B. (1996). Effects of a school-based intervention to reduce cardiovascular disease factors in elementary-school children: The Cardiovascular Health in Children (CHIC) study. *Journal of Pediatrics, 128,* 797–805.

Hayman, L. L. (1988). Measuring lipids, blood pressure, and smoking. *Cardiovascular Nursing, 24,* 49–50.

Hayman, L. L., Meininger, J. C., Coates, P. M., & Gallagher, P. R. (1995). Nongenetic influences of obesity on risk factors for cardiovascular disease during two phases of development. *Nursing Research, 44,* 277–283.

Hayman, L. L., Meininger, J. C., Gallagher, P. R., & Chandler, P. (1992). Gender differences in the lipid profile in two phases of development. *Circulation, 86,* 502.

Hayman, L. L., Meininger, J. C., Stashinko, E. E., Gallagher, P. R., & Coates, P. M. (1988). Type A behavior and physiological cardiovascular risk factors in school-age twin children. *Nursing Research, 37,* 290–296.

Hayman, L. L., & Ryan, E. A. (1991). Cholesterol and cardiovascular risk factors in childhood. *Office Nurse, 4*(1), 4–8.

Hayman, L. L., & Ryan, E. A. (1994). The cardiovascular health profile: Implications for health promotion and disease prevention. *Pediatric Nursing, 20,* 509–515.

Hayman, L. L., Weill, V. A., Tobias, N. E., Stashinko, E. E., & Meininger, J. C. (1988a). Reducing risk for heart disease in children. *MCN: American Journal of Maternal Child Nursing, 13,* 442–448.

Hayman, L. L., Weill, V. A., Tobias, N. E., Stashinko, E. E., & Meininger, J. C. (1988b). Which child is at risk for heart disease? *MCN: American Journal of Maternal Child Nursing, 13,* 328–333.

Heath, G. W., Pratt, M., Waren, C. W., & Kann, L. (1994). Physical activity patterns in American high school students. *Archives of Pediatric and Adolescent Medicine, 148,* 1131–1136.

Horne, P. J., Lowe, C. F., Fleming, P. F. J., & Dowey, A. J. (1995). An effective procedure for changing food preferences in 5–7 year old children. *Proceedings of the Nutrition Society, 54,* 441–452.

Hu, D. J., Covel, R. M., Morgan, J., & Arcia, J. (1989). Health care needs for children of the recently homeless. *Journal of Community Health, 14*(1), 1–8.

Ikeda, J. P., Ceja, D. R., Glass, R. S., & Hardwood, J. O. (1991). Food habits among the Hmong living in Central California. *Journal of Nutrition Education, 23,* 168–175.

Jeffrey, D. B., McLellarn, R. W., & Fox, D. T. (1982). The development of children's eating habits: The role of television commercials. *Health Education Quarterly, 9,* 78–93.

Johnson, D. W., & Johnson, R. T. (1987). Using cooperative learning strategies to teach nutrition. *Journal of the American Dietetic Association, 87*(9 Suppl.), S55–S61.

Johnson, S. R., Schonfeld, D. J., Siegel, D., Krasnovsky, F. M., Boyce, J. C., Saliba, P. A., Boyce, W. T., & Perrin, E. C. (1994). What do minority elementary students understand about the causes of acquired immunodeficiency syndrome, colds, and obesity? *Developmental and Behavioral Pediatrics, 15,* 239–247.

Kaufman, L. (1980). Prime-time nutrition. *Journal of Communication, 30,* 37–45.

Kennedy, C., & Lipsitt, L. P. (1993). Temporal characteristics of non-oral feedings and chronic feeding problems in premature infants. *Journal of Perinatal and Neonatal Nursing, 7,* 77–89.

Kennedy, E. (1996). Healthy meals, healthy food choices, healthy children: USDA's team nutrition. *Preventive Medicine, 25,* 55–60.

Kinneer, M. D., & Beachy, P. (1994). Nipple feeding premature infants in the neonatal intensive-care unit: Factors and decisions. *Journal of Obstetric, Gynecologic, and Neonatal Nursing, 23,* 105–112.

Kotelchuck, M. (1990). Societal trends that affect nutrition status and services for the maternal and child health populations. In C. S. Sharbaugh (Ed.), *Background papers for a call to action: Better nutrition for mothers, children and families* (pp. 23–39). Washington, DC: National Center for Education in Maternal and Child Health.

Kumanyika, S. (1993). Ethnicity and obesity development in children. *Annals of the New York Academy of Sciences, 699,* 81–92.

Kunkel, D., & Gantz, W. (1991). *Television advertising to children: Message content in 1990.* Bloomington, Indiana University: Children's Advertising Review Unit of the National Advertising Division, Council of Better Business Bureaus.

Lauer, R. M., Connor, W. E., Leaverton, P. E., Reiter, M. A., & Clarke, W. R. (1975). Coronary heart disease risk factors in school children: The Muscatine study. *Journal of Pediatrics, 86,* 697–706.

Lewis, C. E. (1988). Disease prevention and health promotion practices of primary care physicians in the United States. *American Journal of Preventive Medicine, 4*(Suppl.), 9–16.

Lewis, M., Brun, J., Talmage, H., & Rasher, S. (1988). Teenagers and food choices: The impact of nutrition education. *Journal of Nutrition Education, 20,* 336–340.

Lewis, M. R., & Meyers, A. (1989). The growth and development status of homeless children entering shelters in Boston. *Public Health Reports, 104,* 247–250.

Luepker, R. V., Perry, C. L., McKinlay, S. M., Nader, P. R., Parcel, G. S., Stone, E. J., Webber, L. S., Elder, J. P., Feldman, H. A., Johnson, C. C., Kelder, S. H., & Wu, M. (1996). Outcomes of a field trial to improve children's dietary patterns and physical activity. The Child and Adolescent Trial for Cardiovascular Health (CATCH). *Journal of the American Medical Association, 275,* 768–776.

Lytle, L., & Achterberg, C. (1995). Changing the diet of America's children: What works and why? *Journal of Nutrition Education, 27,* 250–260.

Mackenzie, M. (1995). The feeding partnership: An anthropological perspective on meals. *Pediatric Basics, 74,* 10–16.

Maloney, M., McGuire, J., Daniels, S., & Specker, B. (1989). Dieting behavior and eating attitudes in children. *Pediatrics, 84,* 482–489.

McCain, G. C. (1995). Promotion of preterm infant nipple feeding with nonnutritive sucking. *Journal of Pediatric Nursing, 10,* 3–8.

McMurray, R. G., Bradley, C. B., Harrell, J. S., Bernthal, P. R., Frauman, A. C., & Bangdiwala, S. I. (1993). Parental influences of childhood fitness and activity patterns. *Research Quarterly for Exercise and Sport, 64,* 249–255.

Mechanic, D. (1979). The stability of health and illness behavior. *American Journal of Public Health, 69,* 1142–1145.

Medoff-Cooper, B. (1991). Changes in nutritive sucking patterns with increasing gestational age. *Nursing Research, 40,* 245–247.

Medoff-Cooper, B., & Gennaro, S. (1996). The correlation of sucking behaviors and Bayley Scales of Infant development at six months of age in VLBW infants. *Nursing Research, 45,* 291–296.

Medoff-Cooper, B., Weininger, S., & Zukowsky, K. (1989). Neonatal sucking as a clinical tool: Preliminary findings. *Nursing Research, 38,* 162–165.

Meier, P., & Anderson, G. C. (1987). Responses of small preterm infants to bottle- and breast-feeding. *MCN: American Journal of Maternal Child Nursing, 12,* 97–105.

Meininger, J. C., Hayman, L. L., Coates, P. M., & Gallagher, P. (1988). Genetics or environment? Type A behavior and cardiovascular risk factors in twin children. *Nursing Research, 37,* 341–346.

Meininger, J. C., Hayman, L. L., Gallagher, P. R., & Coates, P. M. (1992). Stability of genetic influence on cardiovascular disease risk factors during transition from childhood to adolescence. *Circulation, 86,* 502.

Meininger, J. C., Stashinko, E. E., & Hayman, L. L. (1991). Type A behavior in children: Psychometric properties of the Matthews Youth Test for Health. *Nursing Research, 40,* 221–227.

Mennella, J. A., & Beauchamp, G. K. (1996). The early development of human flavor preferences. In E. D. Capaldi (Ed.), *The early development of human flavor preferences* (pp. 83–112). Washington, DC: American Psychological Association.

Miller, D. S., & Lin, E. H. B. (1988). Children in sheltered homeless families: Reported health status and use of health services. *Pediatrics, 81,* 668–673.

Miller, H. D., & Anderson, G. C. (1993). Nonnutritive sucking: Effects on crying and heart rate in intubated infants requiring assisted mechanical ventilation. *Nursing Research, 42,* 305–307.

Moore, M. C., Guenter, P. A., & Bender, J. H. (1986). Nutrition-related nursing research. *IMAGE: Journal of Nursing Scholarship, 18,* 18–21.

Murphy, A. S., Youatt, J. P., Hoerr, S. L., Sawyer, C. A., & Andrews, S. L. (1995). Kindergarten students' food preferences are not consistent with their knowledge of the dietary guidelines. *Journal of the American Dietetic Association, 95,* 219–223.

Nader, P. R. (1993). The role of the family in obesity prevention and treatment. *Annals of the New York Academy of Sciences, 669,* 147–153.

Nader, P. R., Sallis, J. F., & Patterson, T. L. (1989). A family approach to cardiovascular risk reduction: Results from the San Diego Family Health Project. *Health Education Quarterly, 26,* 229–244.

Nader, P. R., Sallis, J. F., Rupp, B. E., Atkins, C., Patterson, T. L., & Abramson, I. S. (1986). San Diego family health project: Reaching families through the schools. *Journal of School Health, 56,* 227–231.

Nader, P. R., Sellers, D. E., Johnson, C. C., Perry, C. L., Stone, E. J., Cook, K. C., Bebchuk, J., & Luepker, R. V. (1996). The effect of adult participation in a school-based family intervention to improve children's diet and physical activity: The child and adolescent trial for cardiovascular health. *Preventive Medicine, 25,* 455–464.

Nader, P. R., Taras, H. L., Sallis, J. F., & Patterson, T. L. (1987). Adult heart disease prevention in childhood: A national survey of pediatricians' practices and attitudes. *Pediatrics, 79,* 843–850.

National Center for Education Statistics. (1984). *The condition of education* (Publication #84-401). Washington, DC: U.S. Government Printing Office.

National Center for Health Statistics. (1995). *Healthy people 2000 review, 1994.* Hyattsville, MD: Public Health Service.

National Commission on Children. (1991). *Beyond rhetoric: A new American agenda for children and families* (p. 127). Washington, DC: The Commission.

National Institute of Child Health and Human Development. (1995). *Child care in the 1990's: The NICHD Study of early child care.* Indianapolis, IN: Society for Research in Child Development (biennial meeting).

Nicklas, T. A., Rarris, R. P., Srinivasan, S. R., Webber, L. S., & Berenson, G. S. (1989). Nutritional studies in children and implications for change: The Bogalusa Heart Study. *Journal of the Advances in Medicine, 2,* 451–474.

Obarzanek, E., Hunsberger, S., Van Horn, L., Hartmuller, V. W., Barton, B. A., Stevens, V. J., Kwiterovich, P. O., Franklin, F. A., Kimm, S. Y. S., Lasser, N. L., Simons-Morton, D. G., & Lauer, R. M. (1997). Safety of a fat-reduced diet: The Dietary Intervention Study in Children (DISC). *Pediatrics, 100,* 51–59.

Office of Disease Prevention and Health Promotion. (1992). *Primary care provider surveys.* Washington, DC: Office of the Assistant Secretary of Health.

Oganov, R. G., Tubol, I. B., Zhukovskii, G. S., Perova, N. V., & Ilchenko, I. N. (1988). Epidemiological characteristics of dyslipoproteinaemia and certain other risk factors of atherosclerosis and aschaemic heart disease in 11- and 14-year children in different climatogeographic zones: Results of a cooperative study. *Cor Vasa, 30,* 248–256.

Olvera-Ezzell, N., Power, T. G., & Cousins, J. H. (1990). Maternal socialization of children's eating habits: Strategies used by obese Mexican-American mothers. *Child Development, 61,* 395–400.

Olvera-Ezzell, N., Power, T. G., Cousins, J. H., Guerra, A. M., & Trujillo, M. (1994). The development of health knowledge in low-income Mexican-American children. *Child Development, 65,* 416–427.

Orem, D. E. (1980). *Nursing: Concepts of practice.* New York: McGraw-Hill.

Parcel, G. S., Edmundson, E., Perry, C. L., Feldman, H. A., O'Hara-Tompkins, N., Nader, P. R., Johnson, C. C., & Stone, E. J. (1995). Measurement of self-efficacy for diet-related behaviors among elementary school children. *Journal of School Health, 65,* 23–27.

Parcel, G. S., Simons-Morton, B. G., O'Hara, N. M., Baranowski, T., Kolbe, L. J., & Bee, D. E. (1987). School promotion of healthful diet and exercise behavior: An integration of organizational change and social learning theory interventions. *Journal of School Health, 57,* 150–156.

Patterson, T. L., Rupp, J. W., Sallis, J. F., Atkins, C. J., & Nader, P. R. (1988). Aggregation of dietary calories, fats, and sodium in Mexican-American and Anglo families. *American Journal of Preventive Medicine, 4*(2), 75–82.

Pearl, D. (1982). *Television and behavior: Ten years of scientific progress and implications for the eighties.* Washington, DC: U.S. Government Printing Office.

Pelchat, M. L., & Pliner, P. (1995). "Try it. You'll like it." Effects of information on willingness to try novel foods. *Appetite, 24,* 153–166.

Pelto, G. H. (1987). Cultural issues in maternal and child health and nutrition. *Social Science and Medicine, 25,* 553–559.

Pender, N. J. (1982). *Health promotion in nursing practice.* Norwalk, CT: Appleton-Century-Crofts.

Perry, C. L., Hearn, M. D., Kelder, S. H., & Klepp, K. I. (1991). The Minnesota heart health program youth program. In D. Nutbeam, B. Haglund, & P. Farley (Eds.), *Youth health promotion: From theory to practice in school and community* (pp. 254–276). Tillgren, PA: Forbes.

Perry, C. L., Luepker, R. V., Murray, D. M., Hearn, M. D., Halper, A., Dudovitz, B., Maile, M. C., & Smyth, M. (1989). Parent involvement with children's health promotion: A one-year follow-up of the Minnesota home team. *Health Education Quarterly, 16,* 171–180.

Perry, C. L., Luepker, R. V., Murray, D. M., Kurth, C., Mullis, R., Crockett, S., & Jacobs, D. R. (1988). Parent involvement with children's health promotion: The Minnesota home team. *American Journal of Public Health, 78,* 1156–1160.

Petchers, M. K., Hirsch, E. Z., & Bloch, B. A. (1987). The impact of parent participation on the effectiveness of a heart health curriculum. *Health Education Quarterly, 14,* 449–460.

Public Health Service. (1990). *Healthy people 2000: National health promotion and disease prevention objectives for the year 2000.* Washington, DC: U.S. Government Printing Office.

Rabbia, F., Veglio, F., Pinna, G., Oliva, S., Surgo, V., Rolando, B., Bessone, A., Melchio, R., & Chiandussi, L. (1994). Cardiovascular risk factors in adolescence: Prevalence and familial aggregation. *Preventive Medicine, 23,* 809–815.

Radius, R. M., Dillman, T. E., & Becker, M. H. (1980). Health beliefs of the school-aged child and their relationship to risk-taking behaviors. *Hygie, 23,* 227–235.

Reeves, B., & Nass, C. (1996). *The media equation: How people treat computers, television, and new media like real people and places.* New York: Cambridge University Press.

Rickard, K. A., Gallahue, D. L., Bewley, N., & Tridle, M. L. (1996). The play approach to learning: An alternative paradigm for healthy eating and active play. *Pediatric Basics, 76,* 2–7.

Robinson, T. N., Hammer, L. D., Killen, J. D., Kraemer, H. C., Wilson, D. M., Hayward, C., & Taylor, C. B. (1993). Does television viewing increase obesity and reduce physical activity? Cross-sectional and longitudinal analyses among adolescent girls. *Pediatrics, 91,* 273–280.

Rosenstock, I. M., Strecher, V. J., & Becker, M. H. (1990). The health belief model: Explaining health behaviors through expectancies. I K. Glanz, F. M. Lewis, & B. K. Rimer (Eds.), *Health belief and health education.* San Francisco: Jossey-Bass.

Ross, J. G., & Gilbert, G. G. (1985). The national children and youth fitness study. A summary of findings. *Journal of Physical Education and Recreational Dance, 56*(1), 45–50.

Ross, J. G., & Pate, R. R. (1987). The national children and youth fitness study II: A summary of findings. *Journal of Physical Education and Recreational Dance, 58*(10), 51–56.

Rozin, P. (1984). The acquisition of food habits and preferences. In J. D. Matarazzo, S. M. Weiss, J. A. Herd, & N. E. Miller (Eds.), *Behavioral health: A handbook of health enhancement and disease prevention* (pp. 590–607). New York: Wiley.

Sallis, J. F., Broyles, S. L., Frank-Spohrer, G., Berry, C. C., Davis, T. B., & Nader, P. R. (1995). Child's home environment in relation to the mother's adiposity. *International Journal of Obesity, 19,* 190–197.

Sallis, J. F., Patterson, T. L., Buona, M. J., & Nader, P. R. (1988). Relation of cardiovascular fitness and physical activity to cardiovascular disease risk factors in children and adults. *American Journal of Epidemiology, 127,* 933–946.

Saltz, K. M., Tamir, I., Erst, N., Kwiterovich, P., Glueck, C., Christensen, B., Larsen, R., Pirhonen, D., Prewitt, T. E., & Scott, L. W. (1983). Selected nutrient intakes of free-living white children ages 6-19 years. The Lipid Research Clinics: Program prevalence study. *Pediatric Research, 17,* 124–130.

Shamir, R., Tershakovec, A. M., Gallagher, P. R., Liacouras, C. A., Hayman, L. L., & Cortner, J. A. (1996). The influence of age and relative weight on the presentation of familial combined hyperlipidemia in childhood. *Atherosclerosis, 121*(1), 85–91.

Shannon, B., & Chen, A. N. (1988). A three-year school-based nutrition education study. *Journal of Nutrition Education, 20,* 114–124.

Sherman, J. B., Alexander, M. A., Clark, L., Dean, A., & Welter, L. (1992). Instruments measuring maternal factors in obese preschool children. *Western Journal of Nursing Research, 14,* 555–569.

Siddell, E. P., & Froman, R. D. (1994). A national survey of neonatal intensive-care units: Criteria used to determine readiness for oral feedings. *Journal of Obstetric, Gynecologic, and Neonatal Nursing, 23,* 783–789.

Signorielli, N., & Lears, M. (1992). Television and children's conceptions of nutrition: Unhealthy messages. *Health Communication, 4,* 245–257.

Singleton, J. C., Achterberg, C. L., & Shannon, B. M. (1992). Role of food and nutrition in the health perceptions of young children. *Journal of the American Dietetic Association, 92*(1), 67–70.

Stark, L. J., Collins, F. L., Osnes, P. G., & Stokes, T. F. (1986). Using reinforcement and cueing to increase healthy snack food choices in preschoolers. *Journal of Applied Behavior Analysis, 19,* 367–379.

Stone, E. J., Perry, C. L., & Luepker, R. V. (1989). Synthesis of cardiovascular behavioral research for youth health promotion. *Health Education Quarterly, 16,* 155–169.

Strasburger, V. C. (1992). Children, adolescents, and television. *Pediatrics in Review, 13,* 144–151.

Sullivan, S. A., & Birch, L. L. (1994). Infant dietary experience and acceptance of solid foods. *Pediatrics, 93,* 271–277.

Swartz, R., Moody, L., Yarandi, H., & Anderson, G. C. (1987). A meta-analysis of critical outcome variables in nonnutritive sucking in preterm infants. *Nursing Research, 36,* 292–295.

Taras, H. L., Sallis, J. F., Patterson, T. L., Nader, P. R., & Nelson, J. A. (1989). Television's influence on children's diet and physical activity. *Developmental and Behavioral Pediatrics, 10,* 176–180.

Tell, G. S. (1982). Factors influencing dietary habits: Experiences of the Oslo Youth Study. In T. J. Coates, A. C. Petersen, & C. Perry (Eds.), *Promoting adolescent health: A dialog on research and practice* (pp. 381–396). New York: Academic Press.

Thelan, M. H., Powell, A. L., Lawrence, C., & Kuhnert, M. E. (1992). Eating and body image concerns among children. *Journal of Clinical Child Psychology, 21*(1), 41 46.

Thuy, T. N., Tam, H. D., Craig, W. J., & Zimmerman, G. (1983). Food habits and preferences of Vietnamese children. *Journal of School Health, 53,* 144–147.

Troiano, R. P., Flegal, K. M., Kuczmarski, R. J., Campbell, S. M., & Johnson, C. L. (1995). Overweight prevalence and trends for children and adolescents. The National Health and Nutrition Examination Surveys, 1963 to 1991. *Archives of Pediatric and Adolescent Medicine, 149,* 1085–1091.

U.S. Bureau of Labor Statistics. (1987). *Statistical abstract of the United States* (107th ed.). Washington, DC: U.S. Department of Commerce.

U.S. Congress, House of Representatives, Committee on Agriculture. (1990). *Hearings on the food stamp program and the community donation program.* Washington, DC: U.S. Government Printing Office.

U.S. Department of Agriculture, & U.S. Department of Health & Human Services. (1990). *Dietary guidelines for Americans.* Washington, DC: U.S. Government Printing Office.

U.S. Department of Health and Human Services. (1992). *Healthy children 2000: National health promotion and disease prevention objectives related to mothers, infants, children, adolescents and youth.* Washington, DC: Health Resources and Services Administration, Maternal and Child Health Bureau.

U.S. Department of Health & Human Services. (1996). *Healthy people 2000. Midcourse review and 1995 revisions.* Washington, DC: U.S. Government Printing Office.

Van Horn, L. V., Stumbo, P., Moag-Stahlberg, A., Obarzanek, E., Hartmuller, V. W., Farris, R. P., Kimm, S. Y. S., Frederick, M., Snetselaar, L., & Liu, K. (1993). The Dietary Intervention Study (DISC): Dietary assessment methods for 8- to 10-year-olds. *Journal of the American Dietetic Association, 93,* 1396–1403.

Wallack, L., & Dorfman, L. (1992). Health messages on television commercials. *American Journal of Health Promotion, 6,* 190–196.

Walter, H. J., Hofman, A., Vaughan, R. D., & Wynder, E. L. (1988). Modification of risk factors for coronary heart disease: Five-year results of a school-based intervention trial. *New England Journal of Medicine, 318,* 1093–1100.

Weaver, K. A., & Anderson, G. C. (1988). Relationship between integrated sucking pressures and first bottle-feeding scores in premature infants. *Journal of Obstetric, Gynecologic, and Neonatal Nursing, 17,* 113–120.

Weiss, E. H., & Kien, C. L. (1987). A synthesis of research on nutrition education at the elementary school level. *Journal of School Health, 57,* 8–13.

Wheeler, R. C., Marcus, A. C., Cullen, J. W., & Konugres, E. (1983). Baseline chronic disease risk factors in a racially heterogeneous elementary school population. The "Know Your Body" program, Los Angeles. *Preventive Medicine, 12,* 569–587.

Who Decides What Kids Eat? (1991, Sept. 17). *Washington Post Weekly,* p. WH5.

Wiecha, J. L., Dwyer, J. T., & Dunn-Strohecker, M. (1991). Nutrition and health services needs among the homeless. *Public Health Reports, 106,* 364–374.

Wilmore, J. H., & McNamara, J. J. (1974). Prevalence of coronary heart disease risk factors in boys, 8 to 12 years of age. *Journal of Pediatrics, 84,* 527–533.

Yip, R., Binkin, N., Fleshood, L., & Trowbridge, F. (1987). Declining prevalence of anemia among low-income children in the United States. *Journal of the American Medical Association, 12,* 1619–1623.

The Writing Group for the DISC Collaborative Research Group. (1995). Efficacy and safety of lowering dietary intake of fat and cholesterol in children with elevated low-density lipoprotein cholesterol. The Dietary Intervention Study in Children (DISC). *Journal of the American Medical Association, 273,* 1429–1435.

Wong, N. D., Hei, T. K., Qaqundah, P. Y., Davidson, D. M., Bassin, S. L., & Gold, K. V. (1992). Television viewing and pediatric hypercholesterolemia. *Pediatrics, 90,* 75–79.

Wood, D. L., Valdez, R. B., Hayashi, T., & Shen, A. (1990). Health of homeless children and housed, poor children. *Pediatrics, 86,* 858–866.

Wright, J. D., & Weber, E. (1987). *Homelessness and health.* Washington, DC: McGraw-Hill.

Chapter 2

Health Care for the School-Age Child

KATHLEEN ANN LONG AND DAVID WILLIAMS
COLLEGE OF NURSING
UNIVERSITY OF FLORIDA

ABSTRACT

The research related to health care for school-age children is reviewed. Two major categories are considered, namely, health-risk behavior and psychosocial health. Research related to the emerging issues of homelessness and AIDS is also reviewed. The research completed to date on school-age children's health care is critiqued with an emphasis on the state of the science in nursing. Recommendations for further research are provided.

Keywords: School-Age Children, Nursing Research, Health Care, Risky Behavior

This chapter focuses on the research literature related to health care for school-age children, identifying recent work relevant to nursing interventions. A series of computerized literature searches was conducted using MEDLINE, the Cumulative Index to Nursing and Allied Health Literature, and PsycINFO to identify child health care studies conducted in the United States from 1985 through 1996. The terms "school age" or "latency age" child were used in conducting searches, and studies were included only if they contained information on children aged 6 through 12 years. Studies with samples including this age group in combination with some younger or older children were reviewed. The initial broad searches provided direction for a series of more targeted searches relating school-age children with the following areas: school health nursing, health education, immunizations and health screening, nutrition, dental health, acute illness, chronic illness, human immunodeficiency virus (HIV) infection, disability, child abuse, substance abuse, depression, suicide, violence, learning disabilities, attention deficit disorders, behavioral disorders, parenting, and homelessness.

Because the overall topic "health care for the school-age child" is quite broad, it was necessary to selectively review certain aspects and specifically exclude others. Several rules guided this process. First, studies that focused primarily on illness or illness care, rather than on *health* care for children were excluded. On this basis, studies related to the care of chronically or acutely ill children were excluded. Second, studies of topical areas that cut across wide age groups not limited to school-age children were generally excluded. For example, there is substantial literature on childhood sexual abuse, but this work focuses on a health problem that spans infancy through late adolescence. A recent review by Kelley (1995) discussed this topic in depth. Thus, studies on child abuse, both physical and sexual, were not included. Certain broad areas, such as childhood alcohol and drug use, were included in a focused, limited way, if studies were located that clearly linked the broad area to health care for school-age children.

A very large number of studies were located on some topics, such as learning disabilities. Only those with clear and specific relevance to nursing interventions were included. For example, studies that focused on examining new screening techniques for use by school psychologists as a part of testing for specific learning disabilities were not included, whereas studies that had implications for nursing interventions with learning-disabled children were.

Numerous articles describing various health screening and immunization programs or procedures are not included for review in this chapter, nor are reviews of health-policy articles. Finally, some relatively new issues and problems affecting the health care of school-age children were identified through the literature searches. The topics of homelessness and HIV infection in families, not traditionally considered a part of school-age children's health care, have been included because recent studies have begun to identify and describe relevant links between these problems and children's health care.

The chapter is divided into four major sections. The first section examines research on health-risk behaviors among children. The next section reviews recent research on psychosocial aspects of child health care. These two areas are not mutually exclusive, nor clearly divisible; the intent, however, is to group studies for the purpose of cogent review. A section is then focused on emerging issues in the field. The final section discusses the state of the science overall, identifying areas needing further research. Recommendations for advancing the knowledge base on school-age children's health care are also provided.

HEALTH-RISK BEHAVIOR

Health-risk behaviors that contribute to the leading causes of mortality, morbidity, and social problems among adults are often established during childhood, extend into adulthood, and are interrelated. A number of researchers have investigated the antecedents of adult health problems in childhood. Research exploring health-risk behavior during the school-age years tends to separate according to two foci. One set of studies focuses on factors that influence how children perceive health, and the second focuses on how children behave with regard to health. The latter further divides into five categories of health-risk behavior among children: dietary behaviors, physical activity, cardiovascular risks, injury, and substance abuse.

Health Perceptions

With few exceptions, studies of school-age children's perceptions of health are descriptive and link demographic variables to perceptions of health. How children view their health is clearly a function of developmental stage. Green and Bird (1986) reported that fifth and seventh graders understood health and illness to be reciprocal aspects of the concept "health" although first and third graders did not. Stember, Stiles, and Rogers (1987) also reported age to be a factor in how children perceived their vulnerability to health problems. Older children felt more vulnerable to childhood injury and younger children felt more vulnerable to adult illness.

The relationship between gender and perceptions of health tends to be somewhat more confusing among school-age children. Graham and Uphold (1992) reported no differences between girls' and boys' perceptions of their own health. In contrast, Farrand and Cox (1993) reported girls to have more positive health self-concepts than boys. Earlier Stember et al. (1987) reported that girls perceived health problems to be more severe and that they were more vulnerable to them than boys.

Farrand and Cox (1993) found health perceptions to be only one of the determinants of health behaviors of 9- and 10-year-old children. Other factors that influenced children's health behavior included health experience, family functioning, self-esteem, and intrinsic motivation. By identifying the interacting variables that contribute to health behavior, Farrand and Cox were able to construct gender-specific models to guide nursing research and to test interventions.

Dietary Behavior

The concern for dietary practices of children is evident in the literature. Nurses have investigated the composition of children's diets, anemia, obesity, and measures to modify children's dietary intake.

As children spend much of their time away from home in the school setting and receive breakfast, lunch, and snacks at school, school dietary programs have been the focus of much research. Farris, Nicklas, Webber, and Berenson (1992) evaluated a school-lunch program by amount of food consumed and recipe analysis. They reported that the school-lunch program contributed less than one third of daily total nutrients, whereas saturated fat, cholesterol, and sodium content were excessive. Hoerr and Louden (1993) evaluated snack selections available to school children from unrefrigerated vending machines. Only 4 of 133 different available snacks met the criterion for nutrient density. Resnicow (1991) found that children who skipped break-fast before school had significantly higher plasma total cholesterol levels.

Anemia has been studied as it relates to learning. Francis, Williams, and Yarandi (1993) reported that anemic children had decreased attentiveness and narrower attention spans in the classroom. Another report suggested that iron deficiency may have some lasting effect on behavior and development (Deinard, List, Lindgren, Hunt, & Chang, 1986). Although there are ethnic differences in incidences of anemia, Jackson and Jackson (1991) suggested that differences in hemoglobin levels were attributable to nutrition rather than any genetic differences.

Much of the research on obesity in children has been conducted in disciplines other than nursing. Sherman and Alexander's (1990) succinct sum-mary, "Obesity in Children: A Research Update," reviewed 35 reports on factors associated with obesity in children. They identified the variables of nutritional knowledge, eating practices, maternal values, and selected sociode-mographic variables including lower socioeconomic status as related to the potential for obesity. Studies on physical activity as a contributing factor to obesity are notably absent from the Sherman and Alexander review.

Muecke, Simons-Morton, Huang, and Parcel (1992) studied the associa-tion between exposure to high-fat foods, low levels of exercise, and obesity. They reported neither high-fat food intake, nor reported level of physical activity were independent risk factors for obesity. They concluded that the two variables may exert a synergistic effect when both are present in the same child.

Research that examined intervention strategies to modify the eating behavior of young children focused on environmental modification and health education. Hoerr and Louden (1993) replaced snack food in school vending machines with nutrient-dense products. Sales from the vending machines dropped until nutrition information was posted on the machines. Based on their analysis of food references in textbooks, D'Onofrio and Singer (1985) recommend better textbook selection to influence children's eating habits.

Health education programs based on social learning theory (Bandura, 1977) have been shown to be effective in altering children's dietary intake and nutrition knowledge. For example, Perry, Mullis, and Maile (1985) tested cartoon role models as vehicles for changing dietary behavior of third- and fourth-grade students. At posttest, students participating in the nutrition education program reported a significant reduction in consumption of foods high in fat and salt and an increase in consumption of complex carbohydrates. Their assessments were confirmed by food-selection measures and by 24-hour diet recalls. Contento, Kell, Keiley, and Corcoran (1992) conducted a formative evaluation of "Changing the Course," a behaviorally oriented, activity-based nutrition education curriculum for elementary students developed by the American Cancer Society. Student achievement results showed most children attained the learning objectives posttest.

Physical Activity

The importance of physical activity in a healthy lifestyle has been recognized for years. Although children represent the fittest and most active section of society, concern exists that children may not be active enough for current or future health benefits (Biddle & Goudas, 1996; Connor et al., 1986). Debate continues about the extent to which children are active (Trost et al., 1996) with some of the differences reflected in measurement problems (Biddle & Goudas, 1996). What seems to be emerging from both anecdotal and scientific reports, however, is that children's activity levels decline with age and that boys are more active than girls (Trost et al., 1996). Whether children are less active now than in previous times cannot be answered with data. This possibility exists, however, due to greater availability of sedentary pursuits and perceived dangers for children active in outdoor environments where physical attack is feared. The following studies illustrate these points and demonstrate the range of inquiry into children's physical activity. Trost and colleagues found gender differences in activity levels and a tendency to overcome exercise barriers in a group of predominantly African American fifth-grade students. Boys demonstrated higher levels of physical fitness, greater self-efficacy in overcoming barriers to physical activity, greater amounts of television watching, and higher levels of participation in community sports and physical activity programs. These investigators suggested that gender differences may reflect a disproportion in community sport and physical activity opportunities for girls. Thus, intervention efforts should be directed toward removing the barriers that prevent girls from participating in community sports and physical activities.

Biddle and Goudas (1996) investigated variables useful in predicting vigorous physical activity for children. Parental support and encouragement were directly related to children's activity levels. This suggests that interventions may need to target multiple generations in order to achieve desired results in children.

Because school-age children are very active, few researchers evaluate the efficacy of physical activity programs. Connor and associates (1986) developed a demonstration project to provide low-cost, heart-health education and physical fitness for third- and fourth-grade children. This was designed to be implemented with minimal training and nominal expenditure for equipment and supplies in after-school programs. Their experimental program was tested against control conditions in four after-school programs. Results indicated significant gains in physical fitness knowledge and changes in attitude and activity in the experimental group.

For the most part, measures of efficacy of physical fitness programs have reported immediate changes in knowledge, attitudes, and activity levels. What is needed are longitudinal studies that will measure the lasting effects of programs implemented in childhood on sustained activity and cardiovascular fitness in adulthood.

Cardiovascular Risk

Research on cardiovascular health risks overlaps research on physical activity and nutrition; however, a growing concern about the early detection and primary prevention of atherosclerotic changes in childhood has focused specific attention on the manifestations of cardiovascular risk in school-age children. Investigations of the physical activity and eating habits of children tended to explore the preventive aspects of cardiovascular risk. At least two other areas of inquiry emerged from the literature. These included a small, but highly significant number of studies focused on identifying the normal physiologic parameters of well children, and those studies that focused on detecting physiological and behavioral risks that predict future disease.

Measurement of changes in heart function in children has traditionally used models derived from adult studies. Grossman (1991) described the characteristics of blood pressure rhythms in school-age children. Although Grossman reported no significant differences in circadian blood pressure rhythms between children of normotensive parents and children of hypertensive parents, Grossman, Jorda, and Farr (1994) reported children's blood pressure rhythms to be ultradian rather than circadian and to be related to height and weight. This research provided the foundation for a better understanding of blood pressure measurement with regard to development and imparted meaning to data describing variations in children's blood pressure.

To examine the predictive value of family history in detecting children with high cholesterol, Davidson et al. (1991) screened children ages 9 to 10 and compared cholesterol levels with family histories of cardiovascular disease events and risk factors. A significant number of children with abnormally high cholesterol levels had no family history of cardiovascular disease. These researchers concluded that adherence to current policies that recommend screening only those children with a positive family history will result in failing to detect a majority of children whose blood cholesterol levels exceed desirable levels.

Several studies of twins have been conducted to determine those risk factors that have the potential to respond to environmental and lifestyle changes. Hayman, Meininger, Stashinko, and Gallagher (1988) studied twins to determine the relationship of type A behavior patterns and its components to physiological cardiovascular disease risk factors of blood pressure, obesity, lipids, and lipoproteins. Although type A behavior and its components were not positively associated with physiological risk factors for cardiovascular disease, the impatience–aggression component is associated with lower levels of atherogenic lipids. From another twin study, Meininger, Hayman, Coates, and Gallagher (1988) reported that type A behavior and its components have a strong genetic basis, but environmental factors interact with biological substrata to produce significant changes in physiological risk factors. Both of these studies provide a basis for focusing nursing interventions on weight, lipid profiles, and blood pressure.

Injury

According to the 1995 "Youth Risk Behavior Surveillance" report, accidental injury constitutes the leading cause of child mortality in the United States

(Kann et al., 1996). Reasons why accidents are such a problem in childhood are not fully understood, however, several probable causes exist. Children have shorter attention spans, and they interpret symbols differently than adults. They also are curious and may not make intelligent decisions about situations related to safety, especially when they are without supervision.

Much of the published research evaluated specific safety projects and reported mixed results. For example, Foss (1989) evaluated a community-wide incentive program to promote safety-restraint use in cars and concluded the program was only minimally effective. Adams (1982) found a school-based seat-belt-restraint program improved children's knowledge of seat belts, but not their attitudes about using seat belts. Adams concluded that parental role models exert more influence than education programs on children's use of seat belts. By contrast, a school-based bicycle-safety project that incorporated interactive education sessions combined with reduced-cost bicycle helmet sales improved helmet use in intervention schools as compared to control schools (Liller, Smorynski, McDermott, Crane, & Weibley, 1995).

The evidence is conflicting regarding "latch-key" children's home-safety behaviors and ability to handle emergency situations. Peterson, Mori, and Scissors (1986) surveyed children regarding home-safety rules that their parents indicated had been taught to them. Correlations of parent–child responses revealed the children were not aware of the safety rules their parents had mentioned as stressed in the home. Frederick and White (1989) surveyed children's responses to descriptions of situations related to stranger safety, fire safety, accident prevention, and first-aid. Students responded appropriately to stranger-safety items, but inappropriately to fire-safety items. Responses to first-aid items were classified as dangerous.

A particularly interesting study of pediatric nurse practitioner safety counseling practices reported that advice about child car restraints and seat belts was routinely given by less than 30% of practitioners (Jones, 1992). Smoke detector and firearm safety in the home were included in counseling even less frequently. This study together with surveys of children's actual behavior illustrate gaps in knowledge and practice with regard to injury prevention.

Substance Abuse

Substance use and abuse, including the use of tobacco, alcohol, prescription and street drugs, is widely recognized as a major health problem among school-age children. Nursing research, however, is only beginning to address this problem; little work has been done testing nursing interventions. This is an area where interdisciplinary interventions may be particularly appropriate, and research from fields related to nursing is relevant. Some examples of such work are provided.

Grube and Wallack (1994) surveyed school children and found that exposure to television beer advertising related positively to stated intentions to drink alcohol. Research by numerous investigators (Backinger, Bruerd, Kinney, & Szpunar, 1993; Binion, Miller, Beauvais, & Oetting, 1988; Oetting, Beauvais, & Edwards, 1988) has documented the increased risk of tobacco, alcohol, and drug abuse by certain vulnerable groups of children, particularly minority children. An interesting study by Klitzner, Bamberger, and Gruencwald (1990) found that parent-led prevention groups, although difficult to establish and currently not prevalent, can be a very effective base for community substance-abuse-prevention programs. Children of alcoholic parents are known to be at high risk for substance abuse. A study by Michaels, Roosa, and Geushiemer (1992) examined a school-based prevention program and found that children of alcoholics were not likely to self-select into the program.

The identification of specific nurse-initiated health care activities to prevent or reduce children's substance use and the design of studies to evaluate the efficacy of these interventions are needed. Nursing research conducted by Long and Boik (1993) provided a basis for developing interventions because they identified specific factors that appear to predict later alcohol use that could be influenced by nursing or interdisciplinary interventions in the early school-age years.

Critique of Health-Risk Behavior Research

In general, studies of health-risk behavior among school-age children are limited to descriptive correlational design and convenience sampling techniques. Because health behavior is most appropriately studied in a natural setting such as the home, community or classroom, research controls are difficult or impossible to introduce. Consequently, it would be erroneous to imply causation in any of the relationships reported.

A few researchers failed to describe the sampling frame (Liller et al., 1995) or to report the number of refusals, withdrawals, or cases lost (Farrand & Cox, 1993; Stember et al., 1987), thus clouding the significance of their results. With the exception of Davidson et al. (1991), ethnicity of subjects was not reported. These errors of omission render the importance of results tenuous at best and attempts at replication impossible.

Formal classroom teaching programs were the most prevalent interventions reported. Noticeably absent from the literature were studies focusing on nursing interventions beyond the classroom. The efficacy of common nursing techniques such as contracting for weight control or dietary change, and family counseling for lifestyle changes and risk reduction have not been studied with school-age children.

PSYCHOSOCIAL HEALTH

There are numerous areas of research that focus specifically or primarily on the psychosocial aspects of health and related health care for school-age children. Because children are uniquely vulnerable to their family, school, and neighborhood environments, much of the research on children's psychosocial health examines approaches to modifying or improving environmental aspects.

Stress and Coping

Most of the research conducted to date in relation to children's stress and coping is descriptive in nature. Although recommendations for health care interventions are frequently derived from the work, very little research has been conducted to test interventions. Stress and coping research falls into two main areas: examination of specific life stressors and their outcomes and descriptions of children's coping responses. The majority of the research completed thus far is in the former category. Numerous studies have examined relationships between children's stress and either specific symptoms (Beautrais, Fergusson, & Shannon, 1986; Cooper, Bawden, Camfield, & Camfield, 1987) or the use of pediatric health services (Grey, 1988; M. A. Lewis & C. E. Lewis, 1985; Schorr; 1986). The relationship between environmental or psychological stressors and both increased physical illness and increased use of pediatric health services appears to be well established. There is also a sizable body of research documenting relationships between stress and psychological and behavioral health problems in children (see Grey, 1993). Luster and McAdoo (1994) found a positive relationship between stressful environmental factors and academic or behavioral problems specifically among African American school children. Webb (1989) examined parental and economic stress and its adverse effects on school-age children's peer relationships.

Other investigators have focused on stressful events within the family and their influence on children's health. Shell, Groppenbacher, Roosa, and Gensheimer (1992) documented increased psychological and behavioral problems among children who had to deal with the stress of parental alcohol abuse. The chronic illness or death of a parent or sibling have also been identified as major stressors and associated with a variety of negative health outcomes (F. M. Lewis, Zahlis, Shands, Simsheimer, & Hammond, 1996; McCown & Davies, 1995; Walker, 1988). Gallo, Breitmayer, Knafe, and Zoeller (1993) emphasized a family context in their research on stress and the school-age child's health. This research yielded specific interventions to be used in supporting parents and promoting children's health.

Grey's (1993) review, "Stressors and Children's Health," provided a comprehensive synopsis of research in the area. She concluded her work by noting that although there is clear evidence to indicate a link between stressful experiences and illnesses of all kinds in children, the nature and strength of the relationship is not clear. Grey emphasized the need for research that will identify the psychophysiological pathways connecting stress with health outcomes.

To date, there is only a small amount of research focused on identifying and describing children's coping responses, although this appears to be a promising direction for enhancing the knowledge base on children's health maintenance and promotion. Walker's (1988) research described children's coping when faced with a sibling with cancer. Ryan (1988) provided a comprehensive review of the state of knowledge regarding coping among school-age children. Sorensen's (1990) work is qualitative and makes a significant contribution by providing a taxonomy of coping strategies as described directly from the perspective of healthy children. Atkins' (1991) integrative review provided information on research conducted prior to Sorensen's work on children's perceptions of stressors and coping strategies. One example of intervention research is provided by the LaMontagne, Mason, and Hepworth (1985) study of relaxation techniques and anxiety reduction in children.

Parenting and Divorce

There is a good deal of overlap between studies on stress and those on parenting as each relates to health care for the school-age child. Hall and Farrel (1988) found a relationship between maternal stress and maternal perception of behavior problems in children. Webster-Stratton and Hammond (1988) found that depressed mothers were more critical of their children; however, the actual behavior of children did not vary significantly based on the affective state of their mothers. Meyers, Taylor, Alvy, Arrington, and Richardson (1992) found a relationship between maternal psychological distress and increased child behavior problems among inner-city African American school children. Moore (1993) conducted research on children's self-care and its relationship to maternal care. She tested aspects of Orem's (1991) Self-Care Theory with children ages 9 to 18 years. Her findings indicated an inverse relationship between children's self-care regarding health and mother's dependent care. Much of this result appeared to be related to the child's age, however, and implications for the health care of school-age children were not clear.

The effects of parental divorce on children's psychosocial health have been studied extensively, resulting in the identification of numerous intervening variables and many recommendations for strategies to promote child health. There has been little research conducted to test the effectiveness of interventions, however, and very little focus in the nursing literature on identifying, examining, or testing nursing interventions to promote psychosocial health among children dealing with parental divorce.

Wallerstein's research on children and divorce (Wallerstein, 1986; Wallerstein, Corbin, & Lewis, 1988) is extensive. It focused on identifying the effects of divorce on critical childhood developmental tasks and on examining the mitigating or exacerbating effects of ongoing parental conflict on children's behavior. Grych and Fincham (1992) developed an overview of interventions designed to support children during divorce and described how these relate to research findings. This very comprehensive work thoroughly reviewed research conducted on the effects of divorce on children, moderating variables, and studies done to evaluate interventions to assist children, couples, and families in dealing with divorce. The consistent finding of a small but reliable negative difference in the adjustment of children from divorced families is noted. The authors stated, "It is apparent that the overlap between basic research on children's adjustment to divorce and child-focused intervention efforts is limited" (Grych & Fincham, 1992, p. 439). They urged a closer relationship between research on the effects of divorce and the design of interventions to promote the psychosocial health of children dealing with parental divorce.

Depression and Anxiety

Much of the nursing care used to prevent depression among children or to assist depressed or anxious children is derived from research conducted in other fields. There is little evidence in the literature that nursing interventions addressing depression or anxiety among school-age children are being tested to determine outcomes. Some descriptive studies with implications for practice have been conducted.

Humphreys (1991) studied children, ages 10 to 17 years, in battered women's shelters. She found that the vast majority expressed numerous worries and concerns. The absence of any control group of children is a notable weakness of the study and is acknowledged by the author. Osofsky (1995) prepared an extensive overview of research examining the effects of exposure to violence on school-age and younger children. She noted that research has documented a variety of depressive, aggressive, and anxious symptoms in children exposed to violence. The degree and type of violence and the interventions of parents are identified as important moderating or mitigating variables.

Nelms (1986) examined parental assessments and child self-assessment of depression among school-age children with diabetes or asthma. Differences between parental perceptions and child self-reports were noted with a tendency for parents to underestimate childhood depression, especially among girls. Kristensen's (1995) phenomenological study of loneliness among school-age children yielded a summary of themes that characterized feeling lonely. This work provides a basis for further study that could lead to the development and testing of nursing interventions to prevent or diminish childhood loneliness and subsequent depression.

Attention Deficit Disorder and Learning Disabilities

There is a great deal of information available regarding attention deficit disorder (ADD), with or without hyperactivity, and learning disabilities. There is a very limited body of literature related to nursing interventions for children with these problems, however. G. K. Lewis' (1991) dissertation research contrasted family functioning among those with a child with ADD, a child with attention deficit hyperactivity disorder (ADHD), and a child with ADHD plus behavioral problems. The family functioning of all those studied was not significantly different from established norms. There were marked differences among the study groups, however. Those families coping with an ADHD child with behavioral problems did less well, as did those with older children. Although nursing implications were discussed, no follow-up work to develop or test interventions could be located. A case study by Brunette (1995) describes ADHD therapies for the disorder and specific interventions to be used by school nurses in working with ADHD children.

No nursing research on health care interventions for learning-disabled children was located. Some research conducted in the fields of psychology and education had implications for nursing practice. For example, Yasutake and Bryan (1995) summarized findings indicating that learning-disabled children are at greater risk for depression and low self-concept and found that improved affect resulted in more positive learning and academic outcomes. Because nurses in school and community settings have numerous opportunities to intervene in order to improve child affect, these results are relevant and could provide a basis for developing and testing nursing interventions. Research by Haager and Vaughn (1995) examined social skills and behavior problems of learning-disabled school children. The findings regarding parental, teacher, peer, and self-perceptions showed a marked difference among these groups with implications for nursing practice and research.

Although neither research based, nor occurring in the United States, it seems important to mention a large body of literature related to the evolving "specialty" of learning-disabilities nursing. This British (English) project and the writings associated with it are described and referenced by Rose and Kay (1995).

Critique of Psychosocial Health Research

Nursing research on the psychosocial health of school-age children is in an early stage. Several quantitative studies have examined the links between stress and psychosocial health outcomes (Webb, 1989; Webster-Stratton & Hammond, 1988), and qualitative work has been done to identify healthy coping responses by children (Sorensen, 1990). There needs to be greater focus on identifying and examining positive influences on children's psychosocial health, such as the ways in which parental actions can promote adaption and adjustment during periods of stress for children. Much of the current nursing-research literature on parenting is focused on the parents' role with either chronically or terminally ill children. Studies focused on the role of parents in maintaining or enhancing the physical and psychosocial health of their children need to be conducted.

Because psychosocial health and adaption to stress are so closely related to a child's developmental level, studies in these areas should be focused on children in a narrow age range, or should clearly identify age as a significant variable. Moore's (1993) research demonstrated the problems associated with testing theoretical constructs in a group of children who vary widely in age.

There are findings from completed studies in other fields that document the effects of psychosocial stressors on children's health (Beautrais et al., 1986; Wallerstein et al., 1988). These can now be used to design nursing interventions to promote or maintain children's psychosocial health, and the testing of these interventions should become the focus of nursing research. In particular, the results of nursing interventions designed to help children cope with parental divorce and school-related problems such as learning disabilities are needed. Nursing actions, programs, or interventions focused on preventing or limiting childhood depression and anxiety disorders also need to be examined and evaluated through well-designed studies that consider efficacy and cost-effectiveness.

EMERGING ISSUES

Homelessness

As homelessness has increased in the United States, its effects on families and children have become more apparent. School-age children are now either not in school, or there only sporadically because of family homelessness. Nursing research is now being conducted to identify, assess, and document the effects of homelessness on the health status and health care of school-age children.

Murata, Mace, Strehlow, and Shuler (1992) compared the health care received by a severely impoverished group of homeless Hispanic children in Los Angeles with that of a national children's sample. As might be expected, the homeless children were found to receive care more often for acute illnesses and injuries and much less often for prevention and screening. A study by Kemsley and Hunter (1993) had somewhat different findings, revealing more treatment for chronic problems such as upper respiratory and skin infections. Although the samples in both studies were homeless children, they were quite different. For example, more than half in the Kemsley and Hunter study had health insurance coverage, whereas none in the Murata and associates study did. The need for precise descriptions of the homeless samples used in future research became increasingly apparent in the course of reviewing current studies. Without such precision, findings will continue to be confounded by numerous other variables. This is well demonstrated in research by Ziesemer, Marcoux, and Marwell (1994). Homeless children and a matched group of mobile, low socioeconomic status children were studied in relation to academic performance and behavior problems. A high rate of academic and behavior problems were found, but no significant differences were identified between the groups. The authors concluded that the variables of poverty, mobility, and lack of social support may be more significant in determining children's performance and well-being than homelessness. Nursing research on the psychosocial health of homeless children is also being reported. An example is work by Wagner and Menke (1991) documenting high levels of depression among homeless school-age children.

To date, nursing research related to homelessness in children is descriptive. This work can provide a basis for the development of nursing interventions and an impetus for the health and social policies needed for broad, large-scale programs of intervention. There is a need for research that critically tests nursing interventions designed to reduce or prevent physical and psychosocial health care problems among homeless school-age children.

AIDS

Acquired immunodeficiency syndrome (AIDS) continues to be an escalating problem with increasing implications for children and their families. Early concerns were for hemophiliac children who acquired the virus from blood-product therapy. As the virus spread in the general population, prenatal transmission of the virus to children became a concern. Recently it is recognized that preadolescents must be prepared to protect themselves from HIV infection by avoiding risky behaviors. An equally growing concern is the number of children who are affected by another member of the family who has HIV/ AIDS. In response to these concerns, numerous articles have been published to provide direction to nursing care of children with HIV/AIDS. The O'Hara and D'Orlando (1996) synopsis published recently in *Nursing Clinics of North America* provides an excellent guide for care.

How to equip children to protect themselves from transmission of HIV prior to engaging in risky behavior has prompted researchers to investigate children's knowledge of HIV/AIDS. Brown, Nassau, and Barone (1990) discovered differences in knowledge and attitudes about HIV/AIDS when personal behavior was implied by survey questions. They concluded that AIDS information widely covered by the media is known by students in all grades, but grades differ in knowledge when students need a conceptual understanding of AIDS to correctly respond to less publicized items. A similar difference between knowledge and understanding has been confirmed by other studies (Obeidallah et al., 1993; Schofeld, Johnson, Perrin, O'Hare, & Cicchetti, 1993). These findings need to be considered when planning and implementing nursing-intervention programs.

Andrews, Williams, and Neil (1993) investigated the nature of the mother–child relationship when the mother is HIV positive. They described the mother–child bond as being strongly attached and as having an element of secrecy. Additionally, children were perceived by their mothers as sources of support as well as sources of stress in the relationship. Many mothers listed children 8 years old or younger as sources of support. The researchers concluded that practice and policy decisions concerning HIV-positive mothers should include emphasis on maintaining the health of the mother–child dyad.

The nursing research conducted thus far on school-age children with HIV/AIDS is descriptive. Further descriptive work is needed to document the ways in which school-age children are affected when parents, siblings, or friends have AIDS. In addition, the nursing interventions being used to protect children from HIV/AIDS and to support children who have the disease complex need to be critically evaluated through well-designed studies.

STATE OF THE SCIENCE

There are several points to be made regarding nursing research methods in the area of health care for the school-age child. The topic area is very broad and a systematic comparison of findings from the studies reviewed was difficult given the variance in design, sampling procedures, sample size, type of data, variables studied, measurement, and data analysis. The majority of studies in the area tended to be discrete and somewhat isolated. Although they contributed to the knowledge base of nursing practice, these contributions were not organized or cumulative. Noticeably absent were interconnected studies that systematically built on one another to form a cohesive foundation on which to base practice and from which to derive theory. Also absent were replications that test and validate previous findings.

In most studies reviewed, sample size was adequate to achieve effect. Given the descriptive nature of the vast majority of studies reviewed, however, several noticeable flaws should be mentioned related to sampling. Many studies reported samples that spanned several age groups, school age and early adolescence, for example, without reporting results according to age or developmental level. Some researchers also neglected to report ethnicity of subjects. Developmental level, as well as ethnicity, are of importance for both building the knowledge base and determining application of findings to practice.

Few well-controlled studies based on large probability samples are represented among the studies reviewed, and nonrandom sampling techniques predominate. Much of the current research relevant to the health of school-age children is preliminary, however. Although highly controlled studies are most useful in determining causality related to single outcome, they rarely provide information about processes children and families experience when they try to manage common health problems. Qualitative methods with small samples of appropriate subjects yield information about these complex processes. The qualitative studies included in this review do provide insight into children's responses to health problems.

An additional point should be made about the generalizability of findings from the studies represented in this review. Although many studies used convenience sampling, large sample sizes may diminish a portion of the possible selection bias rendering results usable with caution.

Further Research Directions

A great deal of work remains to be done in developing the knowledge base for the health care of the school-age child. It appears that much of the current knowledge used to derive nursing interventions is borrowed from the disciplines of psychology, medicine, and to a lesser degree, social work and education. There is an extensive literature regarding health, nursing, and the school-age child. However, the vast majority of it consists of descriptions of practice experiences or the discussion of practice or policy recommendations that are not research based.

There are some well done and comprehensive reviews of research relevant to aspects of the health care of the school-age child. Examples of this are the Grey (1993) review of stressors and children's health and the Sherman and Alexander (1990) review of obesity in children. Implications for nursing practice are derived from these reviews. Nonetheless, one is struck by the lack of an organized knowledge base on children's health care and by the lack of studies designed to test the outcomes of nursing interventions. The nursing-research literature on children's health care, as differentiated from the care of sick children, is primarily descriptive. In some areas such as nutrition, cardiovascular health risk, children's coping, and substance-abuse prevention, there appears to be adequate descriptive work for the generation and testing of specific nursing interventions.

There is an emerging literature regarding school-based health care designed and implemented by nurses. Little research has been conducted on these programs yet, although Rienzo and Button (1993) have reported on a community analysis of responses to such school-based programs. Obviously, research that can clearly document the efficacy and cost-effectiveness of interventions will be critically important as child health services become increasingly selected, controlled, and rationed by managed and capitated care systems.

Review of the literature also revealed that school-age children's health care has received less attention over the past decade than that of adolescents, infants, or preschoolers. The myriad of social and health problems associated with adolescence, for example, sexually transmitted diseases and drug abuse, have brought national focus to the importance of health care for this group. Likewise, the emphasis on early intervention and prevention has brought increased attention to infants and young children. Concomitantly, funding has eroded for public health and especially school-health nursing. This lack of emphasis on school-age children in policy and funding arenas over the past decade may have contributed to less focus on research and knowledge-base development regarding this age group.

As nursing care delivery becomes increasingly community based, the importance of school, neighborhood, and home health care services, especially prevention and health promotion for all children, is reemerging. Thus the next decade should provide impetus and opportunity to build on theory, existing practice, research from other disciplines, and the current descriptive nursing research to further develop a knowledge base on health care for the school-age child. Clear identification of areas of intervention, such as screening, parental teaching, and risk reduction, may facilitate an organized and cumulative development of knowledge. As much of the health care for children in schools is delivered by interdisciplinary teams, it is important to design interdisciplinary research projects that can identify and test child health interventions. Nurse researchers should be active in evolving and verifying how nursing science and nursing practice both contribute to interdisciplinary interventions and make unique contributions.

REFERENCES

Adams, D. (1982). Children's response to a belt restraint program. *Pediatric Nursing, 11,* 28–30.

Andrews, S., Williams, A. B., & Neil, K. (1993). The mother–child relationship in the HIV-1 positive family. *IMAGE: Journal of Nursing Scholarship, 25,* 193–198.

Atkins, F. D. (1991). Children's perspective of stress and coping: An integrative review. *Issues in Mental Health Nursing, 12,* 171–178.

Backinger, C. L., Bruerd, B., Kinney, M. B., & Szpunar, S. M. (1993). Knowledge, intent to use, and use of smokeless tobacco among sixth grade schoolchildren in six selected cities. *Public Health Reports, 108,* 637–642.

Bandura, A. (1977). *Social learning theory.* Englewood Cliffs, NJ: Prentice Hall.

Beautrais, A. L., Fergusson, D. M., & Shannon, F. T. (1986). Life events and child morbidity: A prospective study. *Pediatrics, 70,* 935–940.

Biddle, S., & Goudas, M. (1996). Analysis of children's physical activity and its association with adult encouragement and social cognitive variables. *Journal of School Health, 66,* 75–78.

Binion, A., Miller, C. D., Beauvais, F., & Oetting, E. (1988). Rationales for the use of alcohol, marijuana, and other drugs by eighth-grade Native American and Anglo youth. *International Journal of the Addictions, 23,* 47–64.

Brown, L. K., Nassau, J. H., & Barone, V. J. (1990). Differences in AIDS knowledge and attitudes by grade level. *Journal of School Health, 60,* 270–275.

Brunette, E. A. (1995). Management of ADHD in the school setting—A case study. *Journal of School Health, 11*(3), 33–38.

Connor, M. K., Smith, L. G., Fryer, A., Erickson, S., Fryer, S., & Drake, J. (1986). Future fit: A cardiovascular health education and fitness project in an after-school setting. *Journal of School Health, 56,* 329–333.

Contento, I. R., Kell, D. G., Keiley, M. K., & Corcoran, R. D. (1992). A formative evaluation of the American Cancer Society changing the course nutrition education curriculum. *Journal of School Health, 62,* 411–416.

Cooper, P. J., Bawden, H. N., Camfield, P. R., & Camfield, C. S. (1987). Anxiety and life events in childhood migraine. *Pediatrics, 79,* 999–1004.

Davidson, D. M., Van Camp, J., Iftner, C. A., Landry, S. M., Bradley, B. J., & Wong, N. D. (1991). Family history fails to detect the majority of children with high capillary blood total cholesterol. *Journal of School Health, 61,* 75–80.

Deinard, A., List, A., Lindgren, B., Hunt, J., & Chang, P. (1986). Cognitive deficits in iron-deficient and iron-deficient anemic children. *Journal of Pediatrics, 108,* 681–689.

D'Onofrio, C. N., & Singer, R. (1985). Unplanned nutrition education in the schools: Sugar in elementary reading texts. *Journal of School Health, 53,* 521–526.

Farrand, L. L., & Cox C. L. (1993). Determinants of positive health behavior in middle childhood. *Nursing Research, 42,* 208–213.

Farris, R. P., Nicklas, T. A., Webber, L. S., & Berenson, G. S. (1992). Nutrient contribution of the school lunch program: Implications for *Healthy People 2000*. *Journal of School Health, 62,* 180–184.

Foss, R. D. (1989). Evaluation of a community-wide incentive program to promote safety restraint use. *American Journal of Public Health, 79,* 304–306.

Francis, E., Williams, D., & Yarandi, H. (1993). Anemia as an indicator of nutrition in children. *Journal of Pediatric Health Care, 7,* 156–160.

Frederick, R. A., & White, D. M. (1989). Safety and first aid behavioral intentions of supervised and unsupervised third grade students. *Journal of School Health, 59,* 146–149.

Gallo, A. M., Breitmayer, B. J., Knafe, K. A., & Zoeller, L. H. (1993). Mother's perceptions of sibling adjustment and family life in childhood chronic illness. *Journal of Pediatric Nursing, 8,* 318–324.

Graham, M. V., & Uphold, C. R. (1992). Health perceptions and behaviors of school-age boys and girls. *Journal of Community Health Nursing, 9,* 77–86.

Green, K., & Bird, J. (1986). The structure of children's beliefs about health and illness. *Journal of School Health, 56,* 325–328.

Grey, M. (1988). Stressful life events, absenteeism, and the use of school health services. *Journal of Pediatric Health Care, 2,* 121–127.

Grey, M. (1993). Stressors and children's health. *Journal of Pediatric Nursing, 8,* 85–91.

Grossman, D. G. S. (1991). Circadian rhythms in blood pressure in school-age children of normotensive and hypertensive parents. *Nursing Research, 40,* 28–33.

Grossman, D. G. S., Jorda, M. L., & Farr, L. A. (1994). Blood pressure rhythms in early school-age children of normotensive and hypertensive parents: A replication study. *Nursing Research, 43,* 232–237.

Grube, J. W., & Wallack, L. (1994). Television beer advertising and drinking knowledge, beliefs, and intentions among schoolchildren. *American Journal of Public Health, 84,* 254–259.

Grych, J. H., & Fincham, F. D. (1992). Interventions for children of divorce: Toward greater integration of research and action. *Psychological Bulletin, 3,* 434–454.

Haager, D., & Vaughn, S. (1995). Parent, teacher, peer and self-reports of the social competence of students with learning disabilities. *Journal of Learning Disabilities, 28,* 205–215.

Hall, L. A., & Farrel, A. M. (1988). Maternal stresses and depressive symptoms: Correlates of behavior problems in young children. *Nursing Research, 37,* 156–161.

Hayman, L. L., Meininger, J. C., Stashinko, E. E., & Gallagher, P. R. (1988). Type A behavior and physiological cardiovascular risk factors in school-age twin children. *Nursing Research, 37,* 290–295.

Hoerr, S. M., & Louden, V. A. (1993). Can nutrition information increase sales of healthful vended snacks? *Journal of School Health, 63,* 386–390.

Humphreys, J. (1991). Children of battered women: Worries about their mothers. *Pediatric Nursing, 17,* 342–346.

Jackson, R., & Jackson, F. (1991). Reassessing "heredity" interethnic differences in anemia status. *Ethnicity and Disease, 1,* 26–41.

Jones, N. E. (1992). Injury prevention: A survey of clinical practice. *Journal of Pediatric Health Care, 6,* 182–186.

Kann, L., Warren, C. W., Harris, W. A., Collins, J. L., Williams, B. I., Ross, J. G., & Kolbe, L. J. (1996). Youth risk behavior surveillance—United States, 1995. *Journal of School Health, 66,* 365–377.

Kelley, S. J. (1995). Child sexual abuse: Initial effects. In J. J. Fitzpatrick & J. S. Stevenson (Eds.), *Annual review of nursing research* (Vol. 13, pp. 63–86). New York: Springer Publishing Co.

Kemsley, M., & Hunter, J. K. (1993). Homeless children and families: Clinical and research issues. *Issues in Comprehensive Pediatric Nursing, 16,* 99–108.

Klitzner, M., Bamberger, E., & Gruenewald, P. J. (1990). The assessment of parent-led prevention programs: A national descriptive study. *Journal of Drug Education, 20,* 111–125.

Kristensen, K. L. (1995). The lived experience of childhood loneliness: A phenomenological study. *Issues in Comprehensive Pediatric Nursing, 18,* 125–137.

LaMontagne, L. L., Mason, K. R., & Hepworth, J. T. (1985). Effects of relaxation on anxiety in children: Implications for coping with stress. *Nursing Research, 34,* 289–292.

Lewis, F. M., Zahlis, E. H., Shands, M. E., Simsheimer, J. A., & Hammond, M. A. (1996). The functioning of single women with breast cancer and their school-aged children. *Cancer Practice: A Multidisciplinary Journal of Cancer Care, 4,* 15–24.

Lewis, G. K. (1991). Family functioning as perceived by parents of a child with attention deficit disorder: A nursing study. (Doctoral dissertation, University of Texas at Austin, 1991). *University Microfilms International,* PUZ9128285.

Lewis, M. A., & Lewis, C. E. (1985). Psychological distress and children's use of health services. *Pediatric Annals, 14,* 555, 558–560.
Liller, K. D., Smorynski, A., McDermott, R. J., Crane, N. C., & Weibley, R. E. (1995). The More Health bicycle safety project. *Journal of School Health, 65,* 87–90.
Long, K. A., & Boik, R. J. (1993). Predicting alcohol use in rural children: A longitudinal study. *Nursing Research, 42,* 79–86.
Luster, T., & McAdoo, H. P. (1994). Factors related to the achievement and adjustment of young African American children. *Child Development, 65,* 1080–1094.
McCown, D. E., & Davies, B. (1995). Patterns of grief in young children following the death of a sibling. *Death Studies, 19,* 41–53.
Meininger, J. C., Hayman, L. L., Coates, P. M., & Gallagher, P. (1988). Genetics or environment? Type A behavior and cardiovascular risk factors in twin children. *Nursing Research, 37,* 341–345.
Meyers, H. F., Taylor, S., Alvy, K. T., Arrington, A., & Richardson, M. A. (1992). Parental and family predictors of behavior problems in inner-city black children. *American Journal of Community Psychology, 20,* 557–576.
Michaels, M. L., Roosa, M. W., & Geushiemer, L. K. (1992). Family characteristics of children who self-select into a prevention program for children of alcoholics. *American Journal of Community Psychology, 20,* 663–672.
Moore, J. B. (1993). Predictors of children's self-care performance: Testing the theory of self-care deficit. *Scholarly Inquiry for Nursing Practice, 7,* 199–212.
Muecke, L., Simons-Morton, B., Huang, W., & Parcel, G. (1992). Is childhood obesity associated with high-fat foods and low physical activity? *Journal of School Health, 62,* 19–23.
Murata, J., Mace, J. P., Strehlow, A., & Shuler, P. (1992). Disease patterns in homeless children: A comparison with national data. *Journal of Pediatric Nursing, 7,* 196–204.
Nelms, B. C. (1986). Assessing childhood depression: Do parents and children agree? *Pediatric Nursing, 12,* 23–26.
Obeidallah, D., Turner, P., Iannotti, R. J., O'Brien, R. W., Haynie, D., & Galper, D. (1993). Investigating children's knowledge and understanding of AIDS. *Journal of School Health, 63,* 125–129.
Oetting, E. R., Beauvais, F., & Edwards, R. (1988). Alcohol and Indian youth: Social and psychological correlates and prevention. *Journal of Drug Issues, 18,* 87–99.
O'Hara, M. J., & D'Orlando, D. (1996). Ambulatory care of the HIV-infected child. *Nursing Clinics of North America, 31,* 179–205.
Orem, D. E. (1991). *Nursing concepts of practice.* St. Louis: Mosby-Year Book.
Osofsky, J. D. (1995). The effects of exposure to violence on young children. *American Psychologist, 50,* 782–788.
Perry, C. L., Mullis, R. M., & Maile, M. C. (1985). Modifying the eating behavior of young children. *Journal of School Health, 55,* 399–402.
Peterson, L., Mori, L., & Scissors, C. (1986). Mom or dad says I shouldn't: Supervised and unsupervised children's knowledge of their parents rules for home safety. *Journal of Pediatric Psychology, 11,* 177–188.

Resnicow, K. (1991). The relationship between breakfast habits and plasma cholesterol levels in school children. *Journal of School Health, 61,* 81–85.

Rienzo, B. A., & Button, J. W. (1993). The politics of school-based clinics: A community level analysis. *Journal of School Health, 63,* 266–272.

Rose, S., & Kay, B. (1995). Significant skills. *Nursing Times, 91,* 36, 63–64.

Ryan, N. M. (1988). The stress-coping process in school-age children: Gaps in knowledge needed for health promotion. *Advances in Nursing Science, 11*(1), 1–12.

Schofeld, D. J., Johnson, S. R., Perrin, E. C., O'Hare, L. L., & Cicchetti, D. V. (1993). Understanding of acquired immunodeficiency syndrome by elementary school children—A developmental survey. *Pediatrics, 92,* 389–395.

Schorr, E. L. (1986). Use of health care services by children and diagnoses received during presumably stressful life situations. *Pediatrics, 77,* 834–841.

Shell, R. M., Groppenbacher, N., Roosa, M. W., & Gensheimer, L. K. (1992). Interpreting children's reports of concern about parental drinking: Indicators of risk status? *American Journal of Community Psychology, 20,* 463–489.

Sherman, J. B., & Alexander, M. A. (1990). Obesity in children: A research update. *Journal of Pediatric Nursing, 5,* 161–167.

Sorensen, E. S. (1990). Children's coping responses. *Journal of Pediatric Nursing, 5,* 259–267.

Stember, M. L., Stiles, M. K., & Rogers, S. (1987). Severity of and vulnerability to health problems in school-age children. *Issues in Comprehensive Pediatric Nursing, 10,* 263–272.

Trost, S. G., Pate, R. R., Dowda, M., Saunders, R., Ward, D. S., & Felton, G. (1996). Gender differences in physical activity and determinants of physical activity in rural fifth grade children. *Journal of School Health, 66,* 145–150.

Wagner, J., & Menke, E. (1991). The depression of homeless children: A focus for nursing intervention. *Issues in Comprehensive Pediatric Nursing, 14,* 17–29.

Walker, C. L. (1988). Stress and coping in siblings of childhood cancer patients. *Nursing Research, 37,* 208–212.

Wallerstein, J. S. (1986). Children of divorce. The psychological task of the child. In R. H. Moos (Ed.), *Coping with life crises: An integrated approach* (pp. 35–48). New York: Plenum.

Wallerstein, J. S., Corbin, S. B., & Lewis, J. M. (1988). Children of divorce: A 10-year study. In E. M. Hetherington (Ed.), *Impact of divorce, single parenting, and step-parenting on children* (pp. 197–212). Hillsdale, NJ: Erlbaum.

Webb, A. A. (1989). Parental and economic stress in relation to school-age children's peer relationships and anxiety experiences six years later. (Doctoral dissertation, Wayne State University, 1989), *University Microfilms International,* PUZ9022464.

Webster-Stratton, C., & Hammond, M. (1988). Maternal depression and its relationship to life stress, perceptions of child behavior problems, parenting behaviors, and child conduct problems. *Journal of Abnormal Child Psychology, 16,* 299–315.

Yasutake, D., & Bryan, T. (1995). The influence of affect on the achievement and behavior of students with learning disabilities. *Journal of Learning Disabilities, 28,* 329–334.

Ziesemer, C., Marcoux, L., & Marwell, B. E. (1994). Homeless children: Are they different from other low-income children? *Social Work, 39,* 658–668.

Chapter 3

Childhood Diabetes: Behavioral Research

PATRICIA BRANDT
SCHOOL OF NURSING
UNIVERSITY OF WASHINGTON

ABSTRACT

The major emphasis of behavioral research related to childhood diabetes has been on the child's physical and emotional outcomes, the family's response, and adherence issues. This research review focuses on adherence and related youth and family functioning. Descriptive and intervention studies are critiqued. Common conceptual and methodological issues are discussed with recommendations for future research.

Keyword: Childhood Diabetes

Behavioral research related to childhood diabetes has increased dramatically over the past 10 years. The major emphases of these behavioral investigations have been on the child's physical and emotional outcomes, the family's response, and adherence issues. The populations included in studies have typically been families who have regular access to health services and whose children are school age and preteen. Minimal attention has been devoted to populations of color, the underserved, various socioeconomic classes, or the developmental periods of early childhood and late adolescence.

This research review focuses on adherence and related family and youth functioning. Both descriptive and intervention studies were critiqued. Empirically based work with a positivist perspective framed the predominant orientation found in the literature search. Interpretive perspectives and associated study results were included in the search; however, few were located. Studies reviewed included subjects 18 years of age or younger and their families. Sample sizes ranged from 8 to 270. Nursing, medical, and psychology journals were included in this review. Computer searches from 1985 through 1996 were performed on PsychINFO, Cumulative Index of Nursing and Allied Health Literature, and MEDLINE databases. An ancestry strategy was also used as citations were followed from one publication to another. The review (a) addresses childhood diabetes, its prevalence and challenges; (b) describes the predominant themes found in research related to adherence, family and youth functioning, and analyzes studies as exemplars; (c) identifies common conceptual and methodological research issues; and (d) describes directions for future research.

Nurse researchers have primarily conducted descriptive and cross-sectional studies in respect to children with insulin-dependent diabetes and their families. Behaviorally oriented international nursing studies are seldom published in U.S. journals as investigators from Japan (Nakamura & Kanematsu, 1994), Finland (Hentinen & Kyngas, 1992), and Canada (Hatton, Canam, Thorne, & Hughes, 1995) were the only ones found in the literature search. The majority of nurse investigators used a quantitative and univariate approach in contrast to researchers from other disciplines who conducted multivariate and longitudinal descriptive studies of diabetes during childhood. One qualitative study (Hatton et al., 1995) that used a phenomenological approach was located for this review.

Behaviorally oriented intervention studies related to childhood diabetes are seldom conducted. The few nurse investigators engaged in intervention research primarily have conducted evaluation studies of ongoing clinical programs, such as a diabetes camp program (Zimmerman et al., 1987) and an education program (Brandt & Magyary, 1993). One quasi-experimental study was completed by a nurse investigator, a pilot test of a diabetes self-management program for 8- to 12-year-old children and their parents (McNabb, Quinn, Murphy, Thorp, & Cook, 1994). Treatment-oriented research by researchers from disciplines other than nursing are also few in number and typically involve experimental designs with random assignment of the intervention groups (Boardway, Delameter, Tomakowsky, & Gutai, 1993; Kaplan, Chadwick, & Schimmel, 1985; Satin, La Greca, Zigo, & Skyler, 1989).

PREVALENCE AND CHALLENGES OF CHILDHOOD DIABETES

The onset of insulin-dependent diabetes mellitus (IDDM) in childhood occurs at any time from infancy through adolescence. The highest incidence of IDDM is among youths aged 10 to 14 years; however, diabetes during early childhood has increased dramatically in recent years (Cowie & Eberhardt, 1996). Males and females are about equally affected (Krolewski & Warram, 1985; Sperling, 1996). Although IDDM occurs in most racial and ethnic groups, the evidence at this time indicates that IDDM is primarily a disease of White children and does not vary in the United States according to household income (Kahn & Weir, 1994). The prevalence rate of diabetes in children of color during childhood is 10 per 100,000.

During the first 6 months after the child is diagnosed, the insulin requirements are usually minimal because of the residual functioning of the pancreas (Guthrie, 1988). This is an important period in the family's life as working relationships among members and between the family and health care providers are essential to establish, maintain, and revise the diabetes management plan (Haire-Joshu, 1996).

Normoglycemia (70–180 mg/dl) is the current standard of care, as hyperglycemia is a major factor for long-term complications such as heart disease, retinopathy, and renal disease. Close monitoring of glycemic control typically is prescribed with three to four blood tests and two to three insulin injections daily. Hypoglycemic reactions, which could be expressed as seizure-like behaviors, or the potential of having a reaction creates stress for youths and family members. Some anxiety about hypoglycemia appears to be useful, as researchers (Green, Wysocki, & Reineck, 1990) have found that a minimal level is associated with better control. How anxiety functions within individuals and the dynamics involved in the transition from "useful" anxiety to subclinical or clinical disorders are unclear. Some youths try to prevent hypoglycemia by altering food intake or insulin dosage without family or medical consultation and thus present with poor glycemic control or adherence difficulties.

ADHERENCE WITHIN THE CONTEXT OF THE FAMILY

Youth and family patterns of adherence to the diabetes regimen tend to develop during the diagnostic phase of diabetes and persist into young adulthood. When 95 school-aged youths were followed in a 9-year longitudinal study (Kovacs, Goldston, Obrosky, & Iyengar, 1992), adherence problems were more likely to occur 3 years after the onset of diabetes. About 30% of youths had a serious adherence problem at some time during this study.

Adherence in diabetes is typically measured in the clinical setting by completion of prescribed behavioral tasks: injection, exercise, overall diet, daily blood testing with a memory meter (levels of 80–120 mg/dl are typically recommended), and a laboratory blood assay done quarterly (glycosylated hemoglobin). Good metabolic control is equivalent to an 8% or lower glycosylated hemoglobin level, a cumulative indicator of blood sugar levels over several months (Goldstein et al., 1982; Hanson et al., 1996).

Adherence is a complex, multidimensional construct that consists of both time and content dimensions. Factor analytic results indicated that the *content* dimension of adherence includes five independent components of diabetes management: exercise, injection, diet type, blood testing and frequency, and diet amount. For time dimensions, researchers have found child-oriented adherence measures to be valid and reliable when specific activities are measured within a time-limited context of 24 hours (Johnson, Silverstein, Rosenbloom, Carter, & Cunningham, 1986).

Knowing that adherence is a multidimensional construct has helped investigators focus on the complexities involved in diabetes care. When separate tasks and temporal assessment (within a few days) are used to try and demonstrate linkage to glycemic control as measured by glycosolated hemoglobin, study results are inconclusive, however. Therefore, the content and time dimensions of the adherence construct found in previous research may not fully represent the realities of the child's and family's diabetes experience. Investigators need to develop ways to study the interrelationship of multiple tasks over the same time period using glycemic control as an outcome. Practitioners are presented with similar challenges during periodic clinical evaluations of youths with diabetes.

A recent cross-sectional study (Hanson et al., 1996) was designed to improve the measurement of self-care behaviors to encompass patterns of behaviors across several months. The purpose of this study was to determine which measures of self-care would best predict glycemic control. The participants in the study were 270 youths aged 4 to 20 years and their parents. The investigators found that a semi-structured interview measuring multiple self-care behaviors specific to diabetes over time best predicted glycemic control at both 6-month and 1-year time points. Single measures of diet or exercise did not predict glycemic control. The investigators noted that the study results were "suggestive" as multiple statistical tests were performed, new instruments were used, and a small amount of variance in the outcome was predicted by the best predictor. These limitations are typical of adherence studies conducted within the context of childhood diabetes.

Strong associations between adherence behaviors and glycemic control have been difficult to obtain in longitudinal studies. Results of a longitudinal study (Johnson et al., 1992) during an 18-month time period of 192 youths indicated that 29% of the variance in glycemic control was predicted by eating frequency and insulin dosage. Although the amount of variance explained was significantly higher than in cross-sectional studies, considerable information is unknown. A significant finding of this study was that predictive power was improved when age-homogeneous samples of youth were used. Preadolescents were grouped separately from adolescents in the analyses. Study investigators routinely incorporated a wide distribution of ages in the analyses, which perhaps contributed to the inconsistent and conflicting results obtained. The investigators suggested that physiologic changes and the potential to become "insulin resistant" during puberty may be important mechanisms for explaining the type of associations among adherence behaviors and glycemic control outcomes during that age period. Another major contribution of this study was the testing of a conceptually driven causal model through structural equation analysis. The investigators had believed that a group design was the best approach, as they assumed that adherence and glycemic control were similar across youths. In their summary they questioned this assumption, however, and recommended that future studies incorporate a within-subject design to detect linkages between adherence behavior and diabetes control.

Diabetes education programs and diabetes camps are common avenues for enhancing diabetes self-care behaviors. These interventions differ across agencies and are evaluated rarely, however. In one of the few published evaluations of a diabetes education program, nurse investigators found that the school-aged youth and their mothers who attended the program were more likely to have improved knowledge than skills (Brandt & Magyary, 1993). Significant gains from the diabetes education program were found to be maintained for 3 months for both the children and their mothers. These results may have been influenced by "testing" as a one-group pretest and posttest design was used.

In a study (Zimmerman et al., 1987) of a diabetes camp, a pre–posttest design was used to evaluate outcomes for 63 children with diabetes and 18 without diabetes. Both groups of children aged 8 through 14 gained similar levels of knowledge about diabetes. Limitations of this study included: no evaluation of skill development, imbalance in group size, and covariates were not measured. A major limitation of both the diabetes education and camp studies was that the designs did not include a long-term follow up to determine if gains were maintained over time. In addition, sampling bias may have influenced the results of these two studies, as they both used a convenience sample that had resources and motivation to participate in a program.

One of the findings of the diabetes education study (Brandt & Magyary, 1993) that warrants further investigation was that the direction of the relationship between child learning and the mother–child relationship differed with what the child was learning. A warm mother–child relationship tended to be associated with children who exhibited better problem-solving skills but worse insulin-injection skills. The application of problem-solving skills to diabetes management situations in daily living requires ongoing communication between the parent(s) and the child. In contrast, the technical act of an insulin injection may be accomplished independently and require less communication with a parent. Perhaps, a child who has a problematic relationship with a parent may be motivated to master the skills associated with insulin injection as a means to gain distance and independence, or the parent may have expectations for the child to handle the injection independently. In contrast, children who have a warmer relationship with the parent(s) may have fewer reasons to gain independence through self-management of the insulin injection. Diabetes may be a source of parent–child conflict for many reasons, including the extent of time the parent(s) devotes to the care needed and the degree of interdependence associated with the task (Giordano, Petrila, Banion, & Neuenkirchen, 1992).

Knowledge of diabetes and its associated self-care behaviors have been repeatedly found to be insufficient for explaining health outcomes (Wysocki, Hough, Ward, & Green, 1992). Thus, researchers have turned their attention to other factors that interrelate with adherence behaviors such as youth and family functioning.

Family Functioning

Daily decision making and long-term diabetes management require the family to have over time (a) a knowledge and skill base that changes as needed (Anderson, Auslander, Jung, Miller, & Santiago, 1990); (b) supportive family members that share and adapt responsibilities (Hanson, Henggeler, & Burghen, 1987; Schafer, McCaul, & Glasgow, 1986); and (c) clear, enabling communication among family members (Hauser et al., 1990). The experiences of family members during each developmental phase are likely to contribute toward how the family develops and maintains working relationships with each other.

Little is known about family transitions and diabetes responsibilities during early childhood or young adulthood. There is a known increase for risk of family-relationship difficulties and problematic metabolic control when the youth is between 10 and 15 years of age, however. During this particular transition, youths have marked physical and psychosocial changes that interact with the ongoing family life experiences and dynamics. Youths are encouraged to assume more responsibility as they get older and also tend to have greater adherence problems (Danemen & Frank, 1992). By age 13 or 14 years, youths are likely to perform all the required diabetes behavioral tasks but still need overall parental supervision and assistance in problem solving (Follansbee, 1989). Disagreements about who in the family is or should be assuming responsibility for select tasks are common during adolescence (Anderson et al., 1990).

Adolescents who live in families whose members talk directly to each other about tensions maintain better diabetic control than do adolescents in families that avoid discussions about conflictual issues (Stein, 1989). Exchanges of negative emotions during family problem solving were associated with adjustment problems of youths in the general population (Forgatch, 1989) as well as in populations of youth with insulin-dependent diabetes (Miller-Johnson et al., 1994). It appears to be important for the youth and family to express opinions within a positive emotional family context.

In one of the few longitudinal studies relevant to family dynamics and diabetes (Jacobsen et al., 1994), families with higher levels of verbal expressiveness had youths who were in better glycemic control over a 4-year period. The participants consisted of 61 children aged 9 to 16 years and their families who were within 12 months of the diagnosis of IDDM. The families were serviced by a regional endocrine center. The assessment schedule during the 4 years was based on usual clinical practice. Analyses consisted of a two-step growth-modeling procedure; within- and between-person parameters were estimated. A particular merit of this study was the long-term association found between family communication and glycemic control as reported by the children and mothers. Over time the trajectory of glycemic control differed as the level of expressiveness differed. A hypothesis that may explain these results is that when a family has open communication, the youth may be more comfortable dealing directly with issues and feelings and thus, resolve problematic issues before patterns develop (Saarni & Cowley, 1990). Replica tion of the regression model used in this study needs to be performed to ensure these results are stable as well as useful with different populations.

Parent and adolescent communication, beliefs about the motives of another's behavior, and authority structures are similar in families with adolescents who have diabetes and those families without diabetes (Wysocki, 1993). An example of research designed to identify characteristics of relationships that best predict glycemic control and adherence behaviors was a cross-sectional descriptive study of 115 adolescents and their mothers and fathers (Wysocki, 1993). Using multiple regression, the best predictor of youth adjustment to diabetes was effective problem-solving and conflict resolution skills within the family as reported by the mothers, fathers, and youths. Caution in interpreting these results is needed as family members may endorse negative family dynamics more highly when adolescents have problems with diabetes control than if families have adolescents with better control. Another limitation of this study was that adherence and diabetes control were not measured.

Other resources of family members have been found to be important considerations for behavioral diabetes research (Auslander, Bubb, Rogge, &

Santiago, 1993). Coping of family members appears to have particular relevance for understanding the dynamics involved in these families. Using an in-depth case-study approach, researchers (Hauser, Diplacide, Jacobsen, Willet, & Cole, 1993) found that families whose youth had minimal compliance of self-care behaviors were more likely to employ less active coping than families in which the youth's compliance with the diabetes regimen was high. Coping of mothers of children with diabetes has also been found to be an important variable within family functioning. Although diabetes supervision is increasingly shared among adults in the family, mothers typically assume the primary responsibility (Kovacs et al., 1992). A structural equation model using Lisrel analyses indicated maternal coping was one of the main constructs that predicted depressive symptoms among 52 mothers of children age 4 to 18 with IDDM (Blenkfeld & Holahan, 1994). A major limitation of this study was that the common-method variance potentially shared between the measures of coping and depression was not analyzed. These results suggested that the construct of parental well-being is important to include in future studies. The planning of variables within an overall framework is essential, however.

Intervention research aimed to improve parent–adolescent relationships in families who have a youth with diabetes is rarely conducted. One of the few studies found for this review was a 6-week intervention with 32 families randomly assigned to one of three interventions (Satin et al., 1989). The multifamily treatment approach consisted of 90-minute sessions with three to four families in group meetings aimed to improve diabetes management through problem solving and support from group members. The multifamily-plus-parent-simulation treatment approach consisted of the same strategies with additional opportunities for parents to learn what it was like for the youth to have diabetes by doing the prescribed tasks on themselves. The control group was offered the opportunity to obtain the intervention after the study was completed. No significant group differences were found on gender, age, diabetes duration, or diabetes control. Youths maintained clinically significant improvements in glycemic control for 6 months after completion of the multi-family-plus-parent-simulation-group treatment only. Families in the multifam-ily-plus-simulation-intervention group were more involved in other behavioral interventions in comparison to the other groups. Thus, these families may have differed in motivation and the potential to change. Given the small sample size in each intervention group, this study needs to be replicated.

Youth Functioning

The youth's experience of diabetes develops within an interpersonal system of family, peers, teachers, and health care providers. Gender, emotional regulation, and cognitive competencies influence a youth's ability to benefit from interventions and the ongoing adjustment challenges of living with diabetes (Boardway et al., 1993; Kazak, 1992).

Gender.   Conflicting results were found in the few studies of gender differences of youths who had IDDM and adherence or family impact. One consistent finding was that girls were more likely to have poorer glycemic control than boys (Cruickshanks, Orchard, & Becker, 1985; Wing, Epstein, Nowalt, & Lamparski, 1986). Depression was higher in 12- to 18-year-old girls with diabetes than boys, which may contribute to the increased number of girls with glycemic control problems (La Greca, Swales, Klemp, Madigan, & Skyler, 1995). Investigators need to examine what mechanisms contribute to the association between depression and poor glycemic control in girls. For example, is the linkage biologically or hormonally determined? Are there different levels of physical activity in boys than girls? Are eating disorders indicated in the relationship between depression and glycemic control? There are some indications that eating disorders are higher in adolescent women with IDDM than in the general population (Marcus & Wing, 1990). The design, study methodologies, and small samples have limited these studies, however. Youths in poor metabolic control may use a variety of ways to express an eating disorder such as frequent binge eating or reducing the insulin amount with subsequent glycosuria and weight loss. Thus, individual variations of eating problems need to be included in future studies (La Greca et al., 1995).

Emotion regulation.   Youths who have difficulty adapting to diabetes and its associated management tasks are more likely to have recurrent ketoacidosis (Drotar & Bush, 1985). In particular, youths who have poor adherence to diabetes treatment are more likely to have avoidant coping styles (Hanson et al., 1989). Although having diabetes is not necessarily associated with psychological problems, youths who have difficulties with emotion regulation during the diagnostic phase of diabetes are more likely to have long-term adherence problems (Grey, Cameron, & Thurber, 1991; Jacobsen et al., 1987, 1990).

Cognitive competency/health beliefs.   The youth's cognitive competencies and associated health beliefs are considered major influencing factors on self-care behaviors and diabetes outcome. Although diabetes management requires complex reasoning skills, studies of how cognitive function influences self-care behaviors are nonexistent. Researchers have instead focused on the degree of neuropsychological impairment of children who have diabetes. Children whose diabetes began prior to age 5 are reported to have somewhat poorer attention spans, difficulty completing tasks, and some corresponding minor school difficulties than children without diabetes (Hagen et al., 1990). Overall, the educational problems were found to be minor, subtle, and selective for subgroups of children with diabetes (Rovet, Ehrlich, Czuchta, & Akler, 1993). The results of these studies by Hagen et al. and Rovet et al. need to be interpreted skeptically as correlational and cross-sectional designs are the primary approaches used. Children with diabetes may be at a greater risk for learning disabilities or children with learning problems may be less effective in monitoring their diabetes and subsequently have more negative outcomes.

The studies of health beliefs of children regarding diabetes are preliminary and descriptive. One example of this work is a descriptive study in which school-age children aged 7 to 8 years reported perceptions of susceptibility to diabetes complications as well as perceived benefits of treatment (Charron-Prochownik, Becker, Brown, Liang, & Bennett, 1993). In another study of health beliefs, youths aged 10 to 17 were compliant with the prescribed diabetes regimen when they had low perceived threats to self and perceptions of high benefits of the management plan to low cost ratios (Bond, Aiken, & Somerville, 1992). Poor glycemic control was associated with high perceived susceptibility to threats on health and high cues that action was demanded of them. At this juncture of time, studies of youth health beliefs related to diabetes cannot be compared as different ages, measures, and health belief models have been used in the few studies conducted. Perhaps a focus on health beliefs in future studies will increase the understanding of why adherence typically decreases during adolescence as well as lead toward more effective treatment approaches. Using threats of the long-term consequences of failing to adhere to the diabetes regimen, for example, may negate adherence efforts rather than improve them.

When youths with diabetes develop self-management abilities in the context of parental guidance, the stresses associated with diabetes management are likely to be reduced (Boardway et al., 1993). By developing competencies in self-management of diabetes care, a youth may improve, for example, in error detection through self-observation of responses, glycemic control in relation to daily blood sugar indications, and self-initiated reinforcement for ongoing completion of diabetes tasks (Wiebe, Alderfer, Palmer, Lindsay, & Jarrett, 1994; Wing et al., 1986). By gaining skills in self-management, youths develop self-efficacy (Bandura, 1986). Self-efficacy is the youth's perception that he or she has the ability to participate (as appropriate to age and experience) in the daily challenges of managing diabetes. Research is needed to learn how the youth's self-efficacy improves over time in relation to managing the diabetes tasks and the associated stressors, such as fear of becoming hypoglycemic or being different from peers (Green et al., 1990).

Self-management interventions have been found to improve self-efficacy in respect to the youth's self-monitoring of blood glucose or a behaviorally defined self-care goal (Delameter et al., 1990; Nurick & Johnson, 1991). In a study that compared the standard clinical care approach with a research-based, self-management approach of blood glucose monitoring and problem solving, youths aged 11 to 14 years were able to maintain levels of metabolic control longer in the research-based approach than those receiving the standard care (Anderson, Wolf, Burkhart, Cornell, & Bacon, 1989). Findings from another self-management study (McNabb et al., 1994) indicated that 8- to 12-year-old children who received six 1-hour intervention sessions assumed significantly more responsibility for diabetes self-care than the controls who received the standard clinical care. Although studies on self-management interventions provide future investigators with innovative ideas for designing interventions, they have major limitations. Both the Anderson et al. and McNabb et al. studies used random assignment, but the sample size was small as there were 35 children in the Anderson et al. experimental group and 12 children in the McNabb et al. experimental group. In addition, the investigators did not measure youth or family functioning variables. Ongoing monitoring of treatment integrity was not discussed nor was a follow-up conducted to determine maintenance of change.

The various self-management studies have brought investigators closer to understanding interventions that may enhance family and youth outcomes. In addition, greater knowledge of individual differences is needed to better match interventions to the individual youth and family. As found by Wiebe et al. (1994), youths with diabetes who are prone to anxiety tend to create confusion in respect to their perceptions of symptoms in contrast to youths with diabetes who have low anxiety. Providing the same intervention for adolescents who have differing anxiety levels would not be an effective way to design a study. Furthermore, if single focused interventions such as a blood glucose symptom perception strategy are used as the only approach and the family and professionals involved in the care are not included, the experience of diabetes is oversimplified.

CONCEPTUAL ISSUES IN DIABETES RESEARCH DURING CHILDHOOD

Conceptually based studies that include developmental and family processes are needed to move research to clinical utility. Adherence is not a constant state and neither is childhood, even though the completed studies seldom consider the dynamic transactions that occur in a child's life. Developmental processes that are especially important considerations in childhood diabetes research are the child's cognitive and personal control competencies. Cognitive processes such as memory and the understanding of causality, time, and consequences influence the child's ability to comprehend and follow the complexity of the illness and regimen plans. Motivating factors involved in personal control, particularly the child's autonomy and self-efficacy competencies, have major implications for childhood-based studies of adherence and adjustment to chronic health conditions (Iannotti & Bush, 1993).

Family processes involved in diabetes management need to be addressed in research. For example, how do family members capitalize on the youth's personal motivation to develop his or her own sense of efficacy about each component of diabetes care? How do the family's expectations about what is an acceptable expression of emotion in the family influence the youth's emotional regulation? Does the youth learn to use an "emotional front" to accommodate family expectations? And if so, does this contribute to a building up of negative feelings about diabetes within the youth and subsequent difficulties with adherence? The dynamic nature of the youth and family's interactions and its influence on diabetes are central to clinically relevant research.

The constructs used in childhood diabetes research have evolved primarily from empirical studies in which researchers operationalize the definition and selection of the constructs. These definitions are often "practitioner centered," especially when related to adherence and health outcomes (Karoly, 1993). Thus, the vast majority of research in this field has evolved from a representational model of the professional, either the practitioner or researcher. There has been little emphasis on the interconnectedness of the family, youth, and provider in adherence research or the "goodness of fit" between the diabetic management plan and the family (Karoly, 1993). Diabetes management involves many forms of shared management among the provider, youth, and family. Thus, theoretical models that guide studies need to include the conditions in which diabetes is managed in these various ways, such as joint management among the parent, youth, and provider or, youth management with consultation from the parent and provider.

The reality of the child's and family's experiences from their perspective has seldom been an emphasis of research. In addition, health behaviors mean something different for children and their families at different ages. Instead of conducting studies with adult-oriented health paradigms, a common problem of current research, new paradigms are needed that deal with the interplay of these developmental processes and the child's experiences within the cultural, socioeconomic, health care, and environmental contexts.

METHODOLOGICAL ISSUES OF DIABETES RESEARCH DURING CHILDHOOD

Over the past decade researchers have acknowledged that improvement is needed in the conceptual linkage of theory, design, data collection, and analysis. More recently researchers have been challenged to reflect on how their world views relate to the scholarly inquiry approaches used. To ensure that "reflective consistency" occurs, the investigators need to acknowledge, for example, how the conceptualization of a study and data influence the conclusions (Klein & Jurich, 1993). The current state of research in childhood diabetes consists primarily of a logical positivist perspective as research is primarily empirically driven. In the future, a pluralistic approach is needed so world views are expanded to include such approaches as phenomenological inquiry to draw out the family's knowledge and experience differently and thus, supplement an empirical approach.

Samples for diabetes research also need to be expanded to be population based with various ages and ethnicities of children included. Samples have been predominantly White, school-age children or adolescents from tertiary care centers. With the advent of managed care, it will be important to include the variety of health care sites that serve children.

To move research forward in the field of childhood diabetes, clinically useful investigations are essential. Studies of treatment effects are needed in research-based interventions, ongoing multidisciplinary clinical practice trials, and evaluation of diabetes education programs. Research is needed to test treatments that address the interface of the psychosocial and health components of diabetes. Matching of children and their families to the type of treatment is essential so the best treatment for a particular child and family is identified. An essential question demanding attention is: What specific treatment will prevent or reduce specific problems in specific contexts with certain individuals? (La Greca & Varni, 1993).

Intervention studies are typically focused on improving adherence through knowledge development, self-management, or family communication. These have typically been randomized group designs with small samples of school-age children. Because each treatment group used an average of 14 youths in studies of self-management interventions for youths with diabetes, any differences found would have to be large to be detected (Anderson et al., 1989; Delameter et al., 1990; McNabb et al., 1994; Nurick & Johnson, 1991). Treatments are typically implemented for about 2 months with about 6 months as the usual follow-up period (Delameter, 1993). In future designs, follow up for at least a year is needed to determine whether the effects endure or change over time.

Treatment integrity has been rarely described in studies of children with diabetes. It is critical to determine whether the treatment was implemented as planned. Training of those providing the treatment, manuals, and systematic monitoring of the treatment program's implementation is essential for treatment integrity and future replication (La Greca & Varni, 1993). For research-based interventions, hypothesis-driven experimental design will provide more valid group-comparison results. Few studies of behavior-oriented child diabetes are driven by conceptually based or experimentally designed research. Furthermore, multiple-level interventions that include the treatment team, child, family, and clinical environment will improve these studies as will including quality-of-life outcomes in association with cost-effectiveness (Agras, 1993).

SUMMARY AND FUTURE RESEARCH DIRECTIONS

Children with diabetes are at risk for alterations in attention when diabetes begins prior to age 5 (Hagen et al., 1990), long-term physical complications (Haire-Joshu, 1996), and psychosocial problems (Blanz, Rensch-Rieman, Fritz-Sigmund, & Schmidt, 1993). Thus, prevention research is needed to improve the quality of life for these children and their families. Yet, clinical practice is seldom studied as it naturally occurs. Standard approaches in the clinical field such as promoting independent care by youths are being questioned as further knowledge of the value of cooperative management between the youth and family is gained (Follansbee, 1989).

Existing descriptive and intervention research has improved the understanding of some of the major factors associated with better adherence and metabolic control. There needs to be a shift from reliance on summary variables, however, such as the youth's age and gender or family expressiveness, to the processes and mechanisms of change that dynamically influence the youth and family. For example, what mechanisms are involved in the transfer of responsibilities within a shared management model between the youth and parent(s)? What occurs during transactions with health care providers that influence the youth and parent to assume the prescribed regimen of care? What are the essential developmental processes at each age level that contribute to metabolic control? How does the nurse alter the educational intervention to accommodate the youth's developmental processes such as memory capability and self-efficacy level?

Seligman (1995) challenges the researcher to study clinical practice as it occurs rather than relying predominately on well-controlled intervention studies with samples screened out when any complicating conditions coexist. He notes that randomly assigning participants to treatments, commonly done in "efficacy studies," consumes extensive time and resources and is minimally helpful to clinical practice. Instead, effectiveness studies need to mirror the reality of treatments that are continually altered by clinicians as they work with youths and their families.

By building research programs that are conceptually driven and oriented toward clinical usefulness, the nurse investigator will be able to collaborate more effectively with others in this multidisciplinary practice and research field of childhood diabetes. By expanding world views and methodologies, varying approaches can be explored that potentially will inform the field more fully. Designs, data-collection strategies, and data-analytic techniques that promote the discovery of processes and relationships similar to phenomenologic and ethnographic approaches will add to the field (Wells & Freer, 1994). Single-case and case-study designs would be especially useful to analyze current clinical practices and develop conceptual understanding of the mechanisms involved (Drotar, La Greca, Lemanek, & Kazak, 1995). Randomized clinical trials that test innovative clinical approaches are needed to document the cost-effectiveness of combined psychosocial and physical health approaches. Cost savings should be studied for short- and long-term outcomes as a method of determining the accountability and value of each member's clinical practice within the multidisciplinary team (La Greca & Varni, 1993).

Nurses provide various combinations of interventions to children with diabetes and their families: education, self-management, family counseling, and monitoring of diabetes parameters. Nurse researchers must intensify their contributions to scholarly investigations by dramatically increasing the number of clinically relevant studies in partnership with researchers from other disciplines. The multiple levels required by this complex field demand a collaborative approach across disciplines. Well-planned, conceptually driven work is needed to build the base for new therapeutics and to affirm currently used approaches. The phenomena that are meaningful to the consumers of this research—the child, family, and clinician—need to be a central emphasis. An overall plan to systematically build from conceptualization to intervention within the reality of the clinical world is critical to advance nurse researchers' contributions to childhood diabetes research.

REFERENCES

Agras, W. (1993). Adherence intervention research: The need for a multilevel approach. In N. Krasnegor, L. Epstein, S. B. Johnson, & S. Jaffe (Eds.), *Developmental aspects of health compliance behavior* (pp. 285–301). Hillsdale, NJ: Erlbaum.

Anderson, B., Auslander, W., Jung, K., Miller P., & Santiago, J. (1990). Assessing family sharing of diabetes responsibility. *Journal of Pediatric Psychology, 15,* 477–492.

Anderson, B., Wolf, F., Burkhart, M., Cornell, R., & Bacon, G. (1989). Effects of peer-group intervention on metabolic control of adolescents with IDDM. Randomized outpatient study. *Diabetes Care, 12,* 179–183.

Auslander, W., Bubb, J., Rogge, M. T., & Santiago, J. (1993). Family stress and resources: Potential areas of intervention in children recently diagnosed with diabetes. *Health and Social Work, 18,* 101–113.

Bandura, A. (1986). *Social foundations of thought and action: A social cognitive theory.* Englewood Cliffs, NJ: Prentice Hall.

Blanz, B., Rensch-Rieman, B., Fritz-Sigmund, D., & Schmidt, M. (1993). IDDM is a risk factor for adolescent psychiatric disorder. *Diabetes Care, 16,* 1621–1623.

Blenkfeld, D., & Holahan, C. (1994). Family support, coping strategies, and depressive symptoms among mothers of children with diabetes. *Journal of Family Psychology, 10,* 173–179.

Boardway, R., Delameter, A., Tomakowsky, J., & Gutai, J. (1993). Stress management training for adolescents with diabetes. *Journal of Pediatric Psychology, 18,* 29–45.

Bond, G., Aiken, L., & Somerville, S. (1992). The health belief model and adolescents with insulin-dependent diabetes mellitus. *Health Psychology, 11,* 190–198.

Brandt, P., & Magyary, D. (1993). The impact of a diabetes education program on children and mothers. *Journal of Pediatric Nursing, 8,* 1–10.

Charron-Prochownik, D., Becker, M., Brown, M., Liang, W., & Bennett, S. (1993). Understanding young children's health beliefs and diabetes regimen adherence. *Diabetes Educator, 19,* 409–417.

Cowie, C., & Eberhardt, M. (Eds.). (1996). *Diabetes 1996 vital statistics.* Alexandria, VA: American Diabetes Association.

Cruickshanks, K., Orchard, T., & Becker, D. (1985). The cardiovascular risk profile of adolescents with insulin dependent diabetes. *Diabetes Care, 8,* 118–124.

Danemen, D., & Frank, M. (1992). The adolescent with diabetes. In D. Haire-Joshu (Ed.), *Management of diabetes mellitus* (2nd ed., pp. 685–725). St. Louis: Mosby.

Delameter, A. (1993). Compliance intervention for children with diabetes and other chronic diseases. In N. Krasnegor, L. Epstein, S. B. Johnson, & S. Jaffe (Eds.), *Developmental aspects of health compliance behavior* (pp. 335–353). Hillsdale, NJ: Erlbaum.

Delameter, A., Bubb, J., Davis, S., Smith, J., Schmidt, L., White, N., & Santrage, J. (1990). Randomized perspective study at self-management training with newly diagnosed diabetic children. *Diabetic Care, 13,* 492–498.

Drotar, D., & Bush, M. (1985). Mental health issues and services. In N. Hobbs & J. M. Perrin (Eds.), *Issues in the care of children with chronic illness* (pp. 514–550). San Francisco: Jossey-Bass.

Drotar, D., La Greca, A., Lemanek, K., & Kazak, A. (1995). Case reports in pediatric psychology: Uses and guidelines for authors and reviewers. *Journal of Pediatric Psychology, 20,* 549–565.

Follansbee, D. (1989). Assuming responsibility for diabetes management: What age? What price? *Diabetes Educator, 15,* 347–352.

Forgatch, M. (1989). Patterns and outcome in family problem solving: The disrupting effect of negative emotion. *Journal of Marriage and the Family, 51,* 115–124.

Giordano, B., Petrila, A., Banion, C., & Neuenkirchen, G. (1992). The challenge of transferring responsibility for diabetes management from parent to child. *Journal of Pediatric Health Care, 6,* 235–239.

Goldstein, D., Parker, K., England, J., England, J., Jr., Wiedmeyer, H., Rawlings, S., Hess, R., Little, R., Simonds, J., & Breyfogle, R. (1982). Clinical application of glycosolated hemoglobin measurements. *Diabetes, 31*(suppl. 3), 70–78.

Green, L., Wysocki, T., & Reineck, B. (1990). Fear of hypoglycemia in children and adolescents with diabetes. *Journal of Pediatric Psychology, 15,* 633–641.

Grey, M., Cameron, M., & Thurber, F. (1991). Coping and adaptation in children with diabetes. *Nursing Research, 40,* 144–149.

Guthrie, D. (Ed.). (1988). *Diabetes education: A core curriculum for health professionals.* Alexandria, VA: American Association of Diabetes Education.

Hagen, J., Barclay, C., Anderson, B., Feeman, D., Segal, S., Bacon, G., & Goldstein, G. (1990). Intellective functioning and strategy use in children with insulin dependent diabetes mellitus. *Child Development, 61,* 1714–1727.

Haire-Joshu, D. (1996). *Management of diabetes mellitus: Perspectives of care across the life span.* St Louis, MO: Mosby-Year Book.

Hanson, C., DeGuile, M., Schinkel, A., Kotterman, O., Goodman, J., & Buckingham, B. (1996). Self-care behaviors in insulin-dependent diabetes: Evaluative tools and their associations with glycemic control. *Journal of Pediatric Psychology, 21,* 467–482.

Hanson, C., Harris, M., Relgca, G., Cigrang, J., Carle, D., & Burgher, G. (1989). Coping styles in youth with insulin dependent diabetes mellitus. *Journal of Consulting & Clinical Psychology 57,* 644–651.

Hanson, C., Henggeler, S., & Burghen, G. (1987). Social competence and parental support as mediators of the link between stress and metabolic control in adolescents with insulin dependent diabetes mellitus. *Journal of Consulting & Clinical Psychology, 55,* 529–533.

Hatton, D., Canam, C., Thorne, S., & Hughes, A. (1995). Parents' perceptions of caring for an infant or toddler with diabetes. *Journal of Advanced Nursing, 22,* 569–577.

Hauser, S., Diplacide, J., Jacobsen, A., Willet, J., & Cole, C. (1993). Family coping with an adolescent's chronic illness. *Journal of Adolescence, 16,* 305–329.

Hauser, S., Jacobsen, A., Wertlieb, D., Weiss-Perry, B., Follansbee, D., Wolfsdorf, J., Herskowitz, R., Houlihan, J., & Rajapark, D. (1990). Children with recently diagnosed diabetes: Interactions within families. *Health Psychology, 5,* 273–296.

Hentinen, M., & Kyngas, H. (1992). Compliance of young diabetics with health regimens. *Journal of Advanced Nursing, 17,* 530–536.

Iannotti, R., & Bush, P. (1993). Toward a developmental theory of compliance. In N. Krasnegor, L. Epstein, S. B. Johnson, & S. Jaffe (Eds.), *Development aspects of health compliance behavior* (pp. 53–76). Hillsdale, NJ: Erlbaum.

Jacobsen, A., Hauser, S., Lavori, P., Willett, J., Cole, C., Wolfsdorf, J., Dumont, R., & Wertlieb, D. (1994). Family environment and glycemic control: A four year prospective study of children and adolescents with insulin-dependent-mellitus. *Psychosomatic Medicine, 56,* 401–409.

Jacobsen, A., Hauser, S., Lavori, P., Wolfsdorf, J., Herskowitz, R., Milley, J., Bliss, R., Gelfand, E., Wertlieb, D., & Stein, J. (1990). Adherence among children and adolescents with insulin dependent diabetes mellitus over a four-year longitudinal follow-up: I. The influence of patient coping and adjustment. *Journal of Pediatric Psychology, 15,* 511–526.

Jacobsen, A., Hauser, S., Wolfsdorf, J., Houlihan, J., Milley, J., Herskowitz, R., Wertlieb, D., & Watt, E. (1987). Psychologic predictors of compliance in children with recent onset of diabetes mellitus. *Journal of Pediatrics, 110,* 805–811.

Johnson, S., Silverstein, J., Rosenbloom, A., Carter, R., & Cunningham, W. (1986). Assessing daily management in childhood diabetes. *Health Psychology, 5,* 545–564.

Johnson, S., Kelly, M., Henretta, J., Cunningham, W., Tomer, A., & Silverstein, J. (1992). A longitudinal analysis of adherence and health status in childhood diabetes. *Journal of Pediatric Psychology, 17,* 537–553.

Kahn, C. R., & Weir, G. C. (Eds.). (1994). *Joslin's diabetes mellitus* (13th ed.). Philadelphia: Lea & Febiger.

Kaplan, R., Chadwick, M., & Schimmel, L. (1985). Social learning intervention to promote metabolic control in Type I diabetes mellitus: Pilot experiment. *Diabetes Care, 8,* 152–155.

Karoly, P. (1993). Enlarging the scope of the compliance construct: Toward developmental and motivational relevance. In N. Krasnegor, L. Epstein, S. B. Johnson, & S. Jaffe (Eds.), *Development aspects of health compliance behavior* (pp. 11–27). Hillsdale, NJ: Erlbaum.

Kazak, A. (1992). Stress, change and families: Theoretical and methodological considerations. *Journal of Family Psychology, 6,* 120–124.

Klein, D., & Jurich, J. (1993). Metatheory and family studies. In P. Boss, W. Doherty, R. LaRossa, W. Schumm, & S. Steinmetz (Eds.), *Source book of family theories and methods: A conceptual approach* (pp. 31–67). New York: Plenum.

Kovacs, M., Goldston, D., Obrosky, S., & Iyengar, S. (1992). Prevalence and predictors of pervasive noncompliance with medical treatment among youths with insulin-dependent diabetes mellitus. *Journal of the American Academy of Child & Adolescent Psychiatry, 31,* 1112–1119.

Krolewski, D., & Warram, J. (1985). Epidemiology of diabetes mellitus. In C. R. Kahn & G. C. Weir (Eds.), *Joslin's diabetes mellitus* (13th ed., pp. 12–37). Philadelphia: Lea & Febiger.

La Greca, A., Swales, T., Klemp, S., Madigan, S., & Skyler, J. (1995). Adolescents with diabetes: Gender differences in psychosocial functioning and glycemic control. *Children's Health Care, 24,* 61–78.

La Greca, A., & Varni, A. (1993). Editorial: Interventions in pediatric psychology. A look toward the future. *Journal of Pediatric Psychology, 18,* 667–679.

Marcus, M. O., & Wing, R. (1990). Eating disorder and diabetes. In C. S. Holmes (Ed.), *Neuropsychological and behavioral aspects of diabetes* (pp. 102–121). New York: Springer-Verlag.

McNabb, W., Quinn, M., Murphy, D., Thorp, C., & Cook, S. (1994). Increasing children's responsibility for diabetes: The "In Control" study. *Diabetes Educator, 20,* 121–124.

Miller-Johnson, S., Emery, R., Marvin, R., Clark, W., Lovinger, R., & Marten, M. (1994). Parent–child relationships and the management of insulin-dependent diabetes mellitus. *Journal of Consulting & Clinical Psychology, 62,* 603–610.

Nakamura, N., & Kanematsu, Y. (1994). Coping in relation to self-care behaviors and control of blood glucose levels in Japanese teenagers with insulin-dependent diabetes mellitus. *Journal of Pediatric Nursing, 9,* 427–432.

Nurick, M., & Johnson, S. B. (1991). Enhancing blood glucose awareness in adolescents and young adults with IDDM. *Diabetes Care, 14,* 1–7.

Rovet, J., Ehrlich, R., Czuchta, D., & Akler, M. (1993). Psychoeducational characteristics of children and adolescents with insulin-dependent diabetes mellitus. [Special Series: Pediatric chronic illness]. *Journal of Learning Disabilities, 26,* 7–22.

Saarni, C., & Cowley, M. (1990). The development of emotion regulation: Effects on emotional state and expression. In E. Blechman (Ed.), *Emotions and the family* (pp. 53–73). Hillsdale, NJ: Erlbaum.

Satin, W., La Greca, A., Zigo, M., & Skyler, J. (1989). Diabetes in adolescence: Effects of multi-family group intervention and parent simulation of diabetes. *Journal of Pediatric Psychology, 14,* 259–275.

Schafer, L., McCaul, K., & Glasgow, R. (1986). Supportive and non-supportive family behaviors: Relationships to adherence and metabolic control in persons in Type I diabetes. *Diabetes Care, 9,* 179–185.

Seligman, M. (1995). The effectiveness of psychotherapy. *American Psychologist, 50,* 965–974.

Sperling, M. (1996). *Pediatric endocrinology.* Philadelphia: Saunders.

Stein, J. (1989). *Family interaction and adjustment, adherence and metabolic control in adolescents with insulin-dependent diabetes mellitus.* Unpublished doctoral dissertation, Boston University, Boston.

Wells, K., & Freer, R. (1994). Reading between the lines: The case for qualitative research in intensive family preservation services. *Children and Youth Services Review, 16,* 399–415.

Wiebe, D., Alderfer, M., Palmer, S., Lindsay, R., & Jarrett, L. (1994). Behavioral self-regulation in adolescents with Type I diabetes: Negative affectivity and blood glucose symptom perception. *Journal of Consulting & Clinical Psychology, 62,* 1204–1212.

Wing, R., Epstein, L., Nowalt, M., & Lamparski, D. (1986). Behavioral self-regulation in the treatment of patients with diabetes mellitus. *Psychological Bulletin, 99,* 78–89.

Wysocki, T. (1993). Associations among teen–parent relationships, metabolic control, and adjustment to diabetes in adolescents. *Journal of Pediatric Psychology, 18*, 441–452.

Wysocki, T., Hough, B., Ward, K., & Green, L. (1992). Diabetes mellitus in the transition to adulthood: Adjustments, self-care and health status. *Developmental and Behavioral Pediatrics, 13*, 194–201.

Zimmerman, E., Carter, M., Sears, J., Lawson, J., Howard, C., & Hassanein, R. (1987). Diabetic camping: Effect on knowledge, attitude, and self-concept. *Issues in Comprehensive Pediatric Nursing, 10*, 99–111.

Chapter 4

Prevention of Mental Health Problems in Adolescence

SUSAN KOOLS

SCHOOL OF NURSING

UNIVERSITY OF CALIFORNIA—SAN FRANCISCO

ABSTRACT

Mental health problems in adolescence are noteworthy in that they are outside of the normative adolescent developmental experience. Twenty percent of adolescents in the United States experience significant and persistent mental disorders, which indicates the need for prevention and early intervention. The purpose of this chapter is to review research on the prevention of mental health problems in adolescence. Various sociocontextual factors that place an adolescent at risk for mental health problems are examined. In particular, studies that identify risk factors for problems common to adolescence, including depression, suicide, and disorders of conduct and eating are reviewed. Evaluative research on prevention and early intervention programs in this substantive area are also critically reviewed. A summative report and critique on the state of research in this area is given along with suggestions for future research. A call for the active involvement of nursing in this research agenda is made.

Keywords: Adolescent Mental Health, Adolescent Emotional Problems, Behavioral Problems, Depression, Suicide, Conduct Disorders, Mental Health Promotion

Historically, adolescent mental health has been neglected as an area for scientific inquiry. Traditionally, adolescence has been viewed by developmental theorists as a transitional stage, fraught with erratic behavior, emotional lability, and interpersonal conflict with parents and other authority figures. The behavioral and emotional problems in adolescence were typically viewed as stage specific, time limited, and expected. Recently, however, empirical findings on adolescent development depict a more objective and less dramatic portrayal of adolescence (Brown, 1990; S. S. Feldman & Elliott, 1990; Steinberg, 1990). Most adolescents negotiate this stage with minimal and short-lived difficulty. Thus, when mental health problems occur during adolescence, they are to be considered outside of the norm and seriously addressed.

SCOPE AND PREVALENCE OF MENTAL HEALTH PROBLEMS IN ADOLESCENCE

There is a continuum of mental health problems that may be experienced in adolescence. Problems range from the psychological distress associated with individual traits such as loneliness or low self-esteem to diagnosable clinical disorders such as major depression or conduct disorder. It has been estimated that approximately 20% of adolescents in the United States have suffered from significant mental health problems including disorders of affect, conduct, and personality (Costello, 1989; Institute of Medicine, 1989; Kovacs, Goldston, & Gatsonis, 1993; Zill & Schoenborn, 1990).

The persistence of mental disorders is also noteworthy. Conditions that emerge in childhood, like autism, attention deficit/hyperactivity, and disruptive behavior disorders, continue into adolescence. Others, like depression, schizophrenia, and eating disorders, appear with increased frequency during adolescence and continue into adulthood (Kazdin, 1993). Evidence of this continuity lends strength to the argument that prevention and early identification and treatment of mental disorders are essential to reduce morbidity and mortality in adolescence and to prevent further dysfunction in adulthood (Robins & Rutter, 1990; Zill & Schoenborn, 1990).

Mental health promotion and prevention of mental health problems in adolescence are crucial roles for nursing. The identification of vulnerable populations at risk and creation of promotion and prevention-related interventions and services are integral components of these nursing roles. This chapter reviews nursing research on the prevention of mental health problems in adolescence. Likewise, studies outside the discipline with relevance to nursing science and practice are included in this review. Major topical areas include adolescents at risk for mental health problems and preventive interventions and programs. Computerized searches of nursing, medical, and psychological databases were conducted for the past 20 years, from 1977 to 1997. From this diverse body of literature, studies for this chapter were limited to those that focused on risk and prevention of major clinical dysfunction with the exception of substance-related disorders. Although adolescent substance abuse has a clear overlap with mental health problems, prevention research in this area was excluded as it represents a discreet substantive area that is beyond the scope of this chapter. Likewise, most research on adolescent risk-taking behavior was excluded unless it was focused directly on its relationship to specific emotional and behavioral problems.

ADOLESCENTS AT RISK FOR MENTAL HEALTH PROBLEMS

Multiple, interrelated factors can increase the adolescent's vulnerability for mental health problems. Although individual characteristics like personality traits and cognitive abilities are important influences on mental health, the adolescent is embedded in a social context. The transaction between the individual and his or her experiences and relationships is a more valuable predictor of mental health outcome than a singular focus on person or environment (Sameroff & Fiese, 1989).

Adolescent Emotional and Behavioral Problems

Most of the research in this area took a nonspecific approach to the investigation of adolescent mental health problems; that is, exposure to various risk factors was explored for its relationship to multiple emotional and behavioral symptoms. These studies will be reviewed first, followed by those that focus on the specific mental health problems of depression, suicidal behavior, conduct disorders, and eating disorders. Many of the studies investigated the relationship between variables in the adolescent's social context and mental health status. These variables can be categorized as related to family, peers, school climate, and community.

Family.   It is widely believed that parental loss through death, divorce, or other prolonged absences in childhood is associated with increased psychopathology such as depression, suicidality, substance abuse, and antisocial behavior later in life (Adam, Bouckams, & Streiner, 1982; Dietrich, 1984; Newcomb, Maddahian, & Bentler, 1986). Although most studies of long-term impact have sampled adults, several have attempted to study the effects of loss on adolescents. With a sample of 2,158 adolescents, Raphael, Cubis, Dunne,

Lewin, and Kelly (1990) compared adolescents who had lost a parent (23%) with those who had not (77%). Those who had experienced a loss were more neurotic, introverted, impulsive, and had poor body image. Missing from this cross-sectional data analysis was the consideration of contextual variables that related to the loss such as quality of caregiving, parent–child attachments, and circumstances surrounding a divorce or death. These factors, along with others that affect psychosocial development over time, are variables with the potential for confounding these findings.

Other research, specifically on divorce, has documented higher incidences of antisocial behavior problems such as aggression, acting-out, truancy, and substance abuse (Kalter, Reimer, Brickman, & Chen, 1985; Peck, 1989; Sorosky, 1977). Adolescent girls appear to be more negatively affected by divorce with increased depression, anxiety, behavioral problems, and low self-esteem (Frost & Pakiz, 1990; Hetherington, Cox, & Cox, 1985; Kalter et al., 1985; Wallerstein, 1984). Engagement in antisocial activity, in contrast, was seen more often in adolescent boys (Wallerstein, 1984). There were also age-related differences in effects of divorce. In a longitudinal study of families who had experienced divorce ($N = 30$), adolescents whose parents divorced when they were school aged evidenced more problems than those with parents who divorced during preschool (Wallerstein, 1984). Stein, Marton, Golombek, and Koremblum (1994) reported that early adolescents responded to changes in family structure with emotional and behavioral disturbance such as dysphoria, anxiety, introversion, and pessimism, whereas late adolescents were more likely to be depressed, angry, or suffer from personality disturbance. Middle adolescents demonstrated no significant correlations between loss and affective or personality variables.

With the exception of the Frost and Pakiz (1990) study, which followed a cohort of children ($N = 382$) through adolescence to compare adolescents of divorce with those of intact families, major threats to validity can be found in this body of research. The use of convenience samples and the lack of comparison groups were primary internal validity issues. Potential mediating variables like level of contact with noncustodial parent, social support (e.g., emotional support, financial resources), new parental intimate relationships or remarriage, child personality characteristics (e.g., temperament, coping style), and other historical events with an impact on maturation were not adequately considered.

There are inconsistent findings regarding the differential impact of type of loss. Saucier and Ambert (1983) reported that bereaved adolescents had fewer long-term mental health consequences than those from divorced or separated families, whereas Partridge and Kotler (1987) found them to be more introverted and antisocial. Others found no significant differences between groups based on type of loss (Cooper, Holman, & Braithwaite, 1983; Raphael et al., 1990). Failure to include measures of family cohesion and conflict to describe the context of the loss may have contributed to contradictory results.

The generalizability of the findings from all of these studies on parental loss is limited by the homogeneity of the samples of predominantly White middle-class adolescents and their families. Replication of research with ethnically and socioeconomically diverse families is necessary to address this issue. Based on the sources for access to participants, selection bias may have also skewed the sample by representing only those experiencing overt problems.

It has been well established that parental mental illness increases the likelihood of childhood psychiatric disturbance (R. A. Feldman, Stiffman, & Jung, 1987; Rutter, 1987; Rutter & Quinton, 1984). Although the mechanism of causation is unknown, genetic predisposition, family discord and hostility, attachment difficulties, and abuse have been implicated (Rutter, 1989). No studies were found that specifically focused on the influence of parental mental illness on adolescents, but it was suggested in this literature that risk extends into adulthood. It can be inferred that adolescents continue to be influenced by parental psychopathology, however, more research that specifically investigates its affect on this age group is necessary. It is crucial to develop an understanding of the family factors that are related to negative adolescent effects and the interaction of these factors with individual characteristics of the adolescent that either increase risk or serve as protective mechanisms.

Similarly, parental substance abuse places the adolescent at increased risk for mental health problems. Although many adolescents in substance-abusing families fail to demonstrate significant psychosocial dysfunction, others display the gamut of psychiatric symptoms (Clair & Genest, 1986; Fine, Yudin, Holmes, & Heinemann, 1976; Roosa, Sandler, Beals, & Short, 1988). Researchers are only beginning to identify both risk and protective factors and to develop tentative causative models. In a short-term prospective study, Roosa, Beals, Sandler, and Pillow (1990) tested a model that examined the moderating effects of positive and negative family events on adolescent symptoms. In their small sample of self-identified children of alcoholics ($N = 43$), they reported significantly more negative and less positive events than control adolescents. They also scored higher on measures of depression and anxiety, especially the female subjects. Tomori (1994) found adolescents with an alcoholic parent to have considerably more problems than controls matched for age and gender, including poor self-concept, depression, aggression, anxiety, low future aspirations, and problem drinking. Selection bias was apparent in both studies. Subjects with an alcoholic parent were recruited from a self-help group for children of alcoholics in one and an alcohol treatment setting in the other. There was no way to determine how these individuals were similar to or different from adolescents who did not self-disclose or have parental substance abuse diagnosed. Thus, sample representativeness may be questioned.

The destructiveness of child maltreatment has been well documented. Little is known, however, about the psychosocial correlates of abuse in adolescence. Developmental theory postulates that abuse beginning in adolescence may be related to shifts in the parent–child relationship as the adolescent asserts increasing independence from authority figures in the family or the parents' inability to accommodate to the multiple changes associated with puberty (Garbarino, Sebes, & Schellenbach, 1984; Lourie, 1979).

Using an ecological model, Williamson, Borduin, and Howe (1991) examined relationships between adolescent and family characteristics, stress and social support, and adolescent emotional and behavioral problems. In this well-designed study, researchers considered multiple levels of variables including individual parent and adolescent, family system, and sociocultural variables, thus augmenting knowledge of the complex context of abuse. To strengthen the validity of their findings, they grouped adolescent/parent pairs according to type of maltreatment (neglect, physical, or sexual) and used a comparison group of matched controls. Although there were some commonalities between maltreatment groups (e.g., attention deficits), there were differences in family variables and the influence on adolescent mental health between groups. Sexually abused adolescents reported significantly more emotional symptoms including depression and anxiety, whereas physically abused and neglected groups demonstrated more conduct problems like socialized aggression. The hypothesis that different types of maltreatment lead to differing outcomes may have been supported, but the homogeneity of the groups was uncertain despite the use of specific criteria for group selection. It is common for children to experience more than one type of abuse. Similarly, severity of abuse was not a component of the operational definitions of the categories. These conceptual and measurement issues may have threatened construct validity because of the lack of discreet categories of maltreatment.

Other types of family stress have been shown to be correlated with increased emotional and behavioral problems of adolescents. Conger, Ge, Elder, Lorenz, and Simons (1994) developed and tested a theoretical model which suggested that economic strain resulted in marital conflict, parental irritability, and hostility. This stress is transmitted to the parent–adolescent relationship, is evidenced in struggles over money, and is associated with increases in both internalizing behaviors (depression, anxiety) and externalizing behaviors (aggression, antisocial behavior, hostility) in adolescent females and males, respectively. The 3-year longitudinal design was a strength of the study, but subject attrition, the absence of groups for comparison, and the failure to consider alternate hypotheses to explain adolescent symptoms were validity threats.

The study of adolescent stress is modeled after studies on adults with instruments being modified accordingly. Stressors, problems, and events are typically evaluated by forced choice on a checklist rather than self-generated by adolescent subjects. Family conflicts and other social relationships and experiences have been implicated in increased stress levels and associated mental health problems in adolescents (Puskar & Lamb, 1991; Rae-Grant, Thomas, Offord, & Boyle, 1989; Stark, Spirito, Williams, & Guevremont, 1989). In a longitudinal study, Compas, Howell, Phares, Williams, and Giunta (1989) prospectively explored the relationship between adolescent and parent stress, and emotional/behavioral problems. They found increases in adolescent internalizing behaviors to be related to stressful events and parental psychological symptoms. Though type of stressor was not specified, a distinction was made between daily stressors and major stressful events with everyday, ongoing stress being most predictive of total behavioral problems.

Others have attempted to use structural equation modeling to derive a better understanding of the relationships between variables that appear to affect adolescent mental health. Using multiple informants (parents, teachers, self-report) to evaluate 215 young adolescents, DuBois, Felner, Sherman, and Bull (1994) tested a model that demonstrated direct effects between social support and stressful events and emotional/behavioral problems. Further, they found that self-esteem played a significant role in mediating these effects (normed fit index for the model = 0.94).

These initial efforts to develop causal models that relate stressors to adolescent outcomes have begun to expand the theoretical understanding of adolescent mental health problems. Further research is needed to replicate these studies with diverse populations of adolescents and their families and to explore rival hypotheses to test other models with potential explanatory power.

Peers.   Similar to family dysfunction and parent problems, the quality of peer relationships is thought to increase adolescent risk for emotional and behavioral problems. Problems with friends and girlfriends/boyfriends have been frequently implicated as stressful experiences for adolescents (Puskar & Lamb, 1991; Rae-Grant et al., 1989; Stark et al., 1989). Although characteristics of peer relationships and interactions can place an adolescent at increased risk for psychopathology, others have found them to serve as a protective factor to mediate or reduce risk. In a sample of 3,294 children and adolescents, Rae-Grant et al. (1989) examined the relationship between risk and protective factors and mental disorders in childhood. In a stepwise logistic regression model, they were able to isolate "being a good student" and "getting along with peers" as components of the larger construct of social competence that have particular importance in mediating the impact of family stressors and conflict. The cross-sectional design, however, did not allow the identification of a temporal sequence of risk, protection, and onset or absence of disorder. Hirsch and DuBois (1992) both cross-sectionally and longitudinally documented a strong inverse relationship between peer support and psychiatric symptoms in young adolescents transitioning to middle school ($N = 143$). The inclusion of multiple data points over time strengthened support for this finding.

School climate.   For most adolescents, school is a primary context for psychosocial development. Peer relationships are one major component of this social milieu. For some adolescents, this context may be the source of profound stress. Remafedi (1987) interviewed 29 gay and bisexual adolescent males about the impact of their sexuality on school and peer relationships, among other things. Sixty-nine percent of them revealed school difficulties that they attributed to their sexual orientation including verbal and physical abuse by peers, truancy, and deterioration in academic performance. Despite the lack of representativeness of this small sample that stemmed from recruiting self-identified gay youth, this seminal study laid the groundwork to promote understanding of the impact of negative social experiences on sexual minority male adolescents. More work is needed to expand this substantive knowledge base to include the experiences of lesbian adolescents and those who may be questioning their sexual identities. It is also important to explore the contextual correlates of positive outcomes for sexual minority youth.

Kasen, Johnson, and Cohen (1990) found additional features of the school climate to have an effect on emotional and behavioral problems and alcohol use. Three hundred adolescents attending 250 schools were followed over 2 years. Prevalent dimensions of the school climates were used to develop categorical descriptors of school environments. Adolescents attending high-conflict schools developed more disruptive behavior disorders like attention deficit/hyperactivity, conduct, and oppositional defiant disorders. High conflict was characterized by chaotic classrooms with little teacher control over student behavior, fighting, and vandalism. Higher incidences of anxiety and depression were found over time in schools with a climate of social facilitation where social interactions among students and between students and teachers were fostered. In contrast, schools with a high academic focus had a significant inverse relationship with alcohol use, oppositional defiant, and conduct disorders. Although internal validity may have been affected by the confounding variables of socioeconomic status or other relevant factors in the adolescents' lives, these environmental characteristics may provide direction for preventive efforts.

Community.   There are many anecdotal descriptions of community-level problems (e.g., poverty and crime) and their negative consequences for children, adolescents, and their families. A systematic investigation of specific environmental variables on adolescent mental health has only begun. In their study of 630 urban high-school students, Pastore, Fisher, and Friedman (1996) found a significant association between exposure to violence in their community and emotional problems. Fifty percent of the sample had known a victim of murder and 31% to 61% had witnessed various acts of violence such as stabbing, shooting, or beating. Depression, suicidal behavior, and alcohol abuse were prevalent and significantly related to exposure to violence. Causal relationships cannot be assumed by this cross-sectional study, however, researchers were able to determine relative risk factors using logistic regression analysis.

In summary, a host of sociocontextual variables have been reported to be influential in the development of emotional and behavioral problems in adolescence. Family conflict and dysfunction, stressful peer interactions, a high degree of conflict and chaos in the school environment, and exposure to violence in the neighborhood have been found to contribute to risk and vulnerability. A few studies have begun to identify potential protective or mediating factors such as positive peer relationships and a strong academic focus at school (Hirsch & DuBois, 1992; Kasen et al., 1990; Rae-Grant et al., 1989). It is important to develop transactional or ecological theoretical models to understand the various relationships between contexts and experiences common in adolescence in order to reduce risk and promote resilience.

Adolescent Depression

Depression is the most prevalent mental health problem for adolescents. Twenty percent report at least one diagnosable episode of major depression or dysthymic disorder by age 18 (Clarke, Hawkins, Murphy, & Sheeber, 1993). In school-based clinic studies, the prevalence of depression has ranged from 13% to 59% of adolescent clients (Bartlett, Schleifer, Johnson, & Keller, 1991; Cappelli et al., 1995; Wortman, Donovan, & Woodburn, 1986). Girls represented a disproportionate incidence rate in these samples, which is comparable with epidemiological community studies. There are also high rates of comorbidity of depression with other mental health problems such as suicide, delinquency, eating disorders, and substance abuse (Kovacs, Paulauskas, Gatsonis, & Richards, 1988; Rohde, Lewinsohn, & Seeley, 1991). Further, major depression is the most common psychiatric sequela of exposure of adolescents to suicide among their friends and acquaintances (Brent et al., 1992).

In a random sample of 1,208 adolescents, Gore, Aseltine, and Colton (1992) identified several demographic variables that were associated with a higher incidence of depressive symptoms. Girls appeared to have higher exposure to stress and greater depressive symptoms. Adolescents from single-parent and low socioeconomic backgrounds had a higher vulnerability to stress and symptom level. Although researchers proposed that both stress and support deficits may be linked with these contextual factors, the mechanism of their influence is not well understood from these findings.

The quality of family relationships has been shown to be a significant factor related to adolescent depression. I. Reynolds and Rob (1988) found that adolescents who described their families as less supportive, emotionally close, and affectionate were more depressed and engaged in increased risk-taking behaviors such as substance use and sexual activity. A survey designed by the researchers rather than extant instruments with documented reliability was used. Adequate conceptual definitions for important constructs like family closeness, parental love, and depression itself were lacking.

Aseltine, Gore, and Colten (1994) designed a longitudinal study to examine the interrelationships between personal and social variables and depressive symptoms in 939 high-school students over 2 years. Differences were distinguished between adolescents who were initially asymptomatic and developed depressive symptoms over the course of the study and adolescents who were chronically depressed. Previously asymptomatic youths were negatively affected by family relationship problems and stressful family events, and emotional support from parents was significantly related to lower levels of depression. In contrast, chronically depressed adolescents were less affected by either family stress or support, but were highly influenced by both peer relationship problems and peer support. It was postulated that chronic family stress may lead to an accentuation of the adolescent's distancing from the family and relying on friendships for the primary source of support. This hypothesis warrants further investigation. A strength of this study was its prospective design, however, insufficient data were available about the quality of relationships or individual adolescent attributes and maturation over time for the group of subjects that were determined to be chronically depressed.

These studies have made an important contribution to the knowledge of the context in which adolescent depression occurs. Family relationships and stress are important contributors to the onset of depression, and their influence along with the positive effect of family support may diminish with the persistence of depressive symptomatology.

Suicidal Behavior

Suicide and suicidal behavior is nearly always linked with depression in the literature. Because suicide has risen to the second leading cause of death for adolescents in recent years (National Institute of Mental Health, 1992), health care providers and researchers have engaged in a concentrated effort to identify the risk factors associated with adolescent suicide. Gender, age, and race differences in suicidal behavior are well-known. For example, girls are two to eight times more likely to attempt suicide, whereas boys are three times more successful in their attempts. Suicide rates are highest for Native American and White adolescents. Following puberty, the incidence of suicide continues to rise until it peaks at age 23 (Grossman, Milligan, & Deyo, 1991; Lewinsohn, Rohde, & Seeley, 1994; McIntosh & Jewell, 1986; Shaffer, Garland, Gould, Fisher, & Trautman, 1988).

Using retrospective case analyses for suicide attempters and psychological autopsies for suicide victims, other psychosocial factors have been identified as potential predictive variables or correlates. Individual adolescent variables with strong empirical support have included psychopathology and its comorbidity with substance abuse, impulsivity, and past suicide attempts (Brent et al., 1988; Bukstein et al., 1993; Grossman et al., 1991; Kashden, Fremouw, Callahan, & Franzen, 1993; Lewinsohn et al., 1994). In fact, the vast majority of suicide victims studied had a positive history of psychiatric symptoms or disorders (Shaffer & Gould, 1987). Although depression is the mental health problem most thought to be predictive of suicidal behavior (Martin & Waite, 1994; Thompson, Moody, & Eggert, 1994), some researchers have questioned the assumption of a causal relationship. Morano, Cisler, and Lemerond (1993) noted that not all depressed adolescents demonstrated suicidal behavior and not all victims were known to be seriously depressed prior to committing suicide. In their comparative study of psychiatrically hospitalized attempters and nonattempters, they found that the more specific variable of hopelessness had greater predictive value for suicidal behavior than depression itself.

Other correlates of suicidal behavior that have been validated across studies are parent variables including mental illness, history of suicidal behavior, and substance abuse (Brent et al., 1988, 1994; Bukstein et al., 1993; Shaffer & Gould, 1987), and family stress and discord. Researchers have investigated the relationship between suicide attempts or completions and several family variables indicating dysfunction including parental separation and loss, low family support, interpersonal conflict, physical and sexual abuse, and adolescent alienation (Brent et al., 1988, 1994; Grossman et al., 1991; Morano et al., 1993). Adams, Overholser, and Spirito (1994) found that suicide attempters ($N = 91$) had significantly more acute and chronic stressors than high-school student controls ($N = 155$) with parents being the most frequent source of stress. These stressful experiences were associated with higher levels of depression and suicidal ideation.

Although family psychopathology and conflict are critical risk factors to consider in the evaluation of suicide risk, other social variables are relevant to adolescent suicidal behavior. Interpersonal conflicts and stress with peers (including boyfriend/girlfriend), having a friend attempt or commit suicide, and using social withdrawal as a primary coping mechanism are correlates of suicide that have been found to be developmentally specific to this age group (Adams et al., 1994; Brent et al., 1993; Grossman et al., 1991; Hazell & Lewin, 1993; Spirito, Overholser, & Stark, 1989). This was exemplified in the deAnda and Smith study (1993) in which the researchers compared the characteristics of adult ($N = 246$) versus adolescent ($N = 165$) callers to a suicide help line. Adult suicidal ideation was primarily related to depression, whereas adolescents reported interpersonal problems as precipitating their consideration of suicide.

The preceding studies have illuminated risk factors for adolescent suicide by investigating victims or high-risk adolescents. This raises the threat to external validity by potentially limiting the applicability of the findings to hospitalized adolescents rather than a larger community population. Other methodological issues included inadequate operational definitions of constructs within and across studies like depression (symptoms of versus clinical disorder) and suicidal behavior (ideation, attempt, self-harming, or destructive behavior). Likewise, many of the studies used univariate analyses that often demonstrated significant associations between independent variables and suicidal behavior without accounting for more complex relationships and interactions (Bukstein et al., 1993; deAnda & Smith, 1993; Grossman et al., 1991; Morano et al., 1993). Finally, it was characteristic to rely on retrospective self-report of the adolescents rather than multiple informants to enhance the validity of the findings.

To address the issue of generalizability, other researchers have studied suicide risk in large normative high-school samples ($N = 70$ to 1500) (Choquet, Kovess, & Poutignat, 1993; Lamb & Pusker, 1991; Lewinsohn et al., 1994; Martin, Rozanes, Pearce, & Allison, 1995; Martin & Waite, 1994; Oler et al., 1994; Reifman & Windle, 1995; Reinherz et al., 1993; Rubenstein, Heeren, Housman, Rubin, & Stechler, 1989; Thompson et al., 1994). Rates of suicidal ideation in these community samples were 7% to 25%, and self-harming behavior or suicide attempts were 2% to 15%. Findings were similar to high-risk groups with risk factors including individual psychopathology (especially depression), substance use/abuse, history of previous suicide attempt, and family dysfunction. In a longitudinal study of 385 adolescents, Reinherz et al. (1993) also identified a relationship between gender atypical behavior in preschool (e.g., aggression in girls and excessive dependence in boys) and later suicidal ideation in adolescents. The risk for suicide attempts increased with the number of risk factors that an adolescent experienced (Lewinsohn et al., 1994).

In this body of work, researchers identified several protective factors. Oler et al. (1994) found that the subsample of high-school athletes ($N = 243$) was significantly less depressed and had less suicidal ideation and attempts than its nonathlete peers ($N = 575$). It was speculated that the protective effect of sports participation could be related to biological fitness, peer support, increased self-esteem, and positive perceptions of others. Rubenstein et al. (1989) found that family cohesiveness was associated with less suicidal behavior, and feeling accepted by a peer group had an indirect effect on suicidality by reducing depression. This latter indirect relationship was validated in the findings of Reifman and Windle (1995). Although most of these studies were cross-sectional, three studies were strengthened by their longitudinal, prospective designs (Lewinsohn et al., 1994; Reifman & Windle, 1995; Reinherz et al., 1993), thus increasing predictive validity.

Antisocial Behavior and Conduct Disorder

In contrast to depression, adolescents can also exhibit externalizing behaviors as a manifestation of mental health problems. These include aggressivity, destruction of property, theft, running away, truancy, defiance of authority figures, and substance abuse. Those with a higher degree of clinical dysfunction may be diagnosed with conduct disorder. Conduct disorder in adolescence is characterized by persistent behavior that violates social norms including infringement on the rights of others. Aggressive behavior and poor interpersonal relationships may also be a part of the symptom constellation. It is estimated that 4% to 10% of all children have this disorder (Kazdin, 1986). Conduct disorder has a high comorbidity with other psychiatric disorders such as attention deficit/hyperactivity disorder, learning disorders, and depression. It is more commonly found in boys with a 3:1 male to female ratio, and girls tend to have a later age of onset in early adolescence. Antisocial behavior greatly increases the risk of the adolescent engaging in violence, with its own set of morbidity and mortality issues (Saner & Ellickson, 1996). With the lack of effective treatment, it has a poor prognosis, often continuing into adulthood (Offord, 1989; Rutter & Giller, 1983).

Antisocial behavior and conduct disorder are thought to have their precursors in early childhood. Patterson (1986) developed a model to explain the transactional processes involved in the development of antisocial behavior. When parents consistently respond to a child's disobedient or coercive behavior with harsh discipline, rejection, and a lack of involvement, the antisocial behavior of the child is reinforced and escalates. Likewise, this negative behavioral pattern is reinforced in school as it often results in the lack of peer and teacher acceptance and poor interpersonal relationships.

Given this theoretical understanding of the development of conduct disorder in adolescents, it is clear that the risk factors come into play in early childhood. As a result, much of the research related to risk factors has been conducted with populations of younger children. For example, parent characteristics like mental illness and criminality and parenting practices like harsh discipline, physical abuse, poor supervision, and neglect were identified as correlates to conduct disorder in children (Offord, 1982; Rutter & Giller, 1983). For girls with conduct disorder, there was a high prevalence of sexual abuse (Dryfoos, 1990). Individual child characteristics included hyperactivity, learning problems with secondary poor academic performance, and "troublesomeness," a variable endorsed by peers and teachers as an indicator of the school-aged child's temperament (Farrington, 1986; Offord, Sullivan, & Allen, 1979). Finally, living in impoverished communities with high crime rates increased the likelihood of child participation in antisocial activities (Dryfoos, 1990). These associations were found to be significant, however, their relative importance and interrelationships are unknown.

Some researchers have identified psychosocial correlates of antisocial behavior in adolescence. Tolan (1988) found that poor family functioning, especially a lack of cohesion and social stress, were significantly correlated with antisocial behavior. In a study of 150 Dutch adolescents determined to be at risk for delinquency, Scholte (1992) proposed a socioecological model for understanding the interpersonal and environmental factors contributing to the development of externalizing behaviors. Forty percent of the variance in these behavioral problems was explained by peer group composition and relationships, family relationships and parenting practices, and conflicts within the school environment. Another model was used to test hypotheses about relationships between interparental conflict and adolescent externalizing behaviors (Forehand, Wierson, McCombs, Brody, & Fauber, 1989). Multiple informants, including adolescents, parents, teachers, and trained behavioral observers, were used to strengthen the validity of the findings. In divorced families ($N = 62$), there appeared to be a direct relationship between parent problems and adolescent externalizing behaviors. In two-parent families ($N = 80$), however, the adolescent's perception of the conflict mediated the effects of parent conflict on adolescent behavior.

By identifying the preceding variables as risk factors with potential for predictive value, these researchers have suggested their use as targets for prevention and early intervention. The cross-sectional research design, however, precludes the ability to infer a causal relationship or its direction. One exception was a longitudinal study of 1,167 adolescents which found that earlier onset of sexual activity in adolescence was predictive of increases in other risk-taking behaviors like substance use/abuse and antisocial behavior (Tubman, Windle, & Windle, 1996).

Eating Disorders

Disordered eating in adolescence takes two major forms. Anorexia nervosa is characterized by the adolescent's refusal to maintain a normal body weight (< 85% of expected body weight), an unreasonable fear of gaining weight, and a disturbed body image. A preoccupation with body shape and weight is also a major feature of bulimia nervosa. Other important attributes of the disorder include binge eating patterns and inappropriate means of weight loss such as self-induced vomiting or laxative abuse. Both disorders are more common in females with 90% of anorexia found in females. Prevalence studies on late adolescents and young adults have estimated that 0.5% to 1% of females meet the diagnostic criteria for an eating disorder (American Psychiatric Association, 1994).

Research to identify risk factors for eating disorders has been predominantly conducted with clinical samples of women who reported on their experiences retrospectively. Instruments derived from this work (e.g., Eating Disorders Risk Scale, Eating Attitudes Test) have been used more recently to compare adolescents at high and low risk for developing eating disorders (Garner, Olmstead, & Polivy, 1983; Maloney, McGuire, & Daniels, 1988). High-risk females rated family variables significantly more negatively including family cohesion, satisfaction, and parent–adolescent communication. Teachers rated these girls with a higher degree of internalizing behaviors. No group differences were reported for at-risk males (Leon, Fulkerson, Perry, & Dube, 1994). These findings for girls were validated by Watts and Ellis (1992) with the additional correlates of adolescent risk-taking behaviors (e.g., substance use/abuse, unsafe sexual practices), involvement with substance-abusing peers, and suicidal ideation. A strong association between disturbed patterns of eating and family teasing or criticism about weight or body shape was found in a sample of young adolescent girls. Other aspects of their social context with potential to reinforce poor eating attitudes and behaviors included reading fashion magazines for advice about health and beauty and peer dieting (Levine, Smolak, & Hayden, 1994).

Only one prospective study on a community sample was reviewed. Killen et al. (1994) assessed eating attitudes and behaviors of adolescents over a 3-year period. At baseline, 4% of the sample of 939 was already symptomatic. In a separate analysis, these girls were found to be early maturers based on Tanner self-staging for pubertal development (Killen et al., 1992; Tanner, 1990). Over the course of the study, an additional 4% developed symptoms of an eating disorder. The only factor that was predictive of this outcome was a composite variable referred to as "weight concerns." This variable included a preoccupation with thinness and body shape, fear of weight gain, dieting history, and perceived fatness.

With the exception of the Killen research program, this body of studies has relied predominantly on cross-sectional designs to determine significant correlational relationships between variables. Little understanding has been gained regarding the spectrum of disordered eating, the etiology of eating disorders, or the mechanisms that elevate individual vulnerability or resistance. Prospective, longitudinal studies of community samples are necessary to comprehend how eating disorders develop and therefore, how to target prevention efforts.

PREVENTIVE INTERVENTIONS AND PROGRAMS

As an understanding of the numerous factors that place an adolescent at increased risk for mental health problems has evolved, many authors have proposed interventions based on principles of primary and secondary prevention (Berger & Shechter, 1989; Kazdin, 1993; Rubin, 1986; Wassef, Ingham, Collins, & Mason, 1995). Others have described mental health promotion and prevention programs with interventions derived from theoretical knowledge on adolescent development (e.g., use of peer support, service delivery in high-school settings) (Kisker & Brown, 1996; Niznik, 1994; Puskar, Lamb, & Martsolf, 1990; Scharer, Challberg, & Rearick, 1990). The implementation of preventive interventions, however, has taken precedence over evaluation of effects or outcomes (Peters, 1988). Few attempts have been made to systematically study prevention strategies. Evaluative research on mental health promotion and prevention is only beginning to be conducted. This includes studies on programs that focus on mental health generally and those with a specific problem orientation like depression, suicide, conduct, and eating disorders.

Prevention of Emotional and Behavioral Problems

Programs that target the prevention of emotional and behavioral problems have incorporated the knowledge gained from the evaluation of a larger body of research on substance-abuse prevention in adolescence (Bangert-Drowns, 1988; Tobler, 1986). These earlier efforts based on the assumption that increased factual knowledge would positively change adolescent attitudes and behavior have demonstrated little to no lasting effects (Weissberg, Caplan, & Harwood, 1991). The growing appreciation for the complexity of and interrelationships between mental health problems, along with the heightened awareness of the impact of the relevant social contexts in which they are embedded, has been reflected in the design of programs to enhance mental health in adolescence. Recent interventions have been based on cognitive, affective, and interpersonal approaches to develop psychosocial competence. Promotion of psychosocial competence includes the development of decision-making and problem-solving skills, interpersonal communication and conflict resolution, assertiveness training, stress management, and the promotion of self-esteem and confidence. In addition, an ecological perspective was evidenced in some programs that attempted to incorporate interventions into the adolescent's social world of peers, school, family, and the community.

Hartman (1979) classified 121 asymptomatic adolescents according to risk status for mental health problems based on pretest measures of self-esteem, psychological discomfort, assertiveness, stressful events, and peer ratings. Four levels of risk (from low to high) were identified and adolescents within each level were randomly assigned to intervention or control groups. The intervention consisted of an 8-week interactive training program with components of cognitive restructuring, social skills training, and anxiety and stress management. Its purpose was to teach adolescents new ways of interacting in interpersonal relationships. Posttest measurements were taken at 3-months and 1-year postintervention. Significant main effects for all factors, including self-esteem, level of psychological distress, and assertiveness were found for the intervention groups. Peer ratings at follow up supported the emotional and behavioral gains made from the training. Threats to the validity of the study findings included a moderate subject attrition rate (28%) and the potential influence of extraneous variables including a placebo effect.

In a program of research that focused on the development of social competence in adolescents, Weissberg, Caplan, and their colleagues conducted several studies to assess the behavioral changes attributable to school-based competency-training programs. Weissberg et al. (1991) studied the impact of a middle-school curriculum focusing on impulse control, stress management, problem solving and conflict resolution, and social skills training on 421 early adolescents. They found improvements in problem-solving and conflict-resolution skills, delinquent behavior, and teacher ratings of impulse control and peer sociability after 1 year. Teachers conducted booster training with a subsample of this group over the next year. Only the group that received 2 years of training displayed significant long-term gains in problem-solving skills and psychosocial adjustment as compared with controls. Caplan et al. (1992) evaluated a similar 20-session social-competence training program for 282 inner-city and suburban sixth and seventh graders. Additional components of this program included self-esteem enhancement, information on health and substance use, assertiveness, and social support. Improvements were found for both groups in the areas of conflict resolution, impulse control, coping with anxiety, popularity, and substance use/abuse. These programs were strengthened by an ecological perspective that focused beyond individual adolescent behavior to teacher behavior, adolescent–teacher relationships, and school resources.

Other interventions were designed to provide social support as a mechanism for prevention. Young (1980) evaluated a mandatory, court-ordered 8-week workshop for adolescents ($N = 48$) whose parents were in the process of divorce. The purpose of the workshop was to provide support by giving adolescents the opportunity to talk with peers experiencing similar situations and to sensitize them to personal and parental needs during this stressful time. The intervention consisted of warm-up exercises, a film, and discussion sessions related to the experience of divorce. The study design to evaluate the intervention was weak in that it simply focused on participant satisfaction. Initial attitudes about workshop attendance were primarily negative or neutral (82%). Following attendance, 52% of the sample reported being pleased with the workshop. No behavioral measures were taken pre- or postintervention to determine the impact of adolescent participation, and there was no follow-up regarding potential long-term effects.

Seidl (1982) conducted an evaluation of a small sample of young adolescents and their Big Sisters assigned by an organization ($N = 20$ pairs) to determine the effectiveness of this well-known supportive intervention by laypersons. The referral source was asked to identify target problematic behaviors and assess behavioral change in the adolescent Little Sisters and a matched control group after an 8-week period of participation. Their assessments were rated by trained study personnel. Additionally, each member of the pair was interviewed separately to evaluate the quality of the relationship and Big Sisters were asked to identify strengths and weaknesses of the adolescents. Although the researcher attempted to reduce bias by using a control group, the measurement strategy for treatment outcome was weak. No instruments with documented reliability and validity were used to systematically assess behavioral change from pre- to postintervention. Both groups demonstrated change that could be explained by the Hawthorne effect (Cook & Campbell, 1979), maturation, or statistical regression (Cook & Campbell, 1979).

Outcomes from a secondary prevention intervention were examined by Gutstein, Rudd, Graham, and Rayha (1988). Seventy-five adolescents at risk for psychiatric hospitalization were exposed to a systemic crisis intervention that mobilized their family kinship networks to provide support. At the time of the intervention, adolescents were experiencing psychiatric symptoms including depression, suicidal and self-destructive behavior, and antisocial behavior such as substance abuse and running away. Behavior was evaluated using both parent reports and objective measurements at intake, 3, 6, and 12 to 18 months postintervention. After 3 months, 79% of crises were reported to be resolved, and 74% of the cases were considered to be successful according to criteria reflecting fewer problem behaviors, decreased future crises, and improved family relationships after 12 months. Only five of the adolescents ultimately required hospitalization over the course of the study. Study limitations included bias related to self-selection of participating families and the lack of a control or comparison group. It is also unclear whether adolescent and family improvement was attributable to increased kinship involvement or the result of a competing hypothesis.

These initial programs have begun to address mental health promotion and prevention of mental health problems in a general way. Programs that demonstrated long-term positive outcomes used important strategies such as a booster for the intervention and connection with significant members of the adolescents' social system such as peers and kinship networks (Gutstein et al., 1988; Hartman, 1979; Weissberg et al., 1991). These elements appeared to be influential in the ability to maintain behavioral outcomes and should be replicated in future studies.

Depression Prevention

When depression has been singled out as an area for primary prevention, evaluations of interventions to date have demonstrated minimal evidence of prevention or reduction of depressive symptomatology in adolescents. Several studies investigated the differences between adolescents who received educational and/or behavioral skills training and control groups (Clarke et al., 1993; Klein, Greist, Bass, & Lohr, 1987). Interventions that provided concrete information about depression or strategies to increase pleasurable activities produced no significant long-term benefits in reduction of symptoms, knowledge, and attitudes regarding depression and its treatment, or treatment-seeking behavior. The notable exception was a program that targeted adolescents assessed to be at risk for future depression (Clarke et al., 1995). Subjects with diagnosable affective disorders were referred for treatment, those at risk ($N = 150$) were randomized to either a 15-session group-prevention intervention that focused on the cognitive restructuring of irrational thinking and self-defeating behavior or to a control group. Significant differences between groups were maintained at 12 months with affective disorder incidence rates at 14.5% in the intervention group and 25.7% in the control group. The differences in this intervention that may have contributed to its success were targeting adolescents with identified risk for depression versus asymptomatic adolescents, a longer intervention period, and prevention strategies based on a cognitive theoretical perspective that has documented efficacy in the treatment of depression (Kahn, Kehle, Jenson, & Clark, 1990; Lewinsohn, Clarke, Hops, & Andrews, 1990; M. W. Reynolds & Coats, 1986).

Suicide Prevention

Nurses have had a rich history of involvement in suicide prevention (Fitzpatrick, 1983). Interventions have been linked to a theoretical understanding of suicidal behavior based on its assumed relationship with mental illness (e.g., depression) and crisis theory. With suicide mortality rates for adolescents steadily increasing, suicide prevention programs for this age group have proliferated over the past decade.

Garland, Shaffer, and Whittle (1989) conducted a national survey to ascertain the nature of programs available to adolescents. One hundred and fifteen school-based programs serving approximately 172,000 students were reviewed to determine content, length and methods of intervention, and theoretical orientation. The programs were similar in that nearly all of them provided adolescents with factual information on suicide emphasizing behavioral warning signs and knowledge of the availability and methods of accessing community mental health resources. Eighty-nine percent of the programs trained school personnel, and 71% trained parents in suicide assessment. Two thirds of the programs were didactic and of very short duration (less than 2 hours). All but 4% were based on stress theory, which attributed suicidal behavior to an extreme response to stressors commonly experienced in adolescence. Without the consideration of the strong empirical base of support for the understanding of suicide as a consequence of mental illness, this orientation can be criticized as deficient.

Despite a growing descriptive literature on suicide prevention programs for adolescents, evaluative research on their efficacy has lagged. The few studies that evaluated specific programs used attitudinal change about suicide and help-seeking (Ciffone, 1993; Shaffer, Garland, Underwood, & Whittle, 1987; Shaffer, Garland, Vieland, Underwood, & Busner, 1991) and numbers of mental health referrals (Rustici, 1988) as postintervention outcome criteria. Shaffer et al. (1987, 1991) compared the attitudinal outcomes for adolescent participants in three brief didactic school-based programs with five control groups ($N = 1,000$ 13- to 18-year-olds). At pretest, it was found that most adolescents had an appropriate knowledge base and attitudes regarding suicide including an understanding of the warning signs, the seriousness of threats, and the need for disclosure to and assistance of responsible adults. In all groups, however, there were from 5% to 20% of the subjects who held inappropriate attitudes and beliefs about suicide that were left unchanged following program participation. These high-risk adolescents believed suicide to be a reasonable solution to problems and would be reluctant to reveal or seek assistance for suicidal ideation. Likewise, in a follow-up study 18 months postintervention, there was no evidence of program effect on suicidal or help-seeking behavior (Vieland, Whittle, Garland, Hicks, & Shaffer, 1991).

There is no consensus based on systematic program evaluation that typical forms of suicide prevention targeting all adolescents regardless of risk status are effective in reducing suicidal behavior (Bushong, Coverdale, & Battaglia, 1992; Garland et al., 1989). It has been argued that because universal prevention efforts may actually reach very few who will ultimately commit suicide, adolescents at high risk should be targeted for more intensive secondary or tertiary preventive interventions (Shaffer et al., 1988). Unfortunately, other treatment strategies for adolescents like suicide hot lines, crisis services, and postsuicide interventions to prevent cluster or imitative suicides by other adolescents have been inadequately investigated.

Prevention of Conduct Disorder

Although conduct disorder can have its onset in adolescence, antisocial behaviors typically originate earlier in childhood. Preventive interventions have justifiably targeted either child behavior at earlier stages of development or parenting practices. By enhancing cognitive development and academic achievement, preschool educational interventions have been thought to have indirect benefits on later child and adolescent behavior. In a longitudinal study that followed participants in an intensive 2-year preschool program, subjects demonstrated higher academic achievement and fewer delinquent behaviors at age 19 than controls (Berrueta-Clement, Schweinhart, Barnett, & Weikart, 1986). Similar outcomes were found for children of low-income families who were served for 5 years with structured day care and family support services. Ten years postintervention, only 6% of the sample evidenced antisocial behavior in comparison with 22% of the control group (U.S. Congress, 1988).

Outcome studies of parenting skills training programs have shown short-term skill improvements for parents and decreased aggressive behaviors in school-aged children (Greenwood & Ziming, 1983; Hawkins, Catalano, Jones, & Fine, 1987). These two studies, however, had homogeneous samples of economically privileged participants. Parent training was also found to be ineffective for families with adolescents.

Interventions that focused on curricular development to enhance problem-solving and social skills for school-aged children have evidenced short-term academic and social improvements with less antisocial behavior in the classroom (Michelson, 1986). Similarly, social skills attainment for school-aged children and young adolescents in a nonschool setting was evaluated (Jones & Offord, 1989). Children who participated in sports and recreational activities in their housing project evidenced no significant change in home or school prosocial behavior. Numbers of security reports and criminal charges against juveniles in the housing project were significantly reduced, however, these rebounded to past rates after 1 year. The long-term impact of these programs on adolescent behavior has not been examined.

Few studies were found that specifically addressed the prevention of conduct disorders in adolescent populations. In fact, initial early-intervention efforts that targeted delinquent youth appeared to have an iatrogenic effect. By exposure to peers with similar negative behavioral profiles, antisocial behavior was actually reinforced rather than decreased (O'Donnell, Manos, & Chesney-Lind, 1987). Other school-based strategies that aimed to change characteristics of the school environment and methods to improve academic performance have met with variable success. Hawkins and Lam (1986) found some academic gains but no behavioral change in middle-school students after 1 year of participation in a social development curriculum. Another program that created a cooperative learning environment had a positive affect on antisocial behavior for middle-school but not high-school students (Kimbrough, 1985). Other broader based community interventions have shown promising preliminary results. Dryfoos (1990) reported that by targeting high-risk adolescents for intensive case management, the Boys Club of America has significantly reduced adolescent reinvolvement with the juvenile justice system. Similar programs with multicomponent interventions for high-risk youth have been sponsored by juvenile justice systems in urban areas (L. Feldman, 1988). Positive behavioral changes have been attributed to the adolescent's relationship with a stable adult volunteer who acts as both a role model and advocate.

These findings as a group suggest the need for wider involvement of important members of the adolescent's social network along with ongoing intervention over time. Interventions that are too brief, lacking in reinforcement, and centered on the individual with little regard for the socializing environment have less satisfactory results (Hawkins & Lam, 1986; Jones & Offord, 1989; Michelson, 1986; O'Donnell et al., 1987). There is also empirical support for two major target groups for intensive intervention: younger children and their families (Berrueta-Clement et al., 1986; Kimbrough, 1985; U.S. Congress, 1988) and high-risk adolescents (Dryfoos, 1990; L. Feldman, 1988). Studies of conduct disorder prevention in other adolescent populations has been less promising (Hawkins & Lam, 1986; Kimbrough, 1985).

Prevention of Disordered Eating

Only one study was found that evaluated the outcomes of a long-term prevention curriculum designed to modify eating attitudes and behaviors of young adolescent girls (Killen et al., 1993). Nine hundred sixty-seven girls were randomized into treatment or control groups. The intervention consisted of education regarding nutrition and the harmful effects of unhealthy dieting, development of skills to resist negative cultural influences on body image and dieting, and promotion of good eating and exercise habits. Although the treatment group did show a significant increase in knowledge, positive gains were not seen in physical outcomes (e.g., body-mass-index changes).

These disappointing results are somewhat predictable. With a prevalence rate of approximately 1%, there is actually a very low risk of developing an eating disorder for those in a normative sample. This prevention curriculum might be more appropriate and demonstrate more significant results with a sample of adolescents determined to be at high risk for this problem. Likewise, the assumption that increased knowledge leads to behavioral change has been challenged in many areas of adolescent behavior (e.g., contraception practices, substance use). Further explanation of factors that facilitate or pose barriers for change is needed.

SUMMARY AND FUTURE DIRECTIONS

Researchers have identified many factors that increase the adolescent's risk for mental health problems. It has been well established that several variables from the adolescent's social context, such as problematic relationships and stress within the family, stressors in the school environment, and other detrimental experiences, have a negative effect on the adolescent. The positive qualities of relationships, including family cohesiveness and support by family and peers, have been found to serve as protective factors that may play a role in the prevention of mental health problems. There is, however, only a limited understanding of the complex interrelationships of these multiple positive and negative influences and even less of their mechanisms of causation.

This is due, in part, to several limitations apparent in the studies of risk factors. First, most were cross-sectional, a design that is prohibitive in determining the causal nature of relationships between variables. Likewise, data analyses for many of the studies used univariate methods. Inferences regarding causal influences were made at times without the appropriate level of measurement or analysis to enable this prediction. It was also common to use a singular method of measurement and constructs were often inadequately defined, both threatening the construct validity of the study findings. Finally, data in this body of research were predominantly derived from White adolescents from middle-class families. Racial and ethnic similarities and differences are poorly understood and the confounding nature of socioeconomic status has not been well addressed. With few heterogenous samples, the generalizability of these findings is limited.

Without a complete picture of the etiology of the mental disorders that adolescents experience, it has been difficult to design effective prevention programs. Those that have targeted specific mental health problems, like depression and eating disorders, have demonstrated minimal success. Interventions that have shown more promise are those that are noncategorical in focus with broad mental health objectives.

From the body of work reviewed, two suggested directions for future research may be made. First, the effort to improve the understanding of the etiology of mental health disorders in adolescence must continue. Despite a growing knowledge of the psychobiology of major mental disorders such as depression and eating disorders, there is a wide gap in understanding how biological and psychosocial factors interact to increase or moderate risk. Additionally, developmentally specific risk and protective factors should continue to be elucidated. These factors must be studied within the ecological context of the adolescent in order to adequately comprehend the interrelationships between significant individuals and variables. Qualitative research has the potential to enhance the description of the context of adolescence. Subsequent theory development would be based on a subjective understanding of adolescents range of experiences and the meanings they assign to them. In parallel, the continued development and testing of theoretical models will assist in the effort to identify the causal linkages between risk and protective factors and mental health outcomes. Prospective, longitudinal studies are necessary to achieve this objective.

Second, despite the incomplete knowledge of etiology, prevention programs must continue to be developed and implemented based on the state of empirical knowledge. Previous research supports a focus on nonspecific mental health problems rather than targeting a single disorder. Interventions should be directed at multiple interpersonal and environmental sources of risk along with individual adolescent behavior. Crucial developmental periods like the onset of puberty or transition to middle or high school are important considerations for the timing of interventions. For some problems, like conduct disorder, intervening in adolescence may be far too late to modify established antisocial behavior patterns. There is also support for longer duration interventions with booster periods to maintain positive gains over time. Based on the previous studies, an argument can be made to target interventions to specific high-risk groups of adolescents rather than universally implementing programs for all youth. This must be done with care to avoid the potential stigmatizing effect of singling out individuals for special treatment.

Programs that attempt to prevent mental health problems require rigorous and systematic investigation to evaluate outcomes. Psychometrically sound and culturally sensitive instruments must be used. Instead of relying exclusively on adolescent self-report, including multiple informants and objective measurements can enhance the validity of the findings. Despite the importance of participant satisfaction, knowledge, and attitudes, they are inadequate measures of impact. Behavioral change and decreased incidence of symptoms of psychopathology are critical outcomes to measure over time.

Interventions and research to prevent mental health problems in adolescence fit well within the domain of the nursing discipline. In numerous publications, nurse scholars have written about the roles of nursing in the promotion of mental health and the prevention of mental health problems in this age group. It was poignant that very few of the studies reviewed, however, were conducted by nurses. Research by nurses, both independently and in collaboration with colleagues from other disciplines, must be undertaken to address this gap.

ACKNOWLEDGMENT

The author wishes to acknowledge Ms. Shao-Ti Meredith, RN, MS, former graduate student in advanced practice pediatric nursing at UCSF, for her tremendous assistance in the literature search-and-retrieval process.

REFERENCES

Adam, K. S., Bouckams, A., & Streiner, D. (1982). Parental loss and family stability in attempted suicide. *Archives of General Psychiatry, 39,* 1081–1085.

Adams, D. M., Overholser, J. C., & Spirito, A. (1994). Stressful life events associated with adolescent suicide attempts. *Canadian Journal of Psychiatry, 39,* 43–48.

American Psychiatric Association. (1994). *Diagnostic and statistical manual of mental disorders* (4th ed.). Washington, DC: American Psychiatric Press.

Aseltine, R. H., Jr., Gore, S., & Colten, M. E. (1994). Depression and the social developmental context of adolescence. *Journal of Personality and Social Psychology, 67*, 252–263.

Bangert-Drowns, R. L. (1988). The effects of school-based substance abuse education: A meta-analysis. *Journal of Drug Education, 18*, 243–264.

Bartlett, J. A., Schleifer, S. J., Johnson, R. L., & Keller, S. E. (1991). Depression in inner city adolescents attending an adolescent medicine clinic. *Journal of Adolescent Health, 12*, 316–318.

Berger, R., & Shechter, Y. (1989). Adolescent girls in distress: A high-risk intersection. *Adolescence, 24*, 357–374.

Berrueta-Clement, J., Schweinhart, L., Barnett, W., & Weikart, D. (1986). The effects of early educational intervention on crime and delinquency in adolescence and early adulthood. In J. Burchard & S. Burchard (Eds.), *Prevention of delinquent behavior* (pp. 220–240). Newbury Park, CA: Sage.

Brent, D. A., Perper, J., Moritz, G., Allman, C., Friend, A., Schweers, J., Roth, C., Balach, L., & Harrington, K. (1992). Psychiatric effects of exposure to suicide among the friends and acquaintances of adolescent suicide victims. *Journal of the American Academy of Child and Adolescent Psychiatry, 31*, 629–639.

Brent, D. A., Perper, J. A., Goldstein, C. E., Kolko, D. J., Allan, M. J., Allman, C. J., & Zelenak, J. P. (1988). Risk factors for adolescent suicide. A comparison of adolescent suicide victims with suicidal inpatients. *Archives of General Psychiatry, 45*, 581–588.

Brent, D. A., Perper, J. A., Moritz, G., Allman, C., Schweers, J., Roth, C., Balach, L., Canobbio, R., & Liotus, L. (1993). Psychiatric sequelae to the loss of an adolescent peer to suicide. *Journal of the American Academy of Child and Adolescent Psychiatry, 32*, 509–517.

Brent, D. A., Perper, J. A., Moritz, G., Liotus, L., Schweers, J., Balach, L., & Roth, C. (1994). Familial risk factors for adolescent suicide: A case-control study. *Acta Psychiatrica Scandinavica, 89*, 52–58.

Brown, B. B. (1990). Peer groups and peer cultures. In S. S. Feldman & G. R. Elliott (Eds.), *At the threshold: The developing adolescent* (pp. 171–196). Cambridge, MA: Harvard University Press.

Bukstein, O. G., Brent, D. A., Perper, J. A., Moritz, G., Baugher, M., Schweers, J., Roth, C., & Balach, L. (1993). Risk factors for completed suicide among adolescents with a lifetime history of substance abuse: A case-control study. *Acta Psychiatrica Scandinavica, 88*, 403–408.

Bushong, C., Coverdale, J., & Battaglia, J. (1992). Adolescent mental health: A review of preventive interventions. *Texas Medicine, 88*, 62–68.

Caplan, M., Weissberg, R. P., Grober, J. S., Sivo, P. J., Grady, K., & Jacoby, C. (1992). Social competence promotion with inner-city and suburban young adolescents: Effects on social adjustment and alcohol use. *Journal of Consulting and Clinical Psychology, 60*, 56–63.

Cappelli, M., Clulow, M. K., Goodman, J. T., Davidson, S. I., Feder, S. H., Baron, P., Manion, I. G., & McGrath, P. J. (1995). Identifying depressed and suicidal adolescents in a teen health clinic. *Journal of Adolescent Health, 16,* 64–70.

Choquet, M., Kovess, V., & Poutignat, N. (1993). Suicidal thoughts among adolescents: An intercultural approach. *Adolescence, 28,* 649–659.

Ciffone, J. (1993). Suicide prevention: A classroom presentation to adolescents. *Social Work, 38,* 197–203.

Clair, D. J., & Genest, M. (1986). Variables associated with the adjustment of offspring of alcoholic fathers. *Journal of Studies on Alcohol, 48,* 345–355.

Clarke, G. N., Hawkins, W., Murphy, M., & Sheeber, L. (1993). School-based primary prevention of depressive symptomatology in adolescents: Findings from two studies. *Journal of Adolescent Research, 8,* 183–204.

Clarke, G. N., Hawkins, W., Murphy, M., Sheeber, L. B., Lewinsohn, P. M., & Seeley, J. R. (1995). Targeted prevention of unipolar depressive disorder in an at-risk sample of high school adolescents: A randomized trial of a group cognitive intervention. *Journal of the American Academy of Child and Adolescent Psychiatry, 34,* 312–321.

Compas, B. E., Howell, D. C., Phares, V., Williams, R. A., & Giunta, C. T. (1989). Risk factors for emotional/behavioral problems in young adolescents: A prospective analysis of adolescent and parental stress and symptoms. *Journal of Consulting and Clinical Psychology, 57,* 732–740.

Conger, R. D., Ge, X., Elder, G. H., Jr., Lorenz, F. O., & Simons, R. L. (1994). Economic stress, coercive family process, and developmental problems of adolescents. *Child Development, 65,* 541–561.

Cook, T. D., & Campbell, D. T. (1979). *Quasi-experimentation: Design and analysis issues for field settings.* Chicago: Rand McNally.

Cooper, J. E., Holman, J., & Braithwaite, V. (1983). Self-esteem and family cohesion: The child's perspective. *Journal of Marriage and the Family, 45,* 153–159.

Costello, E. J. (1989). Developments in child psychiatric epidemiology. *Journal of the American Academy of Child and Adolescent Psychiatry, 28,* 836–841.

deAnda, D., & Smith, M. A. (1993). Differences among adolescent, young adult, and adult callers of suicide help lines. *Social Work, 38,* 421–428.

Dietrich, D. R. (1984). Psychological health of young adults who experienced early parent death: MMPI trends. *Journal of Clinical Psychology, 40,* 901–908.

Dryfoos, J. G. (1990). *Adolescents at risk: Prevalence and prevention.* New York: Oxford University Press.

DuBois, D. L., Felner, R. D., Sherman, M. D., & Bull, C. A. (1994). Socioenvironmental experiences, self-esteem, and emotional/behavioral problems in early adolescence. *American Journal of Community Psychology, 22,* 371–397.

Farrington, D. P. (1986). Stepping stones to adult criminal careers. In D. Olweus, J. Block, & M. R. Yarrow (Eds.), *Development of antisocial and prosocial behavior* (pp. 359–384). New York: Academic Press.

Feldman, L. (Ed.). (1988). *Partnerships for youth 2000: A program models manual.* Tulsa, OK: University of Oklahoma, National Resource Center for Youth Services.

Feldman, R. A., Stiffman, A. R., & Jung, K. G. (1987). *Children at risk: In the web of parental mental illness.* New Brunswick: Rutgers University Press.

Feldman, S. S., & Elliott, G. R. (1990). *At the threshold: The developing adolescent.* Cambridge, MA: Harvard University Press.

Fine, E. W., Yudin, L. W., Holmes, J., & Heinemann, S. (1976). Behavioral disorders in children with parental alcoholism. *Annals of the New York Academy of Sciences, 273,* 507–517.

Fitzpatrick, J. J. (1983). Suicidology and suicide prevention: Historical perspectives from the nursing literature. *Journal of Psychosocial Nursing and Mental Health Services, 21*(5), 20–28.

Forehand, R., Wierson, M., McCombs, A., Brody, G., & Fauber, R. (1989). Interparental conflict and adolescent problem behavior: An examination of mechanisms. *Behavioral Research and Therapy, 27,* 365–371.

Frost, A. K., & Pakiz, B. (1990). The effects of marital disruption on adolescents: Time as a dynamic. *American Journal of Orthopsychiatry, 60,* 544–555.

Garbarino, J., Sebes, J., & Schellenbach, C. (1984). Families at risk for destructive parent-child relations in adolescence. *Child Development, 55,* 174–183.

Garland, A., Shaffer, D., & Whittle, B. (1989). A national survey of school-based, adolescent suicide prevention programs. *Journal of the American Academy of Child and Adolescent Psychiatry, 28,* 931–934.

Garner, D. M., Olmstead, M. P., & Polivy, J. (1983). The development and validation of a multidimensional eating disorder inventory for anorexia nervosa and bulimia. *International Journal of Eating Disorders, 2,* 15–34.

Gore, S., Aseltine, R. H., & Colton, M. E. (1992). Social structure, life stress and depressive symptoms in a high school-aged population. *Journal of Health and Social Behavior, 33,* 97–113.

Greenwood, P., & Ziming, F. (1983). *One more chance: The pursuit of promising intervention strategies for chronic juvenile offenders.* Santa Monica, CA: Rand Corporation.

Grossman, D. C., Milligan, B. C., & Deyo, R. A. (1991). Risk factors for suicide attempts among Navajo adolescents. *American Journal of Public Health, 81,* 870–874.

Gutstein, S. E., Rudd, M. D., Graham, J. C., & Rayha, L. L. (1988). Systemic crisis intervention as a response to adolescent crises: An outcome study. *Family Process, 27,* 201–211.

Hartman, L. M. (1979). The preventive reduction of psychological risk in asymptomatic adolescents. *American Journal of Orthopsychiatry, 49,* 121–135.

Hawkins, D., Catalano, R., Jones, G., & Fine, D. (1987). Delinquency prevention through parent training: Results and issues from work in progress. In J. Wilson & G. Loury (Eds.), *Children to citizens: Families, schools, and delinquency prevention* (Vol. 3, pp. 186–204). New York: Springer-Verlag.

Hawkins, D., & Lam, T. (1986). Teacher practices, social development and delinquency. In J. Burchard & S. Burchard (Eds.), *Prevention of delinquent behavior* (pp. 241–274). Newbury Park, CA: Sage.

Hazell, P., & Lewin, T. (1993). Friends of adolescent suicide attempters and completers. *Journal of the American Academy of Child and Adolescent Psychiatry, 32,* 76–81.

Hetherington, E. M., Cox, M., & Cox, R. (1985). Long-term effects of divorce and remarriage on the adjustment of children. *Journal of the American Academy of Child Psychiatry, 24*, 518–530.

Hirsch, B. J., & DuBois, D. L. (1992). The relation of peer social support and psychological symptomatology during the transition to junior high school: A two-year longitudinal analysis. *American Journal of Community Psychology, 20*, 333–347.

Institute of Medicine. (1989). *Research on children and adolescents with mental, behavioral, and developmental disorders.* Washington, DC: National Academy Press.

Jones, M. B., & Offord, D. R. (1989). Reduction of antisocial behavior in poor children by nonschool skill-department. *Journal of Child Psychology and Psychiatry and Allied Disciplines, 30*, 737–750.

Kahn, J. S., Kehle, T. J., Jenson, W. R., & Clark, E. (1990). Comparison of cognitive-behavioral, relaxation, and self-monitoring interventions for depression among middle-school students. *School Psychology Review, 19*, 196–210.

Kalter, N., Reimer, B., Brickman, A., & Chen, J. W. (1985). Implications of parental divorce for female development. *Journal of the American Academy of Child Psychiatry, 24*, 538–544.

Kasen, S., Johnson, J., & Cohen, P. (1990). The impact of school emotional climate on student psychopathology. *Journal of Abnormal Child Psychology, 18*, 165–177.

Kashden, J., Fremouw, W. J., Callahan, T. S., & Franzen, M. D. (1993). Impulsivity in suicidal and nonsuicidal adolescents. *Journal of Abnormal Child Psychology, 21*, 339–353.

Kazdin, A. (1986). *Conduct disorders in childhood and adolescence.* Newbury Park, CA: Sage.

Kazdin, A. E. (1993). Adolescent mental health. Prevention and treatment programs. *American Psychologist, 48*, 127–141.

Killen, J. D., Hayward, C., Litt, I., Hammer, L. D., Wilson, D. M., Miner, B., Taylor, C. B., Varady, A., & Shisslak, C. (1992). Is puberty a risk factor for eating disorders? *American Journal of the Disturbed Child, 146*, 323–325.

Killen, J. D., Taylor, C. B., Hammer, L. D., Litt, I., Wilson, D. M., Rich, T., Hayward, C., Simmonds, B., Kraemer, H., & Varady, A. (1993). An attempt to modify unhealthful eating attitudes and weight regulation practices of young adolescent girls. *International Journal of Eating Disorders, 13*, 369–384.

Killen, J. D., Taylor, C. B., Hayward, C., Wilson, D. M., Haydel, K. F., Hammer, L. D., Simmonds, B., Robinson, T. N., Litt, I., Varady, A., & Kraemer, H. (1994). Pursuit of thinness and onset of eating disorder symptoms in a community sample of adolescent girls: A three-year prospective analysis. *International Journal of Eating Disorders, 16*, 227–238.

Kimbrough, J. (1985). School-based strategies for delinquency prevention. In P. Greenwood (Ed.), *The juvenile rehabilitation reader* (pp. 1–22). Santa Monica, CA: Rand Corporation.

Kisker, E. E., & Brown, R. S. (1996). Do school-based health centers improve adolescents' access to health care, health status, and risk-taking behavior? *Journal of Adolescent Health, 18*, 335–343.

Klein, M. H., Greist, J. H., Bass, S. M., & Lohr, M. J. (1987). Autonomy and self-control: Key concepts for the prevention of depression in adolescents. In R. F. Muñoz (Ed.), *Depression prevention: Research directions* (pp. 103–124). New York: Hemisphere.

Kovacs, M., Goldston, D., & Gatsonis, C. (1993). Suicidal behaviors and childhood onset depressive disorders: A longitudinal investigation. *Journal of the American Academy of Child and Adolescent Psychiatry, 32,* 1–8.

Kovacs, M., Paulauskas, S., Gatsonis, C., & Richards, C. (1988). Depressive disorders in childhood: III. A longitudinal study of comorbidity with and risk for conduct disorders. *Journal of Affective Disorders, 15,* 205–217.

Lamb, J., & Pusker, K. R. (1991). School-based adolescent mental health project survey of depression, suicidal ideation, and anger. *Journal of Child and Adolescent Psychiatric and Mental Health Nursing, 4,* 101–104.

Leon, G. R., Fulkerson, J. A., Perry, C. L., & Dube, A. (1994). Family influences, school behaviors, and risk for the later development of an eating disorder. *Journal of Youth and Adolescence, 23,* 499–515.

Levine, M. P., Smolak, L., & Hayden, H. (1994). The relation of sociocultural factors to eating attitudes and behaviors among middle school girls. *Journal of Early Adolescence, 14,* 471–490.

Lewinsohn, P. M., Clarke, G. N., Hops, H., & Andrews, J. (1990). Cognitive-behavioral group treatment of adolescent depression. *Behavior Therapy, 21,* 385–401.

Lewinsohn, P. M., Rohde, P., & Seeley, J. R. (1994). Psychosocial risk factors for future adolescent suicide attempts. *Journal of Consulting and Clinical Psychology, 62,* 297–305.

Lourie, I. S. (1979). Family dynamics and the abuse of adolescents: A case for a developmental phase specific model of child abuse. *Child Abuse and Neglect, 3,* 967–974.

Maloney, M. J., McGuire, J., & Daniels, S. R. (1988). Reliability testing of a children's version of the Eating Attitudes Test. *Journal of the American Academy of Child and Adolescent Psychiatry, 5,* 541–543.

Martin, G., Rozanes, P., Pearce, C., & Allison, S. (1995). Adolescent suicide, depression and family dysfunction. *Acta Psychiatrica Scandinavica, 92,* 336–344.

Martin, G., & Waite, S. (1994). Parental bonding and vulnerability to adolescent suicide. *Acta Psychiatry Scandinavia, 89,* 246–254.

McIntosh, J. L., & Jewell, B. L. (1986). Sex difference trends in completed suicide. *Suicide and Life-Threatening Behavior, 16,* 16–27.

Michelson, L. (1986). Cognitive-behavioral strategies in the prevention and treatment of antisocial disorders in children and adolescents. In J. Burchard & S. Burchard (Eds.), *Prevention of delinquent behavior* (pp. 275–310). Newbury Park, CA: Sage.

Morano, C. D., Cisler, R. A., & Lemerond, J. (1993). Risk factors for adolescent suicidal behavior: Loss, insufficient familial support, and hopelessness. *Adolescence, 28,* 851–865.

National Institute of Mental Health. (1992). *Suicide fact sheet.* Washington, DC: U.S. Government Printing Office.

Newcomb, M. D., Maddahian, E., & Bentler, P. M. (1986). Risk factors for drug use among adolescents: Concurrent and longitudinal analyses. *American Journal of Public Health, 76*, 525–531.

Niznik, K. (1994). The nurse's role in school-based mental health promotion: Easing the transition into adolescence. *Journal of Child and Adolescent Psychiatric and Mental Health Nursing, 7*, 5–8.

O'Donnell, C., Manos, M., & Chesney-Lind, M. (1987). Diversion and neighborhood delinquency programs in open settings. In E. Morris & C. Braukmann (Eds.), *Behavioral approaches to crime and delinquency* (pp. 251–269). New York: Plenum.

Offord, D. R. (1982). Family backgrounds of male and female delinquents. In J. Gunn & D. P. Farrington (Eds.), *Delinquency and the criminal justice system.* New York: Wiley.

Offord, D. R. (1989). Conduct disorder: Risk factors and prevention. In D. Shaffer, I. Philips, & M. M. Enzer (Eds.), *Prevention of mental disorders, alcohol and other drug use in children and adolescents* (pp. 273–307). Rockville, MD: Office for Substance Abuse Prevention, U.S. Department of Health and Human Services.

Offord, D. R., Sullivan, K., & Allen, N. (1979). Delinquency and hyperactivity. *Journal of Nervous and Mental Disease, 167*, 734–741.

Oler, M. J., Mainous, A. G., Martin, C. A., Richardson, E., Haney, A., Wilson, D., & Adams, T. (1994). Depression, suicidal ideation, and substance use among adolescents. Are athletes at less risk? *Archives of Family Medicine, 3*, 781–785.

Partridge, S., & Kotler, T. (1987). Self-esteem and adjustment in adolescents from bereaved, divorced and intact families: Family type versus family environment. *Australian Journal of Psychology, 39*, 223–234.

Pastore, D. R., Fisher, M., & Friedman, S. B. (1996). Violence and mental health problems among urban high school students. *Journal of Adolescent Health, 18*, 320–324.

Patterson, G. R. (1986). Performance models for antisocial boys. *American Psychologist, 41*, 432–444.

Peck, J. S. (1989). The impact of divorce on children at various stages of the family life cycle. *Journal of Divorce, 12*, 81–106.

Peters, R. D. (1988). Mental health promotion in children and adolescents: An emerging role for psychology. Special Issue: Child and adolescent health. *Canadian Journal of Behavioral Science, 20*, 389–401.

Puskar, K., & Lamb, J. (1991). Life events, problems, stresses, and coping methods of adolescents. *Issues in Mental Health Nursing, 12*, 267–281.

Puskar, K. R., Lamb, J., & Martsolf, D. S. (1990). The role of the psychiatric/mental health nurse clinical specialist in an adolescent coping skills group. *Journal of Child and Adolescent Psychiatric and Mental Health Nursing, 3*, 47–51.

Rae-Grant, N., Thomas, B. H., Offord, D. R., & Boyle, M. H. (1989). Risk, protective factors, and the prevalence of behavioral and emotional disorders in children and adolescents. *Journal of the American Academy of Child and Adolescent Psychiatry, 28*, 262–268.

Raphael, B., Cubis, J., Dunne, M., Lewin, T., & Kelly, B. (1990). The impact of parental loss on adolescents' psychosocial characteristics. *Adolescence, 25,* 689–700.

Reifman, A., & Windle, M. (1995). Adolescent suicidal behaviors as a function of depression, hopelessness, alcohol use, and social support: A longitudinal investigation. *American Journal of Community Psychology, 23,* 329–354.

Reinherz, H. Z., Giaconia, R. M., Pakiz, B., Silverman, A. B., Frost, A. K., & Lefkowitz, E. S. (1993). Psychosocial risks for major depression in late adolescence: A longitudinal community study. *Journal of the American Academy of Child and Adolescent Psychiatry, 32,* 1155–1163.

Remafedi, G. (1987). Adolescent homosexuality: Psychosocial and medical implications. *Pediatrics, 79,* 331–337.

Reynolds, I., & Rob, M. I. (1988). The role of family difficulties in adolescent depression, drug-taking and other problem behaviors. *Medical Journal of Australia, 149,* 250–256.

Reynolds, W. M., & Coats, K. I. (1986). A comparison of cognitive-behavioral therapy and relaxation training for the treatment of depression in adolescents. *Journal of Consulting and Clinical Psychology, 54,* 653–660.

Robins, L. & Rutter, M. (1990). *Straight and devious pathways from childhood to adulthood.* Cambridge, UK: Cambridge University Press.

Rohde, P., Lewinsohn, P. M., & Seeley, J. R. (1991). Comorbidity with unipolar depression: II. Comorbidity with other mental disorders in adolescents and adults. *Journal of Abnormal Psychology, 100,* 214–222.

Roosa, M. W., Beals, J., Sandler, I. N., & Pillow, D. R. (1990). The role of risk and protective factors in predicting symptomatology in adolescent self-identified children of alcoholic parents. *American Journal of Community Psychology, 18,* 725–741.

Roosa, M. W., Sandler, I. N., Beals, J., & Short, J. (1988). Risk status of adolescent children of problem drinking parents. *American Journal of Community Psychology, 16,* 225–229.

Rubenstein, J. L., Heeren, T., Housman, D., Rubin, C., & Stechler, G. (1989). Suicidal behavior in "normal" adolescents: Risk and protective factors. *American Journal of Orthopsychiatry, 59,* 59–71.

Rubin, R. L. (1986). Assisting adolescents toward mental health. *Nursing Clinics of North America, 21,* 439–450.

Rustici, C. J. (1988). Teenline: A CMHC-based adolescent suicide prevention and intervention program. *Journal of Mental Health Administration, 15,* 15–20.

Rutter, M. (1987). Parental mental disorder as a risk factor. In R. E. Hales & A. J. Frances (Eds.), *American Psychiatric Association's annual review, 6.* Washington, DC: American Psychiatric Press.

Rutter, M. (1989). Psychiatric disorder in parents as a risk factor for children. In D. Shaffer, I. Philips, & N. B. Enzer (Eds.), *Prevention of mental disorders, alcohol, and other drug use in children and adolescents* (pp. 157–189). Washington, DC: U.S. Department of Health & Human Services.

Rutter, M., & Giller, H. (1983). *Juvenile delinquency: Trends and prospectives.* New York: Penguin.

Rutter, M., & Quinton, D. (1984). Parental psychiatric disorder: Effects on children. *Psychological Medicine, 14,* 853–880.

Sameroff, A. J., & Fiese, B. H. (1989). Conceptual issues in prevention. In D. Shaffer, I. Philips, & N. B. Enzer (Eds.), *Prevention of mental disorders, alcohol, and other drug use in children and adolescents* (pp. 23–53). Washington, DC: U.S. Department of Health & Human Services.

Saner, H., & Ellickson, P. (1996). Concurrent risk factors for adolescent violence. *Journal of Adolescent Health, 19,* 94–103.

Saucier, J. F., & Ambert, A. M. (1983). Adolescents' self-reported mental health and parents' marital status. *Psychiatry, 46,* 363–369.

Scharer, K., Challberg, C., & Rearick, T. (1990). Young people and AIDS: Mental health promotion in action. *Journal of Child and Adolescent Psychiatric and Mental Health Nursing, 3,* 41–46.

Scholte, E. M. (1992). Prevention and treatment of juvenile problem behavior: A proposal for a socio-ecological approach. *Journal of Abnormal Child Psychology, 20,* 247–262.

Seidl, F. W. (1982). Big sisters: An experimental evaluation. *Adolescence, 17,* 117–128.

Shaffer, D., Garland, A., Gould, M., Fisher, P., & Trautman, P. (1988). Preventing teenage suicide: A critical review. *Journal of the American Academy of Child Adolescent Psychiatry, 27,* 675–687.

Shaffer, D., Garland, A., Underwood, M., & Whittle, B. (1987). *An evaluation of three youth suicide prevention programs in New Jersey:* Report prepared for the New Jersey State Department of Health and Human Services.

Shaffer, D., Garland, A., Vieland, V., Underwood, M., & Busner, C. (1991). The impact of curriculum-based suicide prevention programs for teenagers. *Journal of the American Academy of Child and Adolescent Psychiatry, 30,* 588–596.

Shaffer, D., & Gould, M. (1987). *Study of completed and attempted suicides in adolescents.* Progress Report. Washington, DC: National Institute of Mental Health.

Sorosky, A. (1977). The psychological effects of divorce on adolescents. *Adolescence, 12,* 123–136.

Spirito, A., Overholser, J., & Stark, L. J. (1989). Common problems and coping strategies: II. Findings with adolescent suicide attempters. *Journal of Abnormal Child Psychology, 17,* 213–221.

Stark, L. J., Spirito, A., Williams, C. A., & Guevremont, D. C. (1989). Common problems and coping strategies: I. Findings with normal adolescents. *Journal of Abnormal Child Psychology, 17,* 203–212.

Stein, B. A., Marton, P., Golombek, H., & Korenblum, M. (1994). The relationship between life events during adolescence and affect and personality functioning. *Canadian Journal of Psychiatry, 39,* 354–357.

Steinberg, L. (1990). Autonomy, conflict, and harmony in the family relationship. In S. S. Feldman & G. R. Elliott (Eds.), *At the threshold: The developing adolescent* (pp. 255–276). Cambridge, MA: Harvard University Press.

Tanner, J. M. (1990). Sequence, tempo, and individual variation in growth and development of boys and girls aged twelve to sixteen. In R. E. Muuss (Ed.), *Adolescent behavior and society* (pp. 39–50). New York: McGraw-Hill.

Thompson, E. A., Moody, K. A., & Eggert, L. L. (1994). Discriminating suicide ideation among high-risk youth. *Journal of School Health, 64,* 361–367.

Tobler, N. S. (1986). Meta-analysis of 143 adolescent drug prevention programs: Quantitative outcome results of program participants compared to a control or comparison group. *Journal of Drug Issues, 16,* 537–567.

Tolan, P. (1988). Socioeconomic, family, and social stress correlates of adolescent antisocial and delinquent behavior. *Journal of Abnormal Child Psychology, 16,* 317–331.

Tomori, M. (1994). Personality characteristics of adolescents with alcoholic parents. *Adolescence, 29,* 949–959.

Tubman, J. G., Windle, M., & Windle, R. C. (1996). Cumulative sexual intercourse patterns among middle adolescents: Problem behavior precursors and concurrent health risk behaviors. *Journal of Adolescent Health, 18,* 182–191.

U.S. Congress, House Select Committee on Children, Youth and Families. (1988). *Opportunities for success: Cost-effective programs for children: Update 1988.* Washington, DC: U.S. Government Printing Office.

Vieland, V., Whittle, B., Garland, A., Hicks, R., & Schaffer, D. (1991). The impact of curriculum-based suicide prevention programs for teenagers: An 18-month follow-up. *Journal of the American Academy of Child and Adolescent Psychiatry, 30,* 811–815.

Wallerstein, J. S. (1984). Children of divorce: Preliminary report of a ten-year follow-up of young children. *American Journal of Orthopsychiatry, 54,* 444–458.

Wassef, A., Ingham, D., Collins, M. L., & Mason, G. (1995). In search of effective programs to address students' emotional distress and behavioral problems. Part I: Defining the problem. *Adolescence, 30,* 523–538.

Watts, W. D., & Ellis, A. M. (1992). Drug abuse and eating disorders: Prevention implications. *Journal of Drug Education, 22,* 223–240.

Weissberg, R. P., Caplan, M., & Harwood, R. L. (1991). Promoting competent young people in competence-enhancing environments: A systems-based perspective on primary prevention. [Special Section: Clinical child psychology: Perspectives on child and adolescent therapy.] *Journal of Consulting and Clinical Psychology, 59,* 830–841.

Williamson, J. M., Borduin, C. M., & Howe, B. A. (1991). The ecology of adolescent maltreatment: A multilevel examination of adolescent physical abuse, sexual abuse, and neglect. *Journal of Consulting and Clinical Psychology, 59,* 449–457.

Wortman, R. N., Donovan, D. S., & Woodburn, K. E. (1986). Depression and its relationship to somatic complaints in adolescent patients. *Journal of Adolescent Health Care, 7,* 295.

Young, D. M. (1980). A court-mandated workshop for adolescent children of divorcing parents: A program evaluation. *Adolescence, 15,* 763–774.

Zill, N., & Schoenborn, C. A. (1990). Developmental, learning, and emotional problems. Health of our nation's children, United States, 1988. *Advance Data, 16*(190), 1–18.

Chapter 5

The Development of Sexual Risk Taking in Adolescence

ROSEMARY A. JADACK
COLLEGE OF NURSING
THE OHIO STATE UNIVERSITY

MARY L. KELLER
SCHOOL OF NURSING
UNIVERSITY OF WISCONSIN—MADISON

ABSTRACT

This chapter reviews literature from 1985 to the present that is focused on the development of sexual behaviors in adolescents, decision making about sexual behavior, and sexual risk-taking behaviors. Results show that sexual behavior is part of most people's lives from childhood through adulthood, and that the majority of adolescents begin to engage in sexual behaviors in their teenage years. Synthesis of this large body of research reveals a lack of theoretical frameworks to guide research in sexual risk taking, resulting in an incomplete understanding of the predictors of sexual risk-taking behavior in adolescents. New and broader approaches in the study of sexual risk taking are needed that include consideration of the social and developmental context from which adolescents make decisions about sexual behavior.

Keywords: Adolescence, Sexual Behavior, Sexual Decision Making, Sexual Risk Taking

This chapter reviews research on the development of sexuality and sexual behaviors in adolescents and the subsequent development of sexual risk-taking behaviors. For this report adolescence is defined as persons aged 13 to 19 years, roughly equated with the teenage years. Further, sexual risk taking is defined as those behaviors that are linked to untoward consequences (e.g., sexually transmitted disease, unwanted pregnancy, unprotected sexual activity, unwanted sexual activity). The body of literature addressing sexuality and risk taking is large and is important to nursing. The findings of the research on sexual behavior and risk taking have implications for research on health promotion and disease prevention, areas long recognized as major priorities in nursing research.

The critical review includes a synthesis of the research findings with specific attention to variables that have been addressed and directions for future research. Over the past 20 years, thousands of studies on sexuality and sexual risk taking have been published. This review consists of published peer-reviewed reports of original research and meta-analyses, mainly from 1985 to present, among adolescents and young adults in the United States. Classic works before 1985 are included. To identify studies, computerized searches of MEDLINE, Cumulative Index to Nursing and Allied Health Literature (CINAHL), and PsycINFO databases for the years 1985 to present were done, using combinations of the keywords *sexuality, adolescence*, and *risk taking*. Articles were also identified from review references. The review is organized as follows. First, research on the development of sexuality in adolescence is discussed. Next research addressing the predictors of sexual risk-taking behaviors is explored. Finally, discussion of the findings and limitations of the research is explored.

THE DEVELOPMENT OF SEXUAL BEHAVIOR IN ADOLESCENTS

Humans are sexual beings throughout all the ages and stages of life. Nevertheless, research is limited with respect to describing the normal sexual behaviors of children and adolescents. There are two well-known sources of data available on the sexual behavior of children and adolescents, but both are relatively dated. The best known are the original Kinsey reports (Kinsey, Pomeroy, & Martin, 1948; Kinsey, Pomeroy, Martin, & Gebhard, 1953), the recent studies from the Kinsey Institute (Reinisch & Beasley, 1991), and the Hunt study (1974). In the work of both Kinsey and Hunt, adults were questioned about their childhood sexual behavior. Limitations of these works include accuracy of memory of events that happened long ago and unclear validation of instruments (Sanders, Ziemba-Davis, Hill, & Reinisch, 1991; T. W. Smith, 1991).

An alternative to asking adults about behavior in childhood is to interview children about their sexual behavior or to observe their sexual behavior. Few researchers have done either because of the serious ethical questions that such studies could raise. Published research that is available has been the result of either questionnaires or interviews. Few have made systematic, direct observations of children's sexual behavior.

A surge of sexual interest occurs around puberty and continues through adolescence. This heightened interest in sexuality and subsequent initiation of sexual behaviors are related to a number of factors, including bodily changes (secondary sex characteristics, onset of menarche) (Gargiulo, Attic, Brooks-Gunn, & Warren, 1987; Phinney, Jensen, Olsen, & Cundick, 1990; Schor, 1993), rises in levels of sex hormones (Halpern, Udry, Campbell, & Suchindran, 1993), cultural factors related to sex (Slonim-Nevo, 1992; Wyatt, Peters, & Guthrie, 1988b), and rehearsal for adult gender roles (Bolton & MacEachron, 1988; Jadack, Hyde, & Keller, 1995; Loltes, 1993). In this section, several aspects of sexual behavior in adolescence will be discussed. Because the study of initial sexual behaviors usually begins with the discussion of masturbation, this will be addressed first. Next, the development of sexual orientation in adolescence will be briefly described, followed by research addressing the development of heterosexual behaviors. This includes dating behaviors, initiation of first sexual intercourse, and number of sexual partners.

Masturbation

Evidence of heightened sexuality in adolescence is shown by data on masturbation. Masturbation is a normal and healthy sexual activity that occurs at all ages. Research addressing masturbation since 1985 is limited. Available reports indicate that masturbation often occurs as early as 5 years of age (Arafat & Cotton, 1974; Leitenberg, Detzer, & Srebnik, 1993; Leung & Robson, 1993). According to the Kinsey and Hunt data, there is a sharp increase in masturbation for boys between the ages of 13 and 15 (Hunt, 1974; Kinsey et al., 1948, 1953; Reinisch & Beasley, 1991). Many girls also report beginning to masturbate around age 13; however, research shows that, on average, more girls do not begin to masturbate until later, and many report more guilt associated with masturbation (Davidson & Moore, 1994; Hannonen & Kekki, 1995). Researchers have also reported that among those who report masturbation, adolescent boys report masturbating more often than girls (Leitenberg et al., 1993). Interestingly, significantly more boys learned about masturbation from peers, whereas girls learned of masturbation through self-discovery (Kinsey et al., 1953).

In sum masturbation is a normal and common activity among adolescents. Unfortunately, as children and adolescents learn about the practice of masturbation, they also learn that masturbation is something that should be done privately and not talked about. This is an important point, because at an early age many children learn that aspects of sexuality are not to be discussed.

Sexual Orientation

The development of sexual orientation is beyond the scope of this chapter. Sexual orientation is recognized and mentioned here, however, because data suggest that the development of sexual orientation and to a lesser extent, initiation of homosexual behaviors often occur during the adolescent years (Herdt, 1989). According to data gathered by the Kinsey Institute, by the time boys and girls reach adolescence, their sexual preference is likely to be already determined (Bell, Weinberg, & Hammersmith, 1981). Controversial research has described a biological predisposition to homosexual or heterosexual behavior across the life span (Ellis & Ames, 1987; Hauman, 1995; Roper, 1996). However, current discussion stresses the importance of considering a broader focus on the psychological, sociological, biological, and cultural facets related to the development of sexual orientation and preference rather than a biological focus alone (DeCecco & Parker, 1995). Homosexual feelings are often experienced and explored during the adolescent years. It needs to be recognized that many homosexually inclined adolescents engage in a variety of both homosexual and heterosexual behaviors during this time while a more firmly established sexual orientation develops (Telljohann & Price, 1993).

Heterosexual Behaviors

Dating behaviors.   There is substantial research documenting the sequence of heterosexual behaviors among adolescents that is often included under the category of dating behaviors (DeLamater & MacCorquodale, 1979). Research addressing dating behaviors describes a pattern whereby couples generally embrace and kiss first, then fondle and pet, and subsequently engage in more intimate behaviors that include sexual intercourse. McCabe and Collins (1984) measured the depth of desired and experienced sexual involvement among Australian adolescents during various stages of dating. As the dating relationship becomes more serious and committed, the level of sexual activity increases (G. K. Leigh, Weddle, & Loewen, 1988; Miller, McCoy, & Olson, 1986). Hand holding and embracing are the most frequently occurring behaviors on first dates, whereas genital masturbation and intercourse are much less common.

Several gender comparisons have been made regarding dating behavior. Researchers have reported that adolescent males have more desire for sexual intimacy on a first date than females, but these gender differences decrease as the relationship develops. In general, research reports indicated that young females were less permissive and had a greater commitment to abstinence than their male counterparts (De Gaston, Weed, & Jensen, 1996). Conversely, young males felt more pressured by their peers to engage in sexual activity and less support for delaying sexual intercourse (De Gaston et al., 1996). These gender differences have been shown to narrow as females age and become more committed to their dating relationship, however. Research reports showed that adolescent women who were in steady or committed dating relationships are more likely to engage in sexual behavior then young women who were either not dating or were in new dating relationships (Darling, Davidson, & Passarello, 1992; Thornton, 1990). Gender differences also decreased with age; females showed increasing desire toward sexual intimacy with increase in age (McCabe & Collins, 1984).

Researchers have described racial differences in the sequence of sexual behaviors among adolescents. A longitudinal analysis of the sequence of heterosexual behaviors among younger adolescents in the United States was conducted by Smith and Udry (1985). Dating behaviors were measured every 2 years. After the first data collection point, results for White adolescents aged 12 to 15 showed the expected ordering of heterosexual behavior: necking occurred most often, then feeling breasts through clothing, feeling breasts directly, feeling sex organs directly, feeling penis directly, and finally intercourse (which occurred least often).

The sequence of behaviors for Black adolescents was different from the sequence of behaviors among White adolescents (E. Smith & Udry, 1985). A greater percentage of Black teens indicated that they had engaged in intercourse directly rather than engaging in unclothed petting of breasts, sex organs, or the penis for a period of time before intercourse. Therefore, White teens were more likely than Black teens to engage in a predictable series of noncoital behaviors for a period of time before their first intercourse. In general, however, increases in age and the commitment of the dating relationship are accompanied by an increasing desire for sexual involvement for adolescents, regardless of gender and ethnicity (Darling et al., 1992; Zelnik & Shah, 1983).

In sum, a substantial body of literature exists that describes the onset and sequence of heterosexual dating behaviors among adolescents. Relatively fewer studies focus on the sequencing of dating behaviors in relation to environmental context and psychosocial developmental factors (e.g., gender roles). Future work is needed to better understand the role of adolescent development and societal context on the sequencing of dating behaviors (Foshee & Bauman, 1992; Leigh et al., 1988).

Age at first sexual intercourse.   Data that are available from large national surveys with respect to age of first intercourse show that people in the United States are initiating sexual activity in their adolescent years (Kahn, Kalsbeek, & Hofferth, 1988; B. C. Leigh, Morrison, Trocki, & Temple, 1994; Mott, Fondell, Hu, Kowaleski-Jones, & Menaghan, 1996; Zelnik & Shah, 1983). The total percentage of young women aged 15 to 19 who reported experience with sexual intercourse grew from 47% in 1982 to 53% in 1988 (Hofferth, Kahn, & Baldwin, 1987). Additional data from a survey by the Alan Guttmacher Institute (1994) showed that 42% of teenagers have had sexual intercourse by the age of 16, and 71% by the age of 18. Nationally the average age of first intercourse for young women is 16.2 years, compared to an average age for young men of 15.7 years (Zelnik & Shah, 1983).

The age of first sexual intercourse is related to race, with Black adolescents more likely to report younger ages of first intercourse than White or Hispanic adolescents (Furstenberg, Morgan, Moore, & Peterson, 1987; Mott & Haurin, 1988; Zelnik & Shah, 1983). In the National Survey of Adolescent Males, 20% of Black males said their first intercourse was prior to age 13, compared to only 3% of White and 4% of Hispanic males (Sonenstein, Pleck, & Ku, 1989). These data were consistent with reports of sexual behaviors of persons accessing sexually transmitted disease clinics where a significant number of Black males report age of first intercourse at age 13 or earlier (Zenilman, Weisman, Rompalo, & Ellish, 1995). More current data show the racial gap closing. Comparison of 1988 data from the National Survey of Family Growth with 1982 data indicated that the percentage of women aged 15–19 who have ever had sexual intercourse has increased, and was primarily attributable to increases among White and among nonpoor teenagers (Cooksey, Rindfuss, & Guilkey, 1996; Forrest & Singh, 1990).

Other factors are related to age of first intercourse. Research that addressed age of first intercourse in relation to attitudes and expectations about sexual activity found that earlier age of sexual intercourse was related to more permissive attitudes about sexual activity, depressive symptoms in girls, and lower grade point average (Billy, Landale, Grady, & Zimmerle, 1988). Capaldi, Crosby, and Stoolmiller (1996) longitudinally followed a group of adolescent boys from grades 6 to 12, and found that early initiation of intercourse was related to parental transitions (changes in the parental figures at home). Another longitudinal study of children from birth through adolescence found that the more educated the mother, the later the initiation of intercourse (Udry,

Kovenock, Morris, & van den Berg, 1995). Other important factors that predict early onset of intercourse include adolescent alcohol and other drug use (Capaldi et al., 1996; Dorius, Heaton, & Steffen, 1993; Graves & Leigh, 1995), antisocial behaviors (Tubman, Windle, & Windle, 1996), and early physical maturation (Capaldi et al., 1996; Udry & Billy, 1987). Finally controversial lines of research provide sociobiological explanations for early maturation and onset of sexual intercourse (Belsky, Steinberg, & Draper, 1991). Research findings suggest that family conflict, father absence, and family stress predict sexual maturation and mating behaviors (Dorius et al., 1993; Moffitt, Caspi, Belsky, & Silva, 1992).

There is an alarming trend of initiation of sexual intercourse before the teenage years. A 1992 survey of 2,248 students in grades 6, 8, and 10 from an urban public school district found that 28% of sixth-graders and one half of eighth-graders reported ever having had sexual intercourse (Barone et al., 1996). This is troubling given the unique health risks that pregnancy and sexually transmitted disease pose for female children whose bodies are not fully developed (e.g., immature cervical columnar epithelial cells).

The role of nonconsensual sex on age of first intercourse is unclear in published research. Kinsey and colleagues did not consider the circumstances of the sexual behavior in the original research that reported age of first intercourse (Kinsey et al., 1953). A few published reports do carefully consider age of first voluntary intercourse (Wyatt, Peters, & Guthrie, 1988a, 1988b). These researchers found that mean age of first intercourse dropped when abusive experiences were included in the sample (Moore, Morrison, & Glei, 1995; Wyatt, 1989).

Number of sexual partners.   Rates of sexual intercourse among American adolescents have increased dramatically in the United States (Center for Disease Control [CDC], 1992; Kost & Forrest, 1992, Hofferth et al., 1987). From 1971 to 1988, the proportion of sexually active adolescents and young women aged 15 to 19 years with more than one lifetime sex partner increased nearly 60% (Kost & Forrest, 1992). In the United States, nearly 70% of students in the 12th grade have had sexual intercourse, and 27% of 12th-grade students have had four or more sex partners (CDC, 1995). Furthermore, in another national study, 19% of all teens have had four or more sexual partners, and the number of years an adolescent has been sexually active accounts for the largest percentage of explained variance in the number of sexual partners (Zelnik & Shah, 1983).

In 1988 American adolescents who had sexual intercourse earlier in life reported greater numbers of sex partners (Forrest & Singh, 1990). Among 15- to 19-year-olds who initiated sexual intercourse, 58% reported having had two or more partners; 34% of women aged 18 to 19 and half of all males in this group reported multiple partners in a 1-year period (Forrest & Singh, 1990). Black adolescents report more lifetime partners than White or Hispanic adolescents (Billy, Tanfer, Grady, & Klepinger, 1993; Koniak-Griffin & Brecht, 1995). According to the National AIDS Behavioral Surveys, 15.6% of Hispanics and 22.6% of Blacks have had two or more partners by the time they reach their 20s (Peterson, Catania, Dolcini, & Faigeles, 1993; Sabogal, Faigeles, & Catania, 1993). The high rate of multiple sexual partners in Black youth, particularly males, may be because they report an earlier age of first intercourse.

Gender and the Development of Sexual Behaviors

Researchers and theorists often speculate that adolescent males and females differ widely in their attitudes about sexuality and in their actual behaviors. To address this question comprehensively, Oliver and Hyde (1993) conducted a meta-analysis of gender differences in 177 studies using 21 different measures of sexual attitudes and behaviors. In 44% of the studies the average age of the sample was less than 20 years.

Measures of sexual attitudes included in the meta-analysis related to premarital intercourse, homosexuality, extramarital sex, sexual permissiveness, anxiety about sex, sexual satisfaction, double-standard issues, and masturbation. In general males reported more permissive attitudes on all measures than did females. The greatest gender difference was in the area of attitudes about premarital intercourse, particularly casual intercourse.

Aspects of sexual behavior included in the meta-analysis were incidence of kissing, petting, heterosexual intercourse, masturbation, homosexual behavior, and oral–genital sexual behavior as well as age of first intercourse, number of sexual partners, and frequency of intercourse. Once again, a gender difference emerged with males reporting more frequent behaviors than females. Among all of the variables examined, the largest gender difference occurred in masturbation where males reported much higher rates than females.

Even though these gender differences continue to exist, the researchers noted that the magnitude of differences has narrowed over time probably reflecting true changes in sexual attitudes and behaviors during the past 30 years. Thus, the extent of gender differences in the present adolescent cohort may be minimal. Although research on sexual behavior needs to take gender differences into account, these differences may be much less important than previously thought.

ASSISTING ADOLESCENTS IN THEIR DECISION TO ENGAGE IN SEXUAL BEHAVIORS

Sex and sexuality pervade many aspects of American culture. Although sexuality is recognized as a normal aspect of human development, sexual behavior and the decision to engage in it are often considered private and confidential topics in the United States. This reluctance to discuss matters related to sexual behavior leads to difficulty in openly discussing aspects of sexuality and hinders efforts by some groups to promote open dissemination of information regarding sexuality and its health consequences (Institute of Medicine, 1997).

According to the Committee on Prevention and Control of Sexually Transmitted Diseases, there is a "paradoxical depiction" of sexuality in the United States (Institute of Medicine, 1997, p. 88). According to the committee report, there is consistent saturation and sensationalism of sexual images and messages in the mass media. Yet sexuality remains complex and private with sociocultural taboos and rules of behavior that make talking openly and comfortably about sexuality difficult (Institute of Medicine, 1997; Lear, 1995). The secrecy surrounding sexuality and behaviors linked with sexually transmitted disease (STD) and pregnancy adversely affects STD- and pregnancy-prevention programs. Cultural reluctance to openly discuss sexuality hinders communication between parents and their children about aspects of sexuality (American Social Health Association, 1996), compromises education and counseling activities of health care professionals in a variety of settings (Juhasz, Kaufman, & Meyer, 1986), and results in unbalanced sexual messages in mass media (Strouse, Ruerkel-Rothfuss, & Long, 1995). Because adolescents often spend more time watching television than they do in school (Dietz & Strasburger, 1991), experts agree that the media should be used in positive ways to promote effective and healthy communication among adolescents and children (J. D. Brown, Dykers, Steele, & White, 1994).

Ironically, it may require greater intimacy to discuss sex than to engage in it. The kind of communication that is necessary to explore a partner's sexual history, establish STD risk status, and plan for protection against STDs is made difficult because young persons may not have adequate assertiveness and skills to effectively discuss sex and sexuality (Lear, 1995).

Adolescents are particularly at risk because they are initiating sexual behaviors at a point when developmentally many are finding open communication about dating and other sexual topics difficult. An interesting line of research conducted by Carol Gilligan and her colleagues has suggested that adolescents may differ in their approach to decision making, including those behaviors related to sexuality. According to Gilligan, young females may "lose their voice," thereby finding it more difficult to talk about potentially embarrassing and sensitive topics, while preserving their place and image among their peer group (L. M. Brown & Gilligan, 1992). This inability to discuss concerns related to sexuality can lead to the inability to express one's wishes to delay initiation of sexual activity and relate accurate sexual histories as well as the ability to engage in frank, open discussion about strategies to prevent the negative consequences of unprotected sexual activity (Rosenthal, Burklow, Biro, Pace, & deVellis, 1996; Taylor, Gilligan, & Sullivan, 1995).

Adult role models, parents, and representatives of schools and religious groups often disagree vigorously about the time and place for discussion of sexual behavior. This results in little discussion of sexual behavior during adolescence, promoting secrecy and silence and leaving young people to seek out other sources of information to make sexual decisions that may or may not be accurate and protective (L. Smith & Lanthrop, 1993). Accurate sexual information, given by a variety of sources including schools (Barth, Fetro, Leland, & Volkan, 1992), parents (Handelsman, Cabral, & Weisfeld, 1987; Moore, Peterson, & Furstenberg, 1986; Shoop & Davidson, 1994; Tucker, 1991), and family planning services (Grady, Klepinger, & Billy, 1993) has resulted in safer, more responsible choices on the part of young persons, increased condom use in the event of sexual activity (Mauldon & Luker, 1996), and the acquisition of information that is more accurate.

SEXUAL RISK-TAKING BEHAVIORS IN ADOLESCENCE

Concern about sexual behavior among teenagers is not new. The onset of HIV/AIDS, the rise of other sexually transmitted diseases, and the increase of teen-aged pregnancy have brought new urgency to the study of sexual risk-taking among adolescents, however. There has been an explosion of theorizing about the developmental, social, familial, and hormonal origins of sexual risk taking. In the next section, studies exploring predictors of sexual risk taking are described. Papers that contain unique and interesting views are discussed at the end of the section. Finally, problems with the research and future directions are explored.

Predictors of Sexual Risk Taking

Arguably the greatest focus of research on sexual risk taking has been atheoretical, descriptive studies on correlates of risky sexual behavior among adolescents. In general studies have been focused on the impact of knowledge, attitudes, social norms and peer-group affiliation; perceived susceptibility to

STDs (especially HIV); hormonal and developmental changes; and alcohol and substance abuse. Each of these bodies of research is extensive and will be summarized briefly using representative studies.

In contrast to what might be expected, knowledge about transmission of STDs does not correlate with safer sex practices. Many researchers have demonstrated that adolescents and young adults with high levels of knowledge about STDs (HIV in particular) continue to practice unsafe sex (e.g., Baldwin & Baldwin, 1988; DiClemente, Forrest, Mickler, & Principal Site Investigators, 1990; Goodman & Cohall, 1989; Ramson, Marion, & Mathias, 1993; Walter et al., 1992). The findings appear to extend to all racial groups and both genders. For example, Flaskerud and Nyamathi (1989) failed to find a relationship between knowledge of AIDS and safer sex practices among young Black and Latina women. DiIorio, Parsons, Lehr, Adame, and Carlone (1993) reported similar results among Black males as well as White males and females.

The body of research on attitudes and safer sex practices is difficult to interpret because the attitude variable is frequently not clearly defined or operationalized. Notable exceptions are found in studies that employed a theoretical framework. Using the theory of reasoned action, Jemmott and Jemmott (1991) found that favorable attitudes toward condom use predicted intentions to use this safer sex strategy among Black women. Combining the theory of reasoned action with social cognitive theory, Basen-Enquist and Parcel (1992) demonstrated that a positive attitude toward condoms was a significant predictor of condom-use intentions and frequency among ninth graders.

There is evidence that people who perceive a norm of safer sex behaviors are more likely to protect themselves. In addition to the roles of positive attitudes in the previously mentioned studies it was found that the normative influences of sexual partners and mothers were predictors of condom use (Basen-Enquist & Parcel, 1992; Jemmott & Jemmott, 1991). Further evidence for the effect of norms was found in a study of high-school students; participants whose friends had intercourse and never or almost never used condoms were three times more likely than their peers to demonstrate risky sexual behavior (Walter et al., 1992). Finally, using data from fifth- and eighth-graders, Porter, Oakley, Ronis, and Neal (1996) constructed a path model demonstrating that personal norms about the appropriate age for sexual intercourse indirectly affected sexual debut through an influence on frequency of intimate behaviors (e.g., kissing, touching private parts).

Perceived susceptibility to STDs may increase safer sex practices. A large geographically diverse sample of college students showed a strong association between perceived risk of HIV infection and use of safer sex behaviors (DiClemente et al., 1990). Similar findings were evident in a sample of adolescents (Goodman & Cohall, 1989). It must be noted, however, that some researchers have not found a relationship between perceived susceptibility to HIV and safer sex (Bruce, Shrum, Trefethen, & Slovik, 1990). Furthermore, a review of studies of the relation between perceived vulnerability to HIV and precautionary sexual behavior revealed a number of methodological problems and virtually no relationship between perceived susceptibility to HIV and safer sex behavior (Gerrard, Gibbons, & Bushman, 1996).

Developmental and hormonal changes that accompany adolescence are frequently cited as reasons for sexual risk taking. Adolescents experience tremendous physiological changes; there is some evidence of an association between puberty and onset of sexual activity among males (Halpern, Udry, Campbell, Suchindran, & Mason, 1994; Udry & Billy, 1987). The physiological urge for sexual activity is accompanied by a sense of invulnerability to harm that causes adolescents to believe that STDs, pregnancy, and other negative outcomes will not happen to them. In addition, a drive for increased intimacy and meaningfulness in relationships may make sexual intercourse seem desirable (Grant & Demetriou, 1988).

One variable that has been linked consistently to the practice of risky sex among adolescents is substance use (Fortenberry, 1995). In several surveys of adolescents, a relationship between using drugs or alcohol and engaging in unsafe sex has been established (Feldman, Rosenthal, Brown, & Canning, 1995; Ku, Sonenstein, & Pleck, 1992; Lowry et al., 1994; Mensch & Kandel, 1992). This relationship crosses racial and gender barriers. There is some evidence, however, that White adolescents are at greater risk of unsafe sex while under the influence than are Black adolescents (Cooper, Peirce, & Huselid, 1994).

In sum, despite an enormous amount of effort, very few consistent predictors of sexual risk taking have been identified. There is some evidence of gender differences in attitudes and behavior, but the magnitude of these differences is unclear. Probably attitudes and social norms influence sexual risk taking, but the roles of knowledge and perceived susceptibility to STDs are not substantial. One variable that is clearly correlated with risky behavior is substance use. In many studies, alcohol and drug use were associated with risk taking. Furthermore, when asked about the reasons for having intercourse without using a condom, adolescents identify alcohol use as a reason for this behavior (Jadack et al., 1995).

New Approaches to Understanding Sexual Risk Taking

In this section, studies that represent fruitful avenues for future exploration are described. Most of this research needs further development; it is mentioned here because of its promise and creativity.

An intriguing body of research concerns theorizing and research on factors that are considered to be "protective" during adolescence (Jessor, 1991). Protective factors are conceptualized as decreasing the likelihood of engaging in problem behaviors even when a number of risk factors are present. Three general types of psychosocial protective factors have been defined by Jessor and colleagues: (a) personality system factors (e.g., intolerance of deviant behavior such as theft), (b) perceived environment factors (e.g., positive relations with adults), and (c) behavior system factors (e.g., involvement and time spent with family, volunteer activities) (Jessor, VanDenBos, Vanderryn, Costa, & Turbin, 1995). Using a longitudinal design, Jessor's group conducted a 4-year study of the effect of protective factors on frequency of four problem behaviors (including sexual intercourse) in an urban, racially mixed, young adolescent sample. Both cross-sectional and longitudinal data analyses revealed that protective factors moderated the relationship between risk factors and problem behaviors. The model did not hold up when the sexual intercourse variable was examined alone, however, possibly because it was a dichotomous variable with values of yes (have had sex) or no (never had sex). Despite this finding, the idea of protective factors as important influences on sexual behavior deserves more study as it may explain the behavior of teens who have a number of risk factors but do not engage in risky behaviors.

A second interesting line of research is represented by the work of Sanderson and Cantor (1995) that focuses on the role of predominant developmental goals in sexual behavior. Specifically it is hypothesized that sexual and dating behavior revolve around predominant identity-focused goals or predominant intimacy-focused goals. Adolescents who have predominant identity goals will value independence, self-reliance, and opportunities to try out many different roles or identities. In their dating relationships, they will avoid closeness, may experiment with multiple partners, and will seek pleasure rather than intimacy in sexual experiences. On the other hand, adolescents whose major goal is developing intimacy will seek emotional closeness and mutual dependence in their relationships. Their dating relationships will be marked by intense communications, monogamy, and a view of sexual activities as expressions of emotional intimacy.

In a series of studies conducted with adolescents, Sanderson and Cantor (1995) found the theorized pattern of relationships. Adolescents with predominant identity goals reported more casual dating and sexual partners, whereas those with predominant intimacy goals reported long, emotionally intimate dating relationships.

One implication of this type of theorizing is that interventions to reduce risk should be structured around an individual's goals. Persons who are driven by the need to form an identity may benefit from skill-driven interventions that teach them how to protect themselves. Persons driven by intimacy needs may benefit from interventions that emphasize effective communication, mutual planning, and negotiation with a partner.

Sanderson and Cantor (1995) tested this idea by conducting an experiment to examine the impact of matching subjects' goals with their intervention strategy. Dependent variables included attitudes about condom use, intentions to use condoms, sexual behavior, and perceived susceptibility to HIV. In general subjects who received goal-matched interventions reported greater intentions to use safer sex behaviors than subjects who received nonmatching interventions. More important, at 1-year follow-up, this effect was sustained in reports of actual sexual behavior.

Finally, research focusing on uncovering the thinking of adolescents may offer useful insights (Mathews, Everett, Binedell, & Steinberg, 1995). Using a qualitative approach, a team of researchers examined adolescent thinking about reasons for various sexual choices (Keller, Duerst, & Zimmerman, 1996) and consequences of these choices (Duerst, Keller, Mockrud, & Zimmerman, 1997). In general results of these studies indicated that adolescents identified four interconnected factors as reasons for their sexual decisions: social norms, fear or worry, gratification or pleasure, and availability of condoms. When their perceptions of consequences were explored, some interesting ideas were made explicit. First, adolescents saw the decision to remain abstinent as a threat to the relationship and indicated that it might result in lower self-esteem and insecurity for both partners. On the other hand, use of a condom was viewed as an indication of caring and the result was improvement in the relationship. Interestingly, the identified consequences of unprotected intercourse were almost entirely negative despite the teens' acknowledgment that to engage in unprotected intercourse was the most frequent sexual decision. Themes that emerged from these data can be used to design and test interventions that challenge unhealthy thinking among adolescents and reinforce positive aspects of their decision making.

FINAL COMMENTS ABOUT THE RISK-TAKING LITERATURE

As previously mentioned, the most glaring problem in the literature on sexual risk taking is the lack of theoretical frameworks guiding the research. The result is a rather haphazard look at predictors of behavior with no comprehensive set of variables to guide interventions. Admittedly, sexual behavior is complex, and it is difficult to assess the impact of a large number of variables unless the sample size is very large. It is probably not fruitful to continue the present approach of examining two to three variables in a sample.

As is the case with adults, researchers are also faced with major measurement difficulties. There is no assurance that the behaviors people report are what they actually do, and there is no acceptable method of validating their behaviors. Furthermore, even if adolescents do engage in safer sex behaviors, do they perform them effectively? Langer, Zimmerman, and Cabral (1994) showed a very low correlation between perceived skill with condom use and demonstration of proper technique on a model. Interestingly, men did not have significantly higher skills than women. Problems with accurate measurement and accurate reporting in sensitive areas such as sexuality are major impediments to development of knowledge.

There is a need to question our entire approach to the study of sexual risk taking among adolescents. Ehrhardt (1996) has written of the dangers of focusing on risk behavior without considering the developmental context of adolescence. The implication of much of our research is that sexual behavior during adolescence is "risky" behavior that is unacceptable. Ehrhardt points out that many developed countries of the world view adolescent sexual activity as normal and acceptable. Intervention strategies are directed at preventing unintended negative consequences such as pregnancy but these interventions are framed within a context of acceptance of sexual expression in adolescence. Most of these countries have adolescent pregnancy rates much lower than the United States and are not faced with the enormous economic and social costs of teenaged mother- and fatherhood.

On the other hand, early sexual activity may have serious physiological consequences for girls in particular because the transformation zone of the cervix is quite vulnerable to sexually transmitted diseases in teenaged females. From a physical health perspective, delay of onset of intercourse until females are ready for physical intimacy is desirable. There is evidence that young teen girls do not wish to be sexually active to the point of intercourse but are pressured by older male partners. Theoretically derived educational strategies, such as social inoculation, designed to help them resist pressure may be quite effective if implemented during middle-school years.

Issues surrounding adolescent sexuality and sexual risk taking are obviously complex and controversial. There is ample evidence that adolescents are sexually active and engage frequently in risky sexual behavior. At every turn, they are bombarded by the media with sexually laden messages. In this environment, interventions that assist them to clarify and act on their values regarding sexual behavior are sorely needed.

REFERENCES

Alan Guttmacher Institute. (1994). *Sex and America's teenagers.* New York: Author.

American Social Health Association. (1996). Teenagers know more than adults about STDs, but knowledge among both groups is low. *STD News, 3,* 1–5.

Arafat, I. S., & Cotton, W. L. (1974). Masturbation practices of males and females. *Journal of Sex Research, 10,* 293–307.

Baldwin, J. D., & Baldwin, J. I. (1988). Factors affecting AIDS-related sexual risk-taking behavior among college students. *Journal of Sex Research, 25,* 181–196.

Barone, C., Ickovics, J. R., Ayers, T. S., Katz, S. M., Voyce, C. K., & Weissberg, R. P. (1996). High-risk sexual behavior among young urban students. *Family Planning Perspectives, 28,* 69–74.

Barth, R. P., Fetro, J. V., Leland, N., & Volkan, K. (1992). Preventing adolescent pregnancy with social and cognitive skills. *Journal of Adolescent Research, 7,* 208–232.

Basen-Enquist, K., & Parcel, G. (1992). Attitudes, norms, and self-efficacy: A model of adolescents' HIV-related sexual risk behavior. *Health Education Quarterly, 19,* 263–277.

Bell, A. P., Weinberg, M. S., & Hammersmith, S. K. (1981). *Sexual preference: Its development in men and women.* Bloomington, IN: Indiana University Press.

Belsky, J., Steinberg, L., & Draper, P. (1991). Childhood experience, interpersonal development, and reproductive strategy: An evolutionary theory of socialization. *Child Development, 62,* 647–670.

Billy, J. O., Landale, N. S., Grady, W. R., & Zimmerle, D. M. (1988). Effects of sexual activity on adolescent social and psychological development. *Social Psychology Quarterly, 51,* 190–212.

Billy, J. O. G., Tanfer, K., Grady, W. R., & Klepinger, D. H. (1993). The sexual behavior of men in the United States. *Family Planning Perspectives, 24,* 52–60.

Bolton, F. G., & MacEachron, A. E. (1988). Adolescent male sexuality: A developmental perspective. Special issue: Adolescent sexual behavior. *Journal of Adolescent Research, 3,* 259–273.

Brown, J. D., Dykers, C. R., Steele, J. R., & White, A. B. (1994). Teenage room culture: Where media and identities intersect. Special issue: Methods of observing popular culture. *Communication Research, 21,* 813–827.

Brown, L. M., & Gilligan, C. (1992). *Meeting at the crossroads: Women's psychology and girls' development.* Cambridge, MA: Harvard University Press.

Bruce, K. E., Shrum, J, C., Trefethen, C., & Slovik, L. F. (1990). Students' attitudes about AIDS, homosexuality, and condoms. *AIDS Education and Prevention, 2,* 220–234.

Capaldi, D. M., Crosby, L., & Stoolmiller, M. (1996). Predicting the timing of first sexual intercourse for at-risk adolescent males. *Child Development, 67,* 344–359.

Centers for Disease Control. (1992). Sexual behavior among high school students—United States, 1990. *Morbidity and Mortality Weekly Reports, 40,* 51–52.

Centers for Disease Control. (1995). Trends in sexual risk behavior among high school students—United States, 1990, 1991, and 1993. *Morbidity and Mortality Weekly Reports, 44,* 124–125, 131–132.

Cooksey, E. C., Rindfuss, R. R., & Guilkey, D. K. (1996). The initiation of adolescent sexual and contraceptive behavior during changing times. *Journal of Health & Social Behavior, 37,* 59–74.

Cooper, M., Peirce, R., & Huselid, R. (1994). Substance use and sexual risk taking among Black adolescents and White adolescents. *Health Psychology, 13,* 251–262.

Darling, C. A., Davidson, J. K., & Passarello, L. C. (1992). The mystique of first intercourse among college youth: The role of partners, contraceptive practices, and psychological reactions. *Journal of Youth & Adolescence, 21,* 97–117.

Davidson, J. K., & Moore, N. B. (1994). Masturbation and premarital sexual intercourse among college women: Making choices for sexual fulfillment. *Journal of Sex and Marital Therapy, 20,* 178–199.

DeCecco, J. P., & Parker, D. A. (1995). The biology of homosexuality: Sexual orientation or sexual preference? Special issue: Sex, cells, and same sex desire: The biology of sexual preference: I. *Journal of Homosexuality, 28,* 1–27.

De Gaston, J. R., Weed, S., & Jensen, L. (1996). Understanding gender differences in adolescent sexuality. *Adolescence, 31,* 217–231.

DeLamater, J., & MacCorquodale, P. (1979). *Premarital sexuality: Attitudes, relationships, behavior.* Madison, WI: University of Wisconsin Press.

DiClemente, F. J., Forrest, K. A., Mickler, S., & Principal Site Investigators. (1990). College students' knowledge and attitudes about AIDS and changes in HIV-preventive behaviors. *AIDS Education and Prevention, 2,* 201–212.

Dietz, W. H., & Strasburger, V. C. (1991). Children, adolescents and television. *Current Problems in Pediatrics, 21,* 8–32.

DiIorio, C., Parsons, M., Lehr, S., Adame, D., & Carlone, J. (1993). Factors associated with use of safer sex practices among college freshmen. *Research in Nursing and Health, 16,* 343–350.

Dorius, G. L., Heaton, T. B., & Steffen, P. (1993). Adolescent life events and their association with the onset of sexual intercourse. *Youth & Society, 25,* 3–23.

Duerst, B., Keller, M., Mockrud, P., & Zimmerman, J. (1997). *Consequences of sexual risk-taking: The perceptions of rural adolescents.* Manuscript submitted for publication.

Ehrhardt, A. (1996). Editorial: Our view of adolescent sexuality—A focus on risk behavior without the developmental context. *American Journal of Public Health, 86,* 1523–1525.

Ellis, L., & Ames, M. A. (1987). Neurohormonal functioning and sexual orientation: A theory of homosexuality-heterosexuality. *Psychological Bulletin, 101,* 233–258.

Feldman, S. S., Rosenthal, D. R., Brown, N. C., & Canning, R. D. (1995). Predicting sexual experience in adolescent boys from peer rejection and acceptance during childhood. *Journal of Research on Adolescence, 5,* 387–411.

Flaskerud, J., & Nyamathi, A. (1989). Black and Latina women's AIDS related knowledge, attitudes and practices. *Research in Nursing and Health, 12,* 339–346.

Fortenberry, J. D. (1995). Adolescent substance use and sexually transmitted diseases risk: A review. *Journal of Adolescent Health, 16,* 304–308.

Forrest, J. D., & Singh, S. (1990). The sexual and reproductive behavior of American women, 1982–1988. *Family Planning Perspectives, 22,* 206–214.

Foshee, V. A., & Bauman, K. E. (1992). Gender stereotyping and adolescent sexual behavior: A test of temporal order. *Journal of Applied Social Psychology, 22,* 1561–1579.

Furstenberg, F. F., Morgan, S. P., Moore, K. A., & Peterson, J. L. (1987). Race differences in the timing of adolescent intercourse. *American Sociological Review, 52,* 511–518.

Gargiulo, J., Attic, I., Brooks-Gunn, J., & Warren, M. P. (1987). Girls' dating behavior as a function of social context and maturation. *Developmental Psychology, 23,* 730–737.

Gerrard, M., Gibbons, F. X., & Bushman, B. (1996). Relation between perceived vulnerability to HIV and precautionary sexual behavior. *Psychological Bulletin, 119,* 390–409.

Goodman, E., & Cohall, A. T. (1989). Acquired immunodeficiency syndrome and adolescents: Knowledge, attitudes, beliefs, and behaviors in a New York city adolescent minority population. *Pediatrics, 84*(1), 36–42.

Grady, W. R., Klepinger, D. H., & Billy, J. O. (1993). The influence of community characteristics on the practice of effective contraception. *Family Planning Perspectives, 25,* 4–11.

Grant, J., & Demetriou, E. (1988). Adolescent sexuality. *Pediatric Clinics of North America, 35,* 1271–1289.

Graves, K. L., & Leigh, B. C. (1995). The relationship of substance use to sexual activity among young adults in the United States. *Family Planning Perspectives, 27,* 18–22.

Halpern, C. T., Udry, J. R., Campbell, B., & Suchindran, C. (1993). Testosterone and pubertal development as predictors of sexual activity: A panel analysis of adolescent males. *Psychosomatic Medicine, 55,* 436–447.

Halpern, C. T., Udry, J. R., Campbell, B., Suchindran, C., & Mason, G. (1994). Testosterone and religiosity as predictors of sexual attitudes and activity among adolescent males: A biosocial model. *Journal of Biosocial Science, 26,* 217–234.

Handelsman, C. D., Cabral, R. J., & Weisfeld, G. E. (1987). Sources of information and adolescent sexual knowledge and behavior. *Journal of Adolescent Research, 2,* 455–463.

Hannonen, S., & Kekki, P. (1995). Adolescent readers' responses to the booklet on sex. *Journal of Adolescent Health, 16,* 328–333.

Hauman, G. (1995). Homosexuality, biology, and ideology. [Special Issue: Sex, cells, and same sex desire: The biology of sexual preference I.] *Journal of Homosexuality, 28,* 57–77.

Herdt, G. (1989). Gay and lesbian youth, emergent identities, and cultural scenes at home and abroad. *Journal of Homosexuality, 17,* 1–42.

Hofferth, S. L., Kahn, J. R., & Baldwin, W. (1987). Premarital sexual activity among U.S. teenage women over the past three decades. *Family Planning Perspectives, 19,* 46–53.

Hunt, M. (1974). *Sexual behavior in the 1970s*. Chicago: Playboy Press.

Institute of Medicine. (1997). In T. R. Eng & W. T. Butler (Eds.), *The hidden epidemic: Confronting sexually transmitted diseases*. Washington, DC: National Academy Press.

Jadack, R., Hyde, J., & Keller, M. L. (1995). Gender and knowledge about HIV, risky sexual behavior and safer sex practices. *Research in Nursing and Health, 18,* 313–324.

Jemmott, L. W., & Jemmott, J. B. (1991). Applying the theory of reasoned action to AIDS risk behavior: Condom use among Black women. *Nursing Research, 40,* 228–234.

Jessor, R. (1991). Risk behavior in adolescence: A psychosocial framework for understanding and action. *Journal of Adolescent Health, 12,* 597–605.

Jessor, R., VanDenBos, J., Vanderryn, J., Costa, F., & Turbin, M. (1995). Protective factors in adolescent problem behavior: Moderator effects and developmental change. *Developmental Psychology, 31,* 923–933.

Juhasz, A. M., Kaufman, B., & Meyer, H. (1986). Adolescent attitudes and beliefs about sexual behavior. *Child & Adolescent Social Work Journal, 3,* 177–193.

Kahn, J. R., Kalsbeek, W. D., & Hofferth, S. L. (1988). National estimates of teenage sexual activity: Evaluating the comparability of three national surveys. *Demography, 25,* 189–204.

Keller, M. L., Duerst, B., & Zimmerman, J. (1996). Adolescents' views of sexual decision-making. *IMAGE:The Journal of Nursing Scholarship, 28,* 125–130.

Kinsey, A. C., Pomeroy, W. B., & Martin, C. E. (1948). *Sexual behavior in the human male*. Philadelphia: Saunders.

Kinsey, A. C., Pomeroy, W. B., Martin, C. E., & Gebhard, P. H. (1953). *Sexual behavior in the human female*. Philadelphia: Saunders.

Koniak-Griffin, D., & Brecht, M. L. (1995). Linkages between sexual risk taking, substance use and AIDS knowledge among pregnant adolescents and young mothers. *Nursing Research, 44,* 340–346.

Kost, K., & Forrest, J. D. (1992). American women's sexual behavior and exposure to risk of sexually transmitted diseases. *Family Planning Perspectives, 24,* 244–254.

Ku, L., Sonenstein, F., & Pleck, J. (1992). Patterns of HIV risk and preventive behaviors among teenage men. *Public Health Reports, 107,* 131–138.

Langer, L., Zimmerman, R., & Cabral, R. (1994). Perceived versus actual condom skills among clients at sexually transmitted disease clinics. *Public Health Reports, 109,* 683–687.

Lear, D. (1995). Sexual communication in the age of AIDS: The construction of risk and trust among young adults. *Social Science Medicine, 41,* 1311–1323.

Leigh, B. C., Morrison, D. M., Trocki, K., & Temple, M. T. (1994). Sexual behavior of American adolescents: Results from a U.S. national survey. *Journal of Adolescent Health, 15,* 117–125.

Leigh, G. K., Weddle, K. D., & Loewen, I. R. (1988). Analysis of the timing of transition to sexual intercourse for Black adolescent females. [Special issue: Adolescent sexual behavior.] *Journal of Adolescent Research, 3,* 333–344.

Leitenberg, H., Detzer, M. J., & Srebnik, D. (1993). Gender differences in masturbation experience in preadolescence and/or early adolescence to sexual behavior and sexual adjustment in young adulthood. *Archives of Sexual Behavior, 22,* 87–98.

Leung, A. K., & Robson, W. L. (1993). Childhood masturbation. *Clinical Pediatrics, 32,* 238–241.

Loltes, I. L. (1993). Nontraditional gender roles and the sexual experiences of heterosexual college students. *Sex Roles, 29,* 645–669.

Lowry, R., Holtzman, D., Truman, B., Kann, L., Collins, J., & Kolbe, L. (1994). Substance use and HIV-related sexual behaviors among U.S. high school students: Are they related? *American Journal of Public Health, 84,* 1116–1120.

Mathews, C., Everett, K., Binedell, J., & Steinberg, M. (1995). Learning to listen: Formative research in the development of AIDS education for secondary school students. *Social Science in Medicine, 12,* 1715–1724.

Mauldon, J., & Luker, K. (1996). The effects of contraceptive education on method use at first intercourse. *Family Planning Perspectives, 28,* 19–24.

McCabe, M. P., & Collins, J. K. (1984). Measurement of depth of desired and experienced sexual involvement at different stages of dating. *Journal of Sex Research, 20,* 377–390.

Mensch, B., & Kandel, D. B. (1992). Drug use as a risk factor for premarital teen pregnancy and abortion in a national sample of young white women. *Demography, 29,* 409–429.

Miller, B. C., McCoy, J. K., & Olson, T. D. (1986). Dating age and stage as correlates of adolescent sexual attitudes and behavior. *Journal of Adolescent Research, 1,* 361–371.

Moffitt, T. E., Caspi, A., Belsky, J., & Silva, P. A. (1993). Childhood experience and the onset of menarche: A test of a sociobiological model. *Child Development, 63,* 47–58.

Moore, K. A., Morrison, D. R., & Glei, D. A. (1995). Welfare and adolescent sex: The effects of family history, benefit levels, and community context. *Journal of Family & Economic Issues, 16,* 207–237.

Moore, K. A., Peterson, J. L., & Furstenberg, F. F. (1986). Parental attitudes and the occurrence of early sexual activity. *Journal of Marriage & the Family, 48,* 777–782.

Mott, F. L., Fondell, M. M., Hu, P. N., Kowaleski-Jones, L., & Menaghan, E. G. (1996). The determinants of first sex by age 14 in a high-risk adolescent population. *Family Planning Perspectives, 28,* 13–18.

Mott, F. L., & Haurin, R. J. (1988). Linkages between sexual activity and alcohol and drug use among American adolescents. *Family Planning Perspectives, 20,* 128–136.

Oliver, M. B., & Hyde, J. (1993). Gender differences in sexuality: A meta-analysis. *Psychological Bulletin, 114*(1), 29–51.

Peterson, J. L., Catania, J. A., Dolcini, M. M., & Faigeles, B. (1993). *Family Planning Perspectives, 25,* 263–267.

Phinney, V. G., Jensen, L. C., Olsen, J. A., & Cundick, B. (1990). The relationship between early development and psychosexual behaviors in adolescent females. *Adolescence, 25,* 321–332.

Porter, C., Oakley, D., Ronis, D., & Neal, R. W. (1996). Pathways of influence on fifth and eighth graders reports' about having had sexual intercourse. *Research in Nursing and Health, 19,* 193–204.

Reinisch, J. M., & Beasley, R. (1991). *The Kinsey Institute new report on sex.* New York: St. Martin's Press.

Ramson, D. L., Marion, S. A., & Mathias, R. G. (1993). Changes in university students' AIDS-related knowledge, attitudes and behaviors, 1988 and 1992. *Canadian Journal of Public Health, 84,* 275–278.

Roper, W. G. (1996). The etiology of male homosexuality. *Medical Hypotheses, 46,* 85–88.

Rosenthal, S. L., Burklow, K. A., Biro, F. M., Pace, L. C., & deVellis, R. F. (1996). The reliability of high-risk adolescent girls' report of their sexual history. *Journal of Pediatric Health Care, 10,* 217–220.

Sabogal, F., Faigeles, B., & Catania, J. A. (1993). Multiple sexual partners among Hispanics in high-risk cities. *Family Planning Perspectives, 25,* 257–262.

Sanders, S. A., Ziemba-Davis, M., Hill, C. A., & Reinisch, J. M. (1991). Intent and purpose of the Kinsey Institute/Roper Organization national sex knowledge survey: A rejoinder. *Public Opinion Quarterly, 55,* 458–462.

Sanderson, C., & Cantor, N. (1995). Social dating goals in late adolescence: Implications for safer sexual activity. *Journal of Personality and Social Psychology, 68,* 1121–1134.

Schor, N. (1993). Abortion and adolescence: Relation between the menarche and sexual activity. *International Journal of Adolescent Medicine and Health, 6,* 225–240.

Shoop, D. M., & Davidson, P. M. (1994). AIDS and adolescents: The relation of parent and partner communication to adolescent condom use. *Journal of Adolescence, 17,* 137–148.

Slonim-Nevo, V. (1992). First premarital intercourse among Mexican-American and Anglo-American adolescent women: Interpreting ethnic differences. *Journal of Adolescent Research, 7,* 332–351.

Smith, T. W. (1991). A critique of the Kinsey Institute/Roper Organization national sex knowledge survey. *Public Opinion Quarterly, 55,* 449–457.

Smith, L., & Lanthrop, L. (1993). AIDS and human sexuality. *Canadian Journal of Public Health, 84*(suppl.), S14–S18.

Smith, E., & Udry, J. R. (1985). Coital and non-coital sexual behaviors of White and Black adolescents. *American Journal of Public Health, 75,* 1200–1203.

Sonenstein, F., Pleck, J. H., & Ku, L. C. (1989). Sexual activity, condom use, and AIDS awareness among adolescent males. *Family Planning Perspectives, 21,* 152–158.

Strouse, J. S., Buerkel-Rothfuss, N., & Long, E. C. (1995). Gender and family as moderators of the relationship between music video exposure and adolescent sexual permissiveness. *Adolescence, 30,* 505–521.

Taylor, J. M., Gilligan, C., & Sullivan, A. M. (1995). *Between voice and silence: Women and girls, race and relationship.* Cambridge, MA: Harvard University Press.

Telljohann, S. K., & Price, J. H. (1993). A qualitative examination of adolescent homosexuals' life experiences: Ramifications for secondary school personnel. *Journal of Homosexuality, 26,* 41–56.

Thornton, A. (1990). The courtship process and adolescent sexuality. [Special issue: Adolescent sexuality, contraception, and childbearing.] *Journal of Family Issues, 11,* 239–273.

Tubman, J. G., Windle, M., & Windle, R. C. (1996). Cumulative sexual intercourse patterns among middle adolescents: Problem behavior precursors and concurrent health risk behaviors. *Journal of Adolescent Health, 18,* 182–191.

Tucker, S. K. (1991). The sexual and contraceptive socialization of Black adolescent males. *Public Health Nursing, 8,* 105–112.

Udry, J. R., & Billy, J. (1987). Initiation of coitus in early adolescence. *American Sociological Review, 52,* 841–855.

Udry, J. R., Kovenock, J., Morris, N. M., & van den Berg, B. (1995). Childhood precursors of age at first intercourse for females. *Archives of Sexual Behavior, 24,* 329–337.

Walter, H., Vaughan, R., Gladis, M. M., Ragin, D., Kasen, S., & Cohall, A. T. (1992). Factors associated with AIDS risk behaviors among high school students in an AIDS epicenter. *American Journal of Public Health, 82,* 528–532.

Wyatt, G. E. (1989). Reexamining factors predicting Afro-American and White American women's age at first coitus. *Archives of Sexual Behavior, 18,* 271–298.

Wyatt, G. E., Peters, S. D., & Guthrie, D. (1988a). Kinsey revisited, part I: Comparisons of the sexual socialization and sexual behavior of White women over 33 years. *Archives of Sexual Behavior, 17,* 201–239.

Wyatt, G. E., Peters, S. D., & Guthrie, D. (1988b). Kinsey revisited, part II: Comparisons of the sexual socialization and sexual behavior of Black women over 33 years. *Archives of Sexual Behavior, 17,* 289–332.

Zelnik, M., & Shah, F. K. (1983). First intercourse among young Americans. *Family Planning Perspectives, 15,* 64–70.

Zenilman, J. M., Weisman, C. S., Rompalo, A. M., & Ellish, N. (1995). Condom use to prevent incident STDs: The validity of self-reported condom use. *Sexually Transmitted Diseases, 22,* 15–21.

Chapter 6

Motivation for Physical Activity Among Children and Adolescents

Nola J. Pender
School of Nursing
University of Michigan

ABSTRACT

Assisting children and adolescents in adopting physically active lifestyles is an integral part of the health education and health promotion services provided by nurses in school, family, community, and primary care settings. In order to effectively engage in physical activity counseling, the determinants of physical activity must be understood and integrated into effective interventions for youths. This review of research literature includes a critique of intervention studies aimed at helping children and adolescents adopt active lifestyles that will be sustained throughout life. Social cognitive theory provided the theoretical basis for most of the studies reviewed but specification of how theory concepts were operationalized in the interventions was often unclear. Suggestions for increasing the rigor of theoretically based intervention studies aimed at promoting physical activity are proposed. Models and variables are identified that need further testing to determine their relevance to the promotion of physical activity during childhood and adolescence.

Keywords: Physical Activity, Exercise, Children, Adolescents, Physical Activity Interventions

Childhood and adolescence are critical developmental periods for assisting youths to adopt positive health practices that can become integral aspects of ongoing behavioral patterns and emerging self-identity. Much information already exists about which behaviors promote health and which behaviors compromise health. There is widespread agreement, as noted in the recent report, *Physical Activity and Health: A Report of the Surgeon General* (U.S. Department of Health and Human Services [USDHHS], 1996), that regular moderate or vigorous physical activity contributes to the physical and psychological well-being of children and adolescents through increasing cardiorespiratory fitness and muscle strength, preventing overweight, enhancing self-esteem and self-concept, and lowering anxiety and stress. Further, physical activity has been shown to lessen the risk of chronic disease later in life, including coronary heart disease, by maintaining a favorable lipid profile and decreasing blood pressure (USDHHS, 1996). Unfortunately, physical activity declines at an alarming rate during the late childhood and adolescent years. What is not known and merits the rigorous attention of health scientists is how biobehavioral, developmental, and sociocultural dynamics interact to bring about this decrement and how nurses and other health care professionals can intervene to prevent it.

This chapter reviews what is known about the influences on physical activity of children and adolescents and intervention studies to increase physical activity among youths are critiqued. An analysis of child and adolescent physical activity and exercise research conducted from 1986 to 1997 and indexed in Cumulative Index to Nursing and Allied Health Literature (CI-NAHL), MEDLINE, PsycLit, Educational Resource Information Center (ERIC), and Wilson Indexes was the basis for this review. Studies focused solely on changing the structure of physical education classes to increase physical activity were not included in this review as they are of limited relevance to the education and counseling that nurses provide to children in relation to physical activity.

THE CHALLENGE OF MOTIVATING YOUTHS TO LEAD ACTIVE LIFESTYLES

Evidence is accumulating that youths engaging in regular physical activity reap numerous health benefits (Berlin & Colditz, 1990; Gruber, 1986). Thus, a national goal identified in *Healthy People 2000: National Health Promotion and Disease Prevention Objectives* (USDHHS, 1990) is to increase to at least 75% the proportion of children and adolescents aged 6–17 years who engage in vigorous physical activity that promotes cardiorespiratory fitness 3 days or more per week for 20 minutes or more per occasion. Physical activity is defined as bodily movements produced by skeletal muscle contraction that increase energy expenditure above the basal level. Exercise is more narrowly defined as physical activity that is planned, structured, repetitive, and directed toward improving or maintaining physical fitness (USDHHS, 1996). The 1992 National Health Information Survey–Youth Risk Behavior Survey indicated that 81% and 61% of ninth-grade males and females, respectively, reported a level of activity that would promote fitness, whereas only 67% and 41% of 12th grade males and females, respectively, were at this activity level. Vigorous physical activity was lower in Black and Hispanic than in White adolescents (USDHHS, 1996). Creative interventions by health professionals tailored to the needs and interests of youth from diverse populations are essential to encourage a level of activity conducive to health and well-being

Interventions to promote regular physical activity should be an integral part of health education and health promotion services provided by nurses to children and adolescents for the following reasons: (a) nurses are the health professionals providing care and health guidance most frequently to children and adolescents in schools, primary care clinics, and other community settings; (b) risk factors for chronic disease, including cardiovascular disease, often are detected in early childhood by nurses and may be ameliorated by proactive nursing interventions; (c) chronically ill children who may be particularly prone to inactivity are often under the care of a nurse as primary care provider; (d) nurses have the expertise to assist children and their families in tailoring physical activity to the realities and contexts of their daily lives; and (e) nurses orient their care to the strengths of youths and their potential for healthy living rather than focusing on their deficits. Thus, nurse scientists have a responsibility to contribute to the design and testing of developmentally appropriate physical activity interventions.

It is often assumed that physical education classes meet the needs of youths for physical activity. This is not the case, however. Most schools do not require physical education and even when required, studies indicate that children are provided, on average, with only 3 minutes of moderate or vigorous activity per class (Simons-Morton, Taylor, Snider, & Huang, 1993; Simons-Morton, Taylor, Snider, Huang, & Fulton, 1994). In reality, more than 80% of a child's physical activity takes place outside the school (McGinnis, 1985). Parents, peers, nurses and other health care professionals, and the larger community become major sources of influence on children's physical activity patterns. Thus, health guidance to children and adolescents and their families to establish regular physical activity outside of school hours is critical and must be based on a "state of the science" understanding about what influences participation in physical activity among youths at different developmental stages.

THEORIES AND MODELS APPLIED TO PHYSICAL ACTIVITY OF YOUTHS

Use of various theories and models as frameworks for studying physical activity has escalated in the last decade. Fewer atheoretical studies are appearing in the research literature. A number of theories and models used to explain levels of physical activity among adults appear to have limited applicability to children, however. For example, the health belief model (Janz & Becker, 1984) focuses heavily on susceptibility to disease and seriousness of disease as the primary sources of motivation for health-related behavior. Avoidance of disease several decades hence is too far in the future to be of motivational significance to children. Perceived benefits and barriers, two other key concepts in the model, have been shown to exert some influence on the physical activity of children and adolescents (Sallis et al., 1992). Their affect on motivation to exercise needs further testing as the nature of perceived benefits and barriers may vary according to developmental stage. Protection motivation theory (Rogers, 1975) also has limitations similar to the health belief model when used with youths as there is considerable overlap of key concepts.

The theory of reasoned action has been used in studying influences on exercise among adults (Fishbein & Ajzen, 1975). The theory identifies personal intentions as the immediate determinants of behavior with intentions determined by attitudes and subjective norms. Attitudes are beliefs concerning what the consequences of performing a behavior will be as well as the evaluation of those consequences as either positive or negative. Subjective norms incorporate social influence into the model and consist of what persons think significant others want them to do as well as the extent of motivation to conform to those expectations. Several features of the theory may limit prediction of physical activity among children and adolescents. First, the theory is based on the assumption that deliberative, rational thinking underlies decisions to engage in a behavior. A second assumption is that all behavior is under volitional control of highly independent agents. The critical-thinking skills of youths are not well developed and dependence rather than independence is likely to characterize much of the first and second decades of life. Thus, there may be a lack of fit between the model concepts and the factors most relevant to motivating physical activity among youths.

The transtheoretical model (Prochaska & DiClemente, 1984) based on the stages of behavior change (precontemplation, contemplation, preparation, action, and maintenance) although increasingly popular in studies of adult exercise (Marcus et al., 1992) has not been applied to the study of children's physical activity. This process model was derived from studies of smoking cessation and alcohol abstinence among adults. It has not been determined whether children or adolescents pass through similar stages of behavior change as adults either when discontinuing a negative behavior or adopting a positive behavior. Different change processes may characterize different points in development depending on the level of maturation of abstract thought. This model needs rigorous testing in exercise studies among youths.

Theories of the self-system that focus on self-schematic structures are being increasingly explored among late adolescents and young adults in relation to motivation of exercise behavior (Kendzierski, 1988, 1990). According to the theory, persons schematic for exercise (viewing themselves as athletic or physically active) may be motivated to engage in physical activity to verify their self-image, whereas youth who are schematic for inactivity (view themselves as sedentary) may remain inactive consistent with their self-image. The theory focuses on the self-structure as important in the regulation of behavior and may hold promise for the prediction and motivation of exercise among children and adolescents.

Of the models and theories currently proposed to explain physical activity among children, social cognitive theory (SCT), proposed by Bandura (1986), has received the most attention and empirical testing to date. According to SCT, human behavior is explained by triadic reciprocal determinism with cognition, prior behavior, and the environment operating interactively to influence current behavior. Self-efficacy, a form of self-knowledge defined as judgments of one's ability to perform at a particular level in executing a specific behavior, is identified as a primary cognitive determinant of behavior (Bandura, 1986). According to SCT, efficacy expectations (expectations for successful performance bases on perceptions of personal competency) exert a major influence on behavior. Individuals derive their sense of efficacy in any given area of behavior by evaluating and integrating efficacy information from personal performance experience, physiologic states of arousal that accompany performance, observation of the behavior of others, and persuasion by others of personal capabilities. Efficacious individuals are likely to expend more effort and persist longer in attempts to execute a desired behavior. They are also likely to attribute eventual success to personal effort and skill rather than to luck or chance. Self-efficacy has been manipulated as a cognitive construct in a number of physical activity intervention studies with children and adolescents. An increase in exercise self-efficacy is not always linked to an actual increase in physical activity, however. Other constructs from SCT that have received somewhat less attention than self-efficacy in exercise intervention research with youths include: outcome expectations (anticipated consequences), constraints on behavior (barriers), standards or norms for behavior, and perceived opportunity structures (options) in the environment.

Two models of health-related behavior developed within a nursing perspective need further testing to determine their predictive power for physical activity among children and adolescents: the health promotion model (Pender, 1996) and the interaction model of client health behavior (Cox, 1982). The application of these models in studies of physical activity is discussed next.

The health promotion model (HPM) is intended to predict health behaviors where "threat of illness" is not a primary motivation for action. Constructs from SCT are operationalized in the model: personal factors such as biological, psychological, and sociocultural influences; outcome expectations as perceived benefits; performance constraints as perceived barriers; efficacy expectations as perceived self-efficacy; normative standards as one aspect of interpersonal influences; and perceived opportunity structures as situational influences. The model explained from 21% to 59% of the variance in exercise behavior among adults in a number of studies, but only 19% of the variance in exercise behavior in a study of adolescents (Pender, 1996). In recent revisions of the model, variables with low explanatory power were deleted and new variables were added to enhance the predictive power of the HPM. New concepts included in the model are activity-related affect to recognize the likely influence of the affective domain, commitment to a plan of action, and immediate competing behavioral demands and preferences. The revised HPM is just beginning to be used as a framework for studying physical activity of youths (Garcia et al., 1995; Garcia, Pender, Antonakos, & Ronis, 1997).

The interaction model of client health behavior (IMCHB) is focused on health behavior outcomes such as use of health services and adherence to recommended care regimens, with the latter being expansive enough to include recommended health-promoting behaviors (Cox, 1982). This model, developed within the framework of nursing, has been applied to explain health-promoting behavior including exercise behavior in children and adults (Farrand & Cox, 1993; Hawkes & Holm, 1993). Client background variables (demographic characteristics, social influences, previous health care experiences, and environmental resources) and other elements of client singularity characterizing the individual client (intrinsic motivation, cognitive appraisal, and affective response) are proposed as interfacing with elements of client–professional interaction (affective support, health information, decisional control, and professional/technical competencies) to influence health outcomes. The IMCHB is derived from self-determination theory (Deci & Ryan, 1985). Self-determination is the need for choice or freedom in initiating one's behavior. Intrinsic motivation, operationalized as health self-determinism, is a central construct in the IMCHB. Components of health self-determinism are self-determined health judgments, self-determined health behavior, perceived competence in health matters, and internal and external cue responsiveness. In studying the determinants of a composite of positive health behaviors, including exercise in middle childhood, the model explained 53% of the variance in girls' behavior and 63% of the variance in boys' behavior (Farrand & Cox, 1993). Studies that test the predictive power of the model specific to exercise behavior are needed.

CRITIQUE OF MODELS APPLIED TO PHYSICAL ACTIVITY

The theories and models described share an emphasis on the potential of humans for self-direction and self-influence. In all of the frameworks the human organism is viewed as cognitively active in motivating behavior. Given that youth is a time when decision making and empowerment are salient issues, models applied to youths need to acknowledge the emergence of self-regulation during this developmental period. Cognitions are integral to all of the models. Some psychologists have proposed that affect may be as important as cognition in determining exercise behavior, however (Hardy & Rejecki, 1989; McAuley & Courneya, 1992; Vallerand, 1987). In social cognitive theory, affect is considered to result from varying levels of perceived competence. In the theory of reasoned action, affect is a part of attitude in that it is the evaluation (positive or negative) of the anticipated consequences. In both the health promotion model and in the interaction model of client health behavior, affect is an important model variable. More research is needed that tests the relevance of affect as well as cognition in predicting involvement of youths in physical activity.

In models of exercise behavior for children and adolescents, developmental and cultural perspectives need to be articulated. Exercise behavior may fall under different influences at different levels of maturation and in different sociocultural contexts. Developmental variation in attitudes and subjective norms can be accommodated, in part, by the theory of reasoned action through use of a solicitation process to identify the most salient beliefs and norms at any developmental point to incorporate into physical activity-related measurements. In the IMCHB, the structure of client–professional interaction and its affect on the physical activity of youths may vary developmentally. For younger children, parents are likely to represent the child in interactions with health professionals and be the primary agent of decisional control. In contrast, adolescents are likely to have direct interactions with health professionals. This change in interactional dynamics needs to be considered in application of the model to physical activity among youths.

In relation to social cognitive theory, the question has been raised as to the relative motivational importance of exercise efficacy (competence or mastery) versus experiencing fun and enjoyment from exercise for children and adolescents. What is the optimal balance between feelings of mastery and experiencing fun from activity for youths and does this balance shift throughout maturation? More research is needed to address this theoretically relevant question.

The models described have been developed and tested primarily on European American populations. Their applicability to other race and ethnic groups is questionable until they receive further testing. Theories inductively derived from specific cultural perspectives may best capture the critical constructs for predicting physical activity and developing related interventions for youths from diverse backgrounds. For additional information on theories and models that have been proposed as frameworks for studying exercise and physical activity across varying populations, the reader is referred to other excellent resources (Dishman, 1988, 1994).

ADVANCES IN UNDERSTANDING THE PHYSICAL ACTIVITY BEHAVIORS OF CHILDREN AND ADOLESCENTS

Many studies have focused on identifying the correlates of physical activity in youths. These studies have been primarily cross-sectional rather than prospective in nature and thus cannot address causal influences. Only a few studies of physical activity have been longitudinal, allowing for exploration of developmental variation in influences on physical activity over time. In this section, an integrated review of what is know about the correlates of physical activity among youths is presented.

Current State of Knowledge

Biologic variables.   A number of biologic variables have been shown to affect level of physical activity, but the mechanisms underlying the effects are poorly understood (Blimkie & Bar-Or, 1995; Rowland, 1990). Many studies find that boys are more active than girls (Sallis et al., 1992). This may be due to a larger amount of fat-free mass in boys than girls following puberty, or to the amount of fat-free mass that is muscle. Further, the effects of biologic variables on physical activity may in part be mediated by gender differences in socialization (Eccles & Harold, 1991). That is, boys are socialized to value strength and physical prowess more than girls so they focus on developing competence in sports, which may lead to decreased body fat. Although there is little evidence that high fitness levels "cause" increased participation in physical activity, body mass and extent of body fat appear to affect physical activity with youths of normal weight being more active than obese youths (USDHHS, 1996). Some infants move about more than others but it is not yet known the extent to which genetics predisposes one to differences in activity level. Biologic maturation seems to predispose to inactivity as physical activity in both genders decreases markedly across adolescence. The extent to which biologic variables actually contribute to this decrement and the underlying causal mechanisms need to be explored.

Racial and ethnic background.   The results from the 1990 Youth Risk Behavior Survey (YRBS) of 11,631 American high-school students revealed that in grades 9 through 12, Black students were less likely to be vigorously active than White or Hispanic students (Heath, Pratt, Warren, & Kann, 1994). In another study, African American freshmen at a historically Black southern university were found to have low levels of leisure time physical activity and aerobic fitness and moderately high body fat (Ainsworth, Berry, Schnyder, & Vickers, 1992). To determine if differences by race were consistent across childhood and adolescence and when differences were first detectable, the literature on racial and ethnic differences in physical activity from preschool through college was reviewed. Activity patterns of Anglo and Mexican American preschool children were observed during recess and at home. Mexican American children were less active than Anglo children during the period of observation (McKenzie, Sallis, Nader, Broyles, & Nelson, 1992). Among 2,410 multiethnic third-graders, Black and Hispanic children reported less activity than White children (Simons-Morton et al., 1997). In terms of fitness, Pivarnik, Bray, Hergenroeder, Hill, and Wong (1995) found aerobic fitness to be significantly lower in 11–16-year-old Black girls compared to White girls when body weight was controlled; the authors proposed that differences in fitness performance may be linked to biological factors such as Hispanic and Black girls' fat-free mass (FFM) containing a smaller percentage of skeletal muscle than White girls' FFM. In contrast, Desmond, Price, Lock, Smith, and Stewart (1990) found no differences in physical fitness of 257 Black and White high-school students. The mechanisms underlying racial differences in physical activity and fitness, if differences truly exist, must be understood as sedentary lifestyles that begin very early are likely to predispose to cardiovascular disease and hypertension in later life, problems already prevalent in minority populations. It is possible that socioeconomic status, if not ascertained and controlled in the analyses, may account for some of the observed differences by race and ethnicity.

Behavior-specific cognitions and affect.   Many researchers have explored the influence of behavior-specific cognitions on physical activity in youth. Barriers to exercise, exercise self-efficacy, and intentions to exercise were the cognitions found to correlate most frequently with physical activity in children and adolescents (Sallis et al., 1992). In a study of 286 racially diverse youth, Garcia et al. (1995) found that the extent to which the perceived benefits of exercise outweighed the barriers was a direct determinant of level of physical activity among elementary and junior high school students. Awareness of the benefits of exercise, although a necessary condition for participation, does not appear sufficient itself to motivate physical activity. It is often found to be weakly correlated or uncorrelated with activity among youth. In studying the perceived barriers to exercise among high-school students, Tappe, Duda, and Ehrnwald (1989) found that major barriers were time constraints, lack of interest, unsuitable weather, school, and schoolwork. Time constraints were cited significantly more frequently by the group that was lowest in reported activity compared to the group highest in reported activity. Boys, compared to girls, reported more frequently that use of alcohol or drugs kept them from being active.

According to the theory of reasoned action, intention to be active is the primary determinant of physical activity. In social cognitive theory, efficacy expectations are proposed as major determinants of physical activity. In a group of 743 tenth-grade students, Reynolds et al. (1990) found that when baseline levels of physical activity and body mass index were controlled, intentions to exercise and self-efficacy were associated with physical activity. The two variables accounted for only a modest amount of variance in activity scores. Zakarian, Hovell, Hofstetter, Sallis, and Keating (1994) in studying the correlates of exercise found that self-efficacy predicted vigorous exercise in a low socioeconomic group of 1,634 ninth- and 11th-graders who were predominantly Latino. Their findings provide evidence for the cultural appropriateness of the construct of exercise efficacy in this group. Trost et al. (1996) in studying 334 fifth-grade students who were primarily African American found that physical activity self-efficacy for overcoming barriers was predictive of both moderate and vigorous physical activity for boys and girls. The level of physical activity self-efficacy was higher in boys, however.

Cognitive and affective variables that have received little attention in physical activity studies but merit further exploration among children and adolescents as determinants include: intrinsic motivation, gender-role stereotypes, activity stereotypes, self-schemata, goals, expectations for success, and activity-related affect. Hawkes and Holm (1993) found intrinsic motivation as measured by the health self-determinism index to be directly predictive of exercise. Using the interaction model of client health behavior, Farrand and Cox (1993) investigated the influence of intrinsic motivation on the positive health practices including exercise of 260 preadolescents between 9 and 10 years of age. For girls but not boys, intrinsic motivation was indirectly predictive of health behaviors appearing to be mediated by cognitive appraisal. Intrinsic motivation as an element of client singularity in the IMCHB merits further study to determine its impact on physical activity among youth. Eccles and Harold (1991) have emphasized the importance of looking at gender-role stereotypes and activity stereotypes. Women are often stereotyped as less competent than men in the athletic domain even when they perform equally well. Biased gender-role stereotypes could result in girls having lower physical activity self-concepts than boys. Further, activity stereotypes may connect certain types of sports or exercise with a particular gender. Thus, to act in accordance with what it means to be feminine or masculine, certain activities that could be appropriate across the genders and improve cardiorespiratory fitness may be avoided. Self-schemata are the images that people develop of themselves as to who they are and who they would like to be. Eccles and Harold (1991) have proposed that people select activities that are consistent with or will enhance their self-images and avoid activities inconsistent with these images. The role of self-schematic structures, a part of the self-system, in motivating physical activity merits rigorous attention among youths as the self-system is in a state of emergence during this developmental stage.

Goal setting is integral to a number of the theories and models that have been applied to exercise behavior yet has been given limited attention in empirical studies of physical activity among youth. Particularly for older youth, behavioral goals and expectations for success in achieving them need to be incorporated into exercise studies.

Activity-related affect, defined as subjective feeling states that occur prior to, during, and following a behavior, is stored in memory and associated with subsequent thoughts of the behavior (McAuley & Courneya, 1992). Individuals generally will wish to repeat activities associated with positive affect and avoid those associated with negative affect. The affect associated with exercise reflects a direct emotional response or gut-level reaction to the thought of the behavior as well as a response to self-evaluation of performance. The affective domain may be as important to understanding youths' physical-activity behavior as the cognitive domain. Further exploration is definitely warranted.

Interpersonal influence.   The interpersonal influence of parents on the exercise behavior of children and adolescents has received considerable attention in the research literature (Taylor, Baranowski, & Sallis, 1994). Lau, Quadrel, and Hartman (1990) identified three different mechanisms through which parents can influence the exercise beliefs and behaviors of their off-spring: (a) modeling active lifestyles; (b) discussing exercise beliefs that they hold and why they hold them; and (c) intentionally attempting to transfer exercise beliefs and behaviors through explicit training efforts that may consist of instruction, shared activities, instrumental support, and encouragement. Moore et al. (1991) in studying children 4–7 years of age ($N = 100$), reported a relationship between parents' and children's physical activity levels measured by electronic motion sensors. Children of active mothers were 2.0 times as likely to be active as children with sedentary mothers and children of active fathers were 3.5 times as likely to be active as children of sedentary fathers. When both parents were active, children were 5.8 times as likely to be active as those with inactive parents. Purath, Lansinger, and Ragheb (1995) in study-ing young children in grades 1 to 5 ($N = 357$) also found a correlation between the amount of time that children exercised as reported by their parent and the amount of time that mothers exercised. Because parents, frequently mothers, completed questionnaires for the children as well as for themselves, this relationship could be spurious or inflated in the study.

In contrast, when McMurray et al. (1993) studied parental influences on children between 8 to 10 years of age in terms of activity patterns ($N = 1253$), they found very low correlation between children's and parents' self-reported exercise habits. They did find that parents' perceptions of barriers to physical activity such as lack of time or lack of enjoyment, were related to the child's level of fitness as measured by maximum oxygen consumption (VO_2 max) during testing. Godin and Shephard (1986) in studying older children in seventh and ninth grades, also found no association between parents' and children's activity levels. Failure to find relationships between parents' and older children's activity patterns may indicate that the affect of parental level of activity is more pronounced for younger children. This may be the case because younger children are more likely to actually observe a parent exercis-ing at home or in the community than are older children who are away at school most of the day. No attempt was made in any of the above studies to determine if the children actually observed their parents exercising so modeling could take place.

Lau et al. (1990), in studying the development of exercise behaviors over time in a population of predominately 17- to 19-year-olds ($N = 947$), found that parental modeling had a relatively weak effect on exercise practices at home the year before leaving for college and during the first years of college. Interestingly, they found that the strongest sustained influence on exercise behavior of college students was specific training efforts by parents in earlier years to teach then to exercise. Little attention has been given as to whether there is a developmental gradient for parental influence processes. Both the type and amount of parental influence may vary as a result of the child's stage of development. There may be critical periods during which parents are a particularly potent source of influence on children's physical activity patterns. Attention needs to be given also to the influence of peers on physical activity especially for older children and adolescents for whom peers become increasingly salient in influencing their attitudes and behaviors. Cultural differences in the balance of parental and peer influence across adolescence need to be explored in order to develop appropriate interventions for youth from diverse sociocultural backgrounds.

Environmental or situational influences.   Little research has been focused on the effect of the physical environment in the home, school, neighborhood, and community on physical activity patterns. Environmental influences include options (facilities, equipment), aesthetics (safe, pleasant), and demand characteristics (environmental dictates for specific behaviors) of the surroundings in which children and adolescents live out their daily lives. Seasonal variations are also situational factors that may affect physical activity. Garcia et al. (1995) in studying the leisure time physical activity of fifth-, sixth-, and eighth-graders found that access to exercise and sports facilities directly predicted leisure time physical activity. Level of physical activity also was correlated with seasons; activity level was lower in the winter and higher in the spring and summer in this group of midwestern youth. Among a group of fifth- and sixth-graders, Stucky-Ropp and DiLorenzo (1993) reported that the number of exercise-related items at home (bicycles, balls, jump ropes) was related to level of physical activity for girls but not for boys. In contrast, Zakarian et al. (1994) did not find number of facilities available or neighborhood safety related to physical activity of fifth- and sixth-graders.

Studies of the effects of access to television, generally described as "reported time spent viewing television," on physical activity and fitness of children and adolescents were not definitive. Robinson et al. (1993) reported that among 971 female adolescents, hours of watching television after school was not significantly associated with level of physical activity. It is interesting to note that when metabolic rate during rest and during television viewing were compared, the latter was lower. This may predispose children to obesity who spend lengthy periods viewing television (Klesges, Shelton, & Klesges, 1993).

Few studies have used an ecological approach to examine the child's micro and macro environments to identify the features that predict physical activity or can be altered to increase physical activity. It may be that environmental variables are equally as powerful in motivating and enabling physical activity as variables in the cognitive and affective domains.

MEASUREMENT OF PHYSICAL ACTIVITY AND RELATED VARIABLES

Instrumentation for the measurement of activity in children and adolescents continues to be a challenge to nurses and other scientists, particularly in field studies. Physical activity has three dimensions: duration, frequency, and intensity. It can be measured in a number of ways including energy expenditure, amount of work performed, time period of activity, or as a numerical score derived from questionnaire data.

Direct observation has been used in some field studies to measure physical activity but often is not feasible. Further, children's behavior can be distorted by the presence of observers. Self-report has been used widely but has limitations in terms of accuracy of recall; however, it is the best method for large-scale studies. The frequency of recall affects its accuracy. This author has found daily recall to yield the most accurate data compared to longer recall periods. Physical instrumentation such as accelerometers and actigraphs are being further perfected and are already in use in smaller scale studies or to validate self-report.

A major problem for exercise researchers working with youth is the lack of ways in which to validate the physical activity measures used. Fitness measures are sometimes used but as fitness is affected not only by physical activity but by gender, heredity, age, and weight, fitness measures are not ideal criteria for validating methods for assessing physical activity. Using intercorrelations among methods for measuring physical activity may be problematic as well because there are errors in all methods (Montoye, Kemper, Saris, & Washburn, 1996). Scientists need to continue to work on developing reliable methods for assessing habitual physical activity particularly among children and adolescents. The reader is referred to other resources for further discussion of methods for measurement of physical activity (Docherty, 1996; Garcia, George, Coviak, Antonakos, & Pender, 1997; Leidy, Abbott, & Fedenko, 1997; Mason & Redeker, 1993; Montoye, Kemper, Saris, & Washburn, 1996; Sallis, Buono, Roby, Micale, & Nelson, 1993).

Health-related fitness is the primary goal of physical activity education and counseling by health professionals. Health-related fitness is a multidimensional characteristic of children and adolescents consisting of the dimensions of cardiorespiratory endurance, muscular strength, flexibility, and body composition (Pate & Shephard, 1989). The most frequently used laboratory measure for cardiorespiratory endurance is directly measured maximal aerobic power (VO_2 max). In field studies, distance runs and step tests are most frequently used. In the laboratory, muscle strength is measured by dynamometers and in the field by calisthenic exercises that involve repetitive movements. Flexibility can be measured in the laboratory with a flexibility or goniometer. Sit-and-reach and stand-and-reach are the most common field tests. Body composition has posed particular measurement challenges with laboratory methods including hydrostatic weighing, whole-body radioactive counting of potassium, and dilution techniques with deuterium oxide to estimate total body water (Pate & Shephard, 1989). Some of these techniques have limited applicability to children, thus, measurement of skinfolds at several anatomical sites is used most frequently. Because discussion and critique of measures of physical fitness are beyond the scope of this chapter, suffice it to say that scientists often will need to link measures of physical activity with measures of fitness to determine if activity is adequate to result in health related changes in fitness. It is not yet clear how much activity or what intensity and periodicity is needed by youths to bring about positive changes in health-related fitness. Researchers must be aware of the dimension of fitness that they desire to measure and choose the most valid and reliable method(s) feasible.

ADVANCES IN INTERVENTIONS TO MODIFY PHYSICAL ACTIVITY BEHAVIORS OF YOUTH

Translating what is known into developmentally and culturally appropriate physical activity interventions that can be tested is one of the major challenges facing nurse scientists and other health researchers today. Approximately 20 intervention studies were reported in the literature that were focused on changing physical activity behaviors in youth. Of these studies, 13 are summarized in Table 6.1. Intervention studies not summarized were those in which the study design was described but no outcomes were reported and studies in which recall of physical activity was thought to be highly inaccurate due to the age of the children or the methods used for data collection. Most frequently, the physical activity interventions reviewed were universal (directed to all children), school-based, and part of a more comprehensive intervention aimed at reducing cardiovascular disease risk. Physical activity interventions were frequently coupled with nutrition interventions and occasionally with prevention of smoking interventions as well. To include physical activity as part of a more comprehensive intervention to change the overall health lifestyle is logical. First, when common determinants are involved, interventions that address multiple behaviors are likely to be more effective and efficient in use of resources than targeting one behavior at a time. Second, increasing positive behaviors may be used as leverage to change negative behaviors thus achieving synergy in the intervention. Only two intervention studies were focused solely on increasing physical activity in youth. One was a laboratory study (Epstein, Saelens, Myers, & Vito, 1997) and the other was a home-based activity program (Taggart, Taggart, & Siedentop, 1986). Obese youth were targeted in two of the intervention studies (Epstein et al., 1997; Epstein, Valoski, Wing, & McCurley, 1990).

In a number of studies, researchers combined use of individual behavior-change theories and organizational change theories by embedding school and family interventions in community-wide interventions to change social and family norms. Examples of these studies were the "Class of 89" and "Slice of Life" programs within the Minnesota Heart Health Program (Kelder, Perry, & Klepp, 1993) and the "Heart Smart" program within the Bogalusa Heart Study (Downey et al., 1987). Approaches to organizational change that were used included community outreach through media, restructuring health and physical education curricula, and training teachers in new instructional techniques to promote aerobic activity.

As shown in Table 6.1, social cognitive theory (Bandura, 1986) was the most frequently used theoretical framework for intervention. Multiple variables in cognitive, social, and environmental domains were targeted such as physical activity skills, self-efficacy for physical activity, self-responsibility, and the social environment (family or peer attitudes and behavior) as a means of changing physical activity of youths. Strategies employed included: self-monitoring, parental role modeling, peer role modeling, goal setting, contracts (rewards, reinforcement), self-reinforcement, self-instruction, problem solving, stimulus control, social support, and competition.

Considering the physical activity interventions as a group, they ranged in length from 4 weeks to several years across grades and were offered most frequently to third-graders through 10th-graders. Aerobic activities varied but often included jumping rope to music, aerobic dance, jogging, walking, and biking. Most of the school-based interventions were conducted in health education and physical education classes. Few involved nurses in the intervention. The majority employed a pretest, posttest, control-group design. Two examples of studies with nurses as leaders or members of the investigative team are described here.

Harrell et al. (1996) in the Cardiovascular Health in Children (CHIC) study offered an exercise program within the context of a school-based intervention for 1,274 third- and fourth-grade children to lower cardiovascular disease risk. The investigators employed a randomized, controlled field trial in 12 schools in North Carolina. American Heart Association Lower and Upper Elementary School Program Kits were used to provide instruction on

TABLE 6.1 Overview of Physical Activity Intervention Studies

First author and year[a]	Sample	Design	Intervention	Outcome variables	Results
Connor, 1986	55 3rd- and 4th-graders enrolled in after-school programs 44% Black 44% Hispanic 7% White	Quasi-experimental pretest, posttest control group with random assignment of after-school centers	Future Fit Aerobic Program, 12-week aerobic exercise program with 3 sessions per week	Maintenance of target heart rate during exercise Liking of exercise program Talking to parents about the Future Fit Aerobic Program	Target heart rate not maintained 97% of students reported liking the program 86% of parents reported children talking about program
Taggart, 1986	12 4th-, 5th-, and 6th-graders	Pretest, posttest with no control group	Family training and contracting with parent for activity	Activity points accumulated each week	↑ In activity level time intensity
Killen, 1988	1,447 10th-graders 69% White 2% Black 13% Asian 6% Hispanic	Pretest, posttest control group with random assignment of schools	20 classroom sessions with 4 focused on physical activity (social cognitive theory) • Cognitive and behavioral skills • Skills for resisting social influences • Self-change project	Self-reported physical activity	↑ Reported regular exercise in treatment group compared to control group ↓ Resting heart rate in treatment group ↓ Body mass index and skinfold thickness in treatment group

(continued)

TABLE 6.1 *(continued)*

First author and year[a]	Design	Sample	Intervention	Outcome variables	Results
Patterson, 1988	Randomized controlled trial	60 families 50% Anglo American 50% Mexican American	San Diego Family Health Project (social learning theory) One-year intervention with 12 weeks of intensive program and 6 maintenance sessions • Self-monitoring • Goal setting • Family contract • Social support • Modeling	Physical activity level (observation at zoo) Total distance traveled % of observation intervals physically active Use of escalators	Intervention group walked further and spent more time being physically active (Mexican American families only) Intervention group used escalator less
Nader, 1989	Randomized controlled trial	206 healthy volunteer low- to middle-income Mexican American and Anglo American families with a child in 5th or 6th grade	San Diego Family Health Project (social learning theory) One-year intervention with 12 weeks of intensive program and 6 maintenance sessions · Self-monitoring · Goal setting · Family contract · Social support · Modeling	Self-reported physical activity	↑ Knowledge of skills required to change exercise habits in experimental families No difference in self-reported physical activity No difference in cardiovascular fitness

(continued)

TABLE 6.1 (continued)

Epstein, 1990	76 obese children 6–12 years of age	Prospective, randomized, controlled trial	3 groups • Child and parent target • Child target • Nonspecific target Given information on aerobic exercise start-up Behavioral procedures • Contracting • Self-monitoring • Social reinforcement • Monitoring	Change in percentage of overweight	↓ In percentage of children overweight in group with child and parent as target
Simons-Morton, 1991	3rd- and 4th-graders 62% Anglo American 15% African American 21% Mexican American	Pretest, posttest control group	Go for Health (social cognitive theory) Classroom health education and changes in PE • Physical activity skill development • Fitness development	Time moderate and vigorous physical activity was performed in PE	↑ In moderate and vigorous activity in PE classes in intervention group

(continued)

157

TABLE 6.1 (*continued*)

First author and year[a]	Sample	Design	Intervention	Outcome variables	Results
Arbeit, 1992	556 4th- and 5th-graders 58% White 32% Black	Pretest, posttest control group with random assignment of schools	Heart Smart Cardiovascular School Health Promotion Superkids-Superfit Exercise Program • Benefits of exercise • Physiology of exercise • Exercise skills	1 mile run/walk time	↓ Time by 1.3 minutes (boys only) in intervention group ↓ Systolic BP and skinfold thickness among those who ↓ run/walk time
Kelder, 1993	2,376 8th- and 10th-graders predominantly White	Pretest, posttest with intervention and reference community	Minnesota Heart Health Program—Class of 1989—Community and school intervention (social learning theory) • Knowledge • Self-efficacy • Skills • Goals • Social support • Barriers	Hours per week of exercise Physical activity score (frequency and intensity)	↑ Self-reported physical activity (females only) in intervention group

(continued)

TABLE 6.1 (*continued*)

Edmundson, 1996	6,956 3rd-, 4th-, and 5th-graders 67% White 14% African American 14% Hispanic	Randomized intervention trial with 4 sites; 14 intervention schools and 10 comparison schools per site	Child Adolescent Trial for Cardiovascular Health (CATCH) (social cognitive theory) • Class curriculum • CATCH PE • Family activity packets Target variables • Enactment learning • Role modeling • Peer support • Goal setting	Perceived reinforcement of physical activity Physical activity self-efficacy	↑ Perceived positive reinforcement of activity in intervention group ↑ Physical activity self-efficacy in intervention group No added effects of family intervention over school intervention
Harrell, 1996	1,274 3rd- and 4th-graders in 12 schools 74% White 20% Black	Randomized controlled field trial	Cardiovascular Health in Children (CHIC)—classroom-based intervention to ↓ CVD risk factors (Bruhn and Parcel Development of Positive Behavior Model)—8-week exercise program, American Heart Association Kits used	Physical activity Blood pressure Aerobic power Skinfolds Body mass index	↑ Self-reported physical activity

(*continued*)

TABLE 6.1 (*continued*)

First author and year[a]	Sample	Design	Intervention	Outcome variables	Results
Luepker, 1996	5,106 3rd-, 4th-, and 5th-graders	Randomized intervention trial with 4 sites; 14 intervention schools and 10 comparison schools per site	Child Adolescent Trial for Cardiovascular Health (CATCH) (social cognitive theory) • Class curriculum • CATCH PE • Family activity packets Target variables • Enactment learning • Role modeling • Peer support • Goal setting	Amount of moderate to vigorous physical activity performed in PE Leisure time physical activity	↑ In moderate to vigorous activity in PE classes in intervention group ↑ Self-report of leisure time physical activity in intervention group

(continued)

TABLE 6.1 (continued)

| Epstein, 1997 | 37 obese children
8–12 years old
33 White
4 African American | Pretest, posttest control group with random assignment of children | 3 intervention groups (behavioral economic theory)
• Positive reinforcement for not engaging in sedentary activities
• Punishment for engaging in sedentary activities
• Access to sedentary activities restricted | Number of 30-second intervals spent in physically active and sedentary activities | Reinforcement and punishment group more physically active on intervention days but no difference post intervention

Liking for sedentary activity ↓ in the reinforcement group and ↑ in the restriction group |

aComplete citations for all studies appear in the list of references.

161

the importance of getting regular physical exercise. Children received a physical activity intervention three times a week for 8 weeks. This intervention included a brief warm-up, 20 minutes of fun, noncompetitive aerobic activities (jumping rope, relays, games, and aerobic dance), and a cool-down period. A strength of the study was that both school-level and individual-level analyses were conducted. In school-level analyses, children in the intervention group had a significant increase in self-reported activity compared to children in the control group. In individual-level analyses, posttest knowledge about physical activity was significantly greater in the intervention as compared to the control group. There was a trend in the intervention group toward lower total serum cholesterol, decreased body fat, and increased aerobic power. Also, the diastolic blood pressure of children in the intervention group did not increase as much as for children in the control group. Although it is not possible to separate out the specific effects of the exercise program from the effects of the intervention components focused on diet and smoking, the exercise program in combination with other program components did have a positive effect on knowledge, behavior, and cardiovascular risk factors. Additional strengths of this study were use of a randomized, controlled clinical-trial design, identification of the theoretical framework for the study, and the inclusion of physiologic measures linked to reduced cardiovascular disease (CVD) risk in the outcome measures. Study limitations were the moderate level of precision with which physical activity was measured, the potential confounding effects of seasonal variation in physical activity among youths (higher in spring and summer, lower in winter), and the lack of clear specification of how the model variables were operationalized in the study consistent with the parent theory. This study is one of only a few intervention studies focused on increasing physical activity among youth that have been led by nurse investigators.

"Future Fit" was developed to provide a low-cost, after-school heart health education and fitness program to third- and fourth-grade students. Four sites in which the program was offered were randomly assigned to experimental and control groups (Connor et al., 1986). A quasi-experimental pretest, posttest design was used. An interdisciplinary team of clinicians from the medical center in the region met with parents to orient them to the program and conducted the screening of participants. The study sample was small with a total of 55 children participating in the study. The study group was primarily African American and Hispanic. American Heart Association resource materials were used, and nutrition, smoking, and handling stress were addressed in addition to physical activity in the after-school program delivered by teachers. Three 45-minute exercise sessions were conducted each week for a period of 12 weeks with warm-up, aerobic activity, and cool-down by trained aerobic instructors. Children helped lead the exercise activities. At the end of the session, results indicated that children had a positive attitude toward the exercise program and that they would like to be in the exercise program again the next time it was offered. Parents reported that their children were enthusiastic about the program, often talked about it at home, and were exercising more. Postprogram physical activity was not specifically measured, however. Enjoyment of the program may have been one of the most important outcomes as the children were favorably predisposed toward continuing exercise and future program participation. Strengths of the study included use of a randomized, controlled trial design, and collaboration of nurses, teachers, and parents in development of the curriculum. A major limitation of this study was reliance on global parental report rather than use of a systematic approach for assessing physical activity following the program. Further, the very small sample size limited the statistical power of the study and thus confidence in study results.

Two of the studies reported (Connor et al., 1986; Edmundson et al., 1996) did not attempt to measure physical activity as an outcome. Instead, the outcomes measured were changes in cognitions or related behaviors including reported liking for the physical activity program and willingness to participate again, discussion of program with parents, perceived positive reinforcement for physical activity, and physical activity self-efficacy. These studies provide support for the fact that interventions can change activity-related cognitions and affect but do not address the important questions of whether such changes actually mediate changes in exercise activity.

Of the seven intervention studies that measured physical activity as an outcome (see Table 6.1), six showed an increase in reported or observed physical activity. The one exception was in the San Diego Family Health Project (Nader et al., 1989) in which no difference in self-reported physical activity was apparent between children in the experimental and control families. In studies where no behavioral effect is apparent, probing may reveal dimensions of the intervention that are ineffectual or have not been rigorously implemented. Madsen et al. (1993) conducted a probe in the San Diego Family Health Project and found that intervention process variables such as attendance at sessions, adherence to self-monitoring, achievement of physical activity goals, and attitudes toward the program partially mediated intervention effects. Lack of sensitivity of physical activity measures to small or moderate changes in level of activity may also be a problem. The transtheoretical model (Prochaska & DiClemente, 1984; Prochaska, Norcross, & DiClemente, 1994) offers a staging paradigm for exercise behavior that, if developmentally appropriate for children, may provide a means of identifying more sensitive stage-specific outcomes throughout exercise adoption.

Physiological parameters relevant to CVD risk were clearly incorporated as outcome measures in four of the studies in Table 6.1. Three of the studies

(Arbeit et al., 1992; Epstein et al., 1990; Killen et al., 1988) found decreases in CVD risk factors such as resting heart rate, body mass index, skinfold thickness, systolic blood pressure, and 1 mile run/walk time (aerobic power). Harrell et al. (1996) reported no significant changes in cardiovascular disease risk factors such as lowered blood pressure, decreased body mass index or skinfolds, or increased aerobic power from the physical activity interventions, although there was a trend in the positive direction. The lack of change in cardiovascular disease risk factors in intervention studies with youth may be due to inadequate intensity, duration, or frequency of the physical activity intervention to effect cardiorespiratory fitness, premature cessation of the intervention, short follow-up periods, or confounding of the effect of activity on risk-reduction measures by gender, heredity, age, and other health behaviors. Scientists need to address all of these issues in the conduct of rigorous intervention studies on the effects of physical activity.

A major criticism of all of the interventions reviewed is that they seldom built in measures to determine if the variables targeted for manipulation and thought to affect physical activity actually changed as a result of the intervention. For example, interventions often attempted to increase exercise self-efficacy, lower perceived barriers to participation, or increase intentions to exercise as a means of increasing physical activity. It was alarming to see that little attention was given to actually measuring whether changes in the proposed mediating variables had occurred, however. Pre- and post-intervention measures were not reported. Thus, data did not exist to determine if changes in the proposed mediating variables (variables built into the intervention) were actually responsible for the observed changes in physical activity. Although measuring mediating variables raises issues concerning the subject burden of instrumentation, collection of these data is essential to understand the process of exercise adoption among children and adolescents.

Exercise is a behavior that must occur with regularity throughout the life span to have optimum health benefits. A major dilemma in child and adolescent physical activity interventions is how long and with what periodicity should one intervene to get children to adopt patterns of regular exercise and maintain them. Intervention studies need to be conducted that compare programs of varying lengths and tract physical activity levels over extended periods of time to ascertain the dose–response relationship between length and periodicity of intervention efforts and maintaining habitual physical activity.

PHYSICAL ACTIVITY COUNSELING BY NURSES

Little research has been focused on the physical activity counseling behaviors of nurses. Brown and Waybrant (1988) examined the health promotion counseling activities of 110 nurse practitioners in primary care settings. When asked if they had provided counseling concerning physical activity and exercise to any clients on the prior day, 76.4% said that they had. Physical activity counseling was the third most frequently reported counseling activity, surpassed only by counseling in relation to screening and nutrition. No specific information was available on the content of the counseling activities. Further, it could not be ascertained as to whether such counseling was provided to children and adolescents. Holcomb and Mullen (1986) examined the health promotion counseling practices in a random sample of 250 nurse midwives, and found that the nurse midwives were less likely to ask patients about their level of physical activity than about smoking, weight, and alcohol intake. Of the midwives, 72% reported that health promotion counseling was an important part of their professional role. Midwives can provide valuable physical activity counseling to pregnant adolescents yet the potential of this area of counseling has not been explored by nurse scientists in rigorously designed intervention studies.

As knowledge is gained concerning the determinants of physical activity, nurse scientists need to conduct intervention studies in primary care settings to find out what works to promote physical activity among children and adolescents at different developmental stages and in different life circumstances. The Physician-Based Assessment and Counseling for Exercise (PACE) program provides an example of an intervention specifically developed for use by physicians in primary care. The testing of this protocol by Calfas et al. (1996) is reported elsewhere. Interventions incorporating the educative/developmental approach that nurses use in providing primary care to youth need to be developed and tested. Further, interventions that work must be incorporated into the health-counseling strategies of nurses who provide primary care and health education to youths and their families. Scientists must not only empirically evaluate interventions but take responsibility for seeing that society is well served by the integration of effective interventions into nursing activities aimed at increasing physical activity among children and adolescents.

FUTURE ADVANCES IN PHYSICAL ACTIVITY PROMOTION THEORY AND RESEARCH FOR YOUTHS

Exploration of the determinants of physical activity in children and adolescents is in the early stages. Given the low prevalence of moderate to vigorous physical activity among youths despite its documented positive effects on physical and mental health, the research agenda in this area is most pressing.

Not only does physical activity improve health but there is accumulating evidence that it may also deter involvement in health-compromising behaviors. Most of the research conducted to date has been cross-sectional. Major advances in theory and research will only result through more prospective, longitudinal, and intervention studies, however. These studies should explore multimodal interventions in which families, schools, communities, and primary care settings all are built into the intervention to provide consistent messages that encourage and reinforce physical activity. The next generation of intervention studies should also explore the integration of peer leadership into physical activity promotion interventions. With the increasing influence of peers throughout childhood and adolescence, positive use of peer influence should be tested in physical activity interventions. Given the many differences in exercise-related cognitions, affect and exercise behaviors between boys and girls, gender-specific interventions may need to be developed to optimally promote physical activity in child and adolescent populations.

Physical activity intervention studies should be designed around particular theories or models. Further, not only must the theory inform the intervention, the theoretical variables proposed as mediating physical activity must be measured. For example, did an intervention directed toward improving physical activity by decreasing barriers or increasing self-efficacy actually affect these mediating variables? Unless changes in mediating variables are substantiated, other intervening variables unknown to the investigators may be responsible for change. It is also important that the models be tested with instruments that are psychometrically sound. There is a need to develop more reliable and valid measures of physical activity as well as of variables proposed as determinants of physical activity for use with children and adolescents. Instruments that have been developed for adults, if adapted for children and adolescents, must be validated to determine their applicability in younger age groups. Also, efforts should be made to develop exercise-related instrumentation inductively from the physical activity experiences of children and adolescents. Measures that can be used to assess risk for inactivity, particularly in young children, need to be developed so that interventions can begin to affect lifelong physical activity patterns during "critical windows of opportunity."

Studies that test models proposed from a nursing perspective as explanations of health behaviors are important in determining the utility of the models in predicting physical activity of youths and in successfully intervening to increase level of activity. The models developed within the perspective of nursing integrate concepts from multiple behavioral theories and thus may provide the basis for more powerful interventions than reliance on a single theory. Only through testing can it be determined whether these nursing models are sufficiently useful in predicting and modifying physical activity of youths or whether there is a need to develop new models.

Intervention studies are needed that assess whether increasing physical activity can decrease health-compromising behaviors such as binge eating and purging to reduce weight. Studies show that adolescents, particularly girls, have major concerns about weight and often exhibit a high level of body dissatisfaction (Kolody & Sallis, 1995; Wadden, Foster, Stunkard, & Linowitz, 1989; Wardle & Marsland, 1990). Body image is also likely to be a concern for boys with a tendency to be overweight. Physical activity interventions should capitalize on major preadolescent and adolescent concerns to promote active lifestyles. Another health-compromising behavior that may be addressed through physical activity interventions is smoking initiation. A study funded by the National Cancer Institute is already under way at the University of Michigan to determine whether an after-school physical activity program can decrease the incidence of smoking initiation (A. Garcia, personal communication, September 20, 1996). Such studies need to be conducted not only in schools but for street youths and homeless populations, who are at high risk for health-damaging behaviors with negligible opportunities to adopt and maintain health-promoting behaviors.

In summary, there are many research challenges for nurse scientists who invest their energies in contributing to the knowledge base for promoting physical activity among children and adolescents. New scientific discoveries are critical to enhance the effectiveness of physical activity counseling by nurses in primary care as well as the physical activity promotion programs for families, schools, and communities in which nurses collaborate with other health professionals.

ACKNOWLEDGMENT

The technical assistance of Karen McIlroy, Administrative and Research Associate, Child and Adolescent Health Behavior Research Center, School of Nursing, University of Michigan, in preparing this review is acknowledged.

REFERENCES

Ainsworth, B. E., Berry, C. B., Schnyder, V. N., & Vickers, S. R. (1992). Leisure-time physical activity and aerobic fitness in African-American young adults. *Journal of Adolescent Health, 13,* 606–611.

Arbeit, M. L., Johnson, C. C., Mott, D. S., Harsha, D. W., Nicklas, T. A., Webber, L. S., & Berenson, G. S. (1992). The heart smart cardiovascular school health promotion: Behavior correlates of risk factor change. *Preventive Medicine, 21,* 18–32.

Bandura, A. (1986). *Social foundations of thought and action: A social cognitive theory.* Englewood Cliffs, NJ: Prentice Hall.

Berlin, J. A., & Colditz, G. A. (1990). A meta-analysis of physical activity in the prevention of coronary heart disease. *American Journal of Epidemiology, 132,* 612–628.

Blimkie, C. J. R., & Bar-Or, O. (1995). *New horizons in pediatric exercise science.* Champaign, IL: Human Kinetics.

Brown, M. A., & Waybrant, K. M. (1988). Health promotion, education, counseling and coordination in primary health care nursing. *Public Health Nursing, 5,* 16–23.

Calfas, K. J., Long, B. J., Sallis, J. F., Wooten, W. J., Pratt, M., & Patrick, K. (1996). A controlled trial of physician counseling to promote the adoption of physical activity. *Preventive Medicine, 25,* 225–233.

Connor, M. K., Smith, L. G., Fryer, A., Erickson, S., Fryer, S., & Drake, J. (1986). Future Fit: A cardiovascular health education and fitness project in an after-school setting. *Journal of School Health, 56,* 329–333.

Cox, C. (1982). An interaction model of client health behavior: Theoretical prescription for nursing. *Advances in Nursing Science, 5,* 41–56.

Deci, E. L., & Ryan, R. M. (1985). *Intrinsic motivation and self-determinism in human behavior.* New York: Plenum.

Desmond, S. M., Price, J. H., Lock, R. S., Smith, D., & Stewart, P. W. (1990). Urban Black and White adolescents' physical fitness status and perceptions of exercise. *Journal of School Health, 60,* 220–226.

Dishman, R. K. (Ed.). (1988). *Exercise adherence: Its impact on public health.* Champaign, IL: Human Kinetics.

Dishman, R. K. (Ed.). (1994). *Advances in exercise adherence.* Champaign, IL: Human Kinetics.

Docherty, D. (Ed.). (1996). *Measurement in pediatric exercise science.* Champaign, IL: Human Kinetics.

Downey, A. M., Frank, G. C., Webber, L. S., Harsha, D. W., Virgilio, S. J., Franklin, F. A., & Berenson, G. S. (1987). Implementation of "Heart Smart:" A cardiovascular school health promotion program. *Journal of School Health, 57,* 98–104.

Eccles, J. S., & Harold, R. D. (1991). Gender differences in sports involvement: Applying the Eccles' expectancy-value model. *Journal of Applied Sport Psychology, 3,* 7–35.

Edmundson, E., Parcel, G. S., Perry, C. L., Feldman, H. A., Smyth, M., Johnson, C. C., Layman, A., Bachman, K., Perkins, T., Smith, K., & Stone, E. (1996). The effects of the child and adolescent trial for cardiovascular health intervention on psychosocial determinants of cardiovascular disease risk behavior among third-grade students. *American Journal of Health Promotion, 10,* 217–225.

Epstein, L. H., Saelens, B. E., Myers, M. D., & Vito, D. (1997). Effects of decreasing sedentary behaviors on activity choice in obese children. *Health Psychology, 16,* 107–113.

Epstein, L. H., Valoski, A., Wing, R. R., & McCurley, J. (1990). Ten-year follow-up of behavioral, family-based treatment for obese children. *Journal of the American Medical Association, 264,* 2519–2523.

Farrand, L. L., & Cox, C. L. (1993). Determinants of positive health behavior in middle childhood. *Nursing Research, 42,* 208–213.

Fishbein, M., & Ajzen, I. (1975). *Belief, attitude, intention and behavior: An introduction to theory and research.* Reading, MA: Addison-Wesley.

Garcia, A. W., George, T. R., Coviak, C., Antonakos, C., & Pender, N. J. (1997). *The child/adolescent activity log: A comprehensive and feasible measure of leisure-time physical activity.* Manuscript submitted for publication.

Garcia, A. W., Norton-Broda, M. A., Frenn, M., Coviak, C., Pender, N. J., & Ronis, D. L. (1995). Gender and developmental differences in exercise beliefs among youth and prediction of their exercise behavior. *Journal of Adolescent Health, 65,* 213–319.

Garcia, A. W., Pender, N. J., Antonakos, C. L., & Ronis, D. L. (1997). *Changes in exercise beliefs and behaviors of adolescents across the elementary to junior high transition.* Manuscript submitted for publication.

Godin, G., & Shephard, R. J (1986). Psychosocial factors influencing intentions to exercise of young students from grades 7 to 9. *Research Quarterly for Exercise and Sport, 57,* 41–52.

Gruber, J. J. (1986). Physical activity and self-esteem development in children: A meta-analysis. In G. Stull & H. Eckert (Eds.), *Effects of physical activity on children: American Academy of Physical Education papers, 19,* (pp. 30–48). Champaign, IL: Human Kinetics.

Hardy, C. J., & Rejecki, W. J. (1989). Not what, but how one feels: The measurement of affect during exercise. *Journal of Sports and Exercise Psychology, 11,* 304–317.

Harrell, J. S., McMurray, R. G., Bangdiwala, S. I., Frauman, A. C., Gansky, S. A., & Bradley, C. B. (1996). The effects of a school-based intervention to reduce cardiovascular disease risk factors in elementary school children: The Cardiovascular Health in Children (CHIC) study. *Journal of Pediatrics, 128,* 797–805.

Hawkes, J. M., & Holm, K. (1993). Gender differences in exercise determinants. *Nursing Research, 42,* 166–172.

Heath, G. W., Pratt, M., Warren, C. W., & Kann, L. (1994). Physical activity patterns in American high school students. *Archives of Pediatric and Adolescent Medicine, 148,* 1131–1136.

Holcomb, J. D., & Mullen, P. D. (1986). Certified nurse-midwives and health promotion and disease prevention: Results of a national survey. *Journal of Nurse Midwifery, 31,* 141–148.

Janz, N. K., & Becker, M. H. (1984). The health belief model: A decade later. *Health Education Quarterly, 11,* 1–47.

Kelder, S. H., Perry, C. L., & Klepp, K. I. (1993). Community-wide youth exercise program: Long-term outcomes of the Minnesota Heart Health Program and the Class of 1989 study. *Journal of School Health, 63,* 218–223.

Kendzierski, D. (1988). Self-schemata and exercise. *Basic and Applied Social Psychology, 9,* 45–59.

Kendzierski, D. (1990). Exercise self-schemata: Cognitive and behavioral correlates. *Health Psychology, 9,* 69–82.

Killen, J. D., Telch, M. J., Robinson, T. N., Maccoby, N., Taylor, B., & Farquhar, J. W. (1988). Cardiovascular disease risk reduction for tenth graders: A multiple-factor school-based approach. *Journal of the American Medical Association, 260,* 1728–1733.

Klesges, R. C., Shelton, M. L., & Klesges, L. M. (1993). Effects of television on metabolic rate: Potential implications for childhood obesity. *Pediatrics, 91,* 281–286.

Kolody, B., & Sallis, J. F. (1995). A prospective study of ponderosity, body image, self-concept, and psychological variables in children. *Developmental and Behavioral Pediatrics, 16,* 1–5.

Lau, R. R., Quadrel, M. J., & Hartman, K. A. (1990). Development and change of young adults' preventive health beliefs and behaviors: Influence from parents and peers. *Journal of Health and Social Behavior, 31,* 240–259.

Leidy, N. K., Abbott, R. D., & Fedenko, K. M. (1997). Sensitivity and reproducibility of the dual-mode actigraph under controlled levels of activity intensity. *Nursing Research. 46,* 5–11.

Luepker, R. V., Perry, C. L., McKinlay, S. M., Nader, P. R., Parcel, G. S., Stone, E. J., Webber, L. S., Elder, J. P., Feldman, H. A., Johnson, C. C., Kelder, S. H., & Wu, M. (1996). Outcomes of a field trial to improve children's dietary patterns and physical activity: The child and adolescent trial for cardiovascular health (CATCH). *Journal of the American Medical Association, 275,* 768–776.

Madsen, J., Sallis, J. F., Rupp, J. W., Senn, K. L., Patterson, T. L., Atkins, C. J., & Nader, P. R. (1993). Process variables as predictors of risk factor changes in a family health behavior change program. *Health Education Research, 8,* 193–204.

Marcus, B. H., Rossi, J. S., Selby, V. C., Niaura, R. S., & Abrams, D. B. (1992). The stages and processes of exercise adoption and maintenance in a worksite sample. *Health Psychology, 11,* 386–395.

Mason, D. J., & Redeker, N. (1993). Measurement of activity. *Nursing Research, 42,* 87–92.

McAuley, E., & Courneya, K. S. (1992). Self-efficacy relationships with affective and exertional responses to exercise. *Journal of Applied Social Psychology, 22,* 312–326.

McGinnis, J. M. (1985). The national children and youth fitness study: Introduction. *Journal of Physical Education, Recreation and Dance, 56*(1), 44.

McKenzie, T. L., Sallis, J. F., Nader, P. R., Broyles, S. L., & Nelson, J. A. (1992). Anglo- and Mexican-American preschoolers at home and at recess: Activity patterns and environmental influences. *Journal of Developmental and Behavioral Pediatrics, 13,* 173–180.

McMurray, R. G., Bradley, C. B., Harrell, J. S., Bernthal, P. R., Frauman, A. C., & Bangidawala, S. I. (1993). Parental influences on childhood fitness and activity patterns. *Research Quarterly for Exercise and Sport, 64,* 249–255.

Montoye, H. J., Kemper, H. C. G., Saris, W. H. M., & Washburn, R. A. (1996). *Measuring physical activity and energy expenditure.* Champaign, IL: Human Kinetics.

Moore, L. L., Lombardi, D. A., White, M. J., Campbell, J. L., Oliveria, S. A., & Ellison, R. C. (1991). Influence of parents' physical activity levels on activity levels of young children. *Journal of Pediatrics, 118,* 215–219.

Nader, P. R., Sallis, J. F., Patterson, T. L., Abramson, I. S., Rupp, J. W., Senn, K. L., Atkins, C. J., Roppe, B. E., Morris, J. A., Wallace, J. P., & Vega, W. A. (1989). A family approach to cardiovascular risk reduction: Results from the San Diego Family Health Project. *Health Education Quarterly, 16,* 229–244.

Pate, R. R., & Shephard, R. J. (1989). Characteristics of physical fitness in youth. In C. V. Gisolfi & D. R. Lamb (Eds.), *Perspectives in exercise science and sports medicine: Youth, exercise, and sport* (Vol. 2, pp. 1–45). Carmel, IN: Cooper.

Patterson, T. L., Sallis, J. F., Nader, P. R., Rupp, J. W., McKenzie, T. L., Roppe, B., & Bartok, P. W. (1988). Direct observation of physical activity and dietary behaviors in a structured environment: Effects of a family-based health promotion program. *Journal of Behavioral Medicine, 11,* 447–458.

Pender, N. J. (1996). *Health promotion in nursing practice* (3rd ed.). Stanford, CT: Appleton & Lange.

Pivarnik, J. M., Bray, M. S., Hergenroeder, A. C., Hill, R. B., & Wong, W. W. (1995). Ethnicity affects aerobic fitness in U.S. girls. *Medicine and Science in Sports and Exercise, 27,* 1635–1638.

Prochaska, J. O., & DiClemente, C. C. (1984). *The transtheoretical approach: Crossing traditional boundaries of change.* Homewood, IL: Dow Jones-Irwin.

Prochaska, J. O., Norcross, J. C., & DiClemente, C. C. (1994). *Changing for good.* New York: Avon.

Purath, J., Lansinger, T., & Ragheb, C. (1995). Cardiac risk evaluation for elementary school children. *Public Health Nursing, 12,* 189–195.

Reynolds, K. D., Killen, J. D., Bryson, S. W., Maron, D. J., Taylor, C. B., Maccoby, N., & Farquhar, J. W. (1990). Psychosocial predictors of physical activity in adolescents. *Preventive Medicine, 19,* 541–551.

Robinson, T. N., Hammer, L. D., Killen, J. D., Kraemer, H. C., Wilson, D. M., Hayward, C., & Taylor, C. B. (1993). Does television viewing increase obesity and reduce physical activity? Cross-sectional and longitudinal analyses. *Pediatrics, 91,* 273–280.

Rogers, R. W. (1975). A protection motivation theory of fear appeals and attitude change. *Journal of Psychology, 91,* 93–114.

Rowland, T. W. (1990). *Exercise and children's health.* Champaign, IL: Human Kinetics.

Sallis, J. F., Buono, M. J., Roby, J. J., Micale, F. G., & Nelson, J. A. (1993). Seven-day recall and other physical activity self-reports in children and adolescents. *Medicine and Science in Sports and Exercise, 25,* 99–108.

Sallis, J. F., Simons-Morton, B. G., Stone, E. J., Corbin, C. B., Epstein, L. H., Faucette, N., Iannotti, R. J., Killen, J. D., Klesges, R. C., Petray, C. K., Rowland, T. W., & Taylor, W. C. (1992). Determinants of physical activity and interventions in youth. *Medicine and Science in Sports and Exercise, 24,* S248–S257.

Simons-Morton, B. G., McKenzie, T. J., Stone, E., Mitchell, P., Osganian, V., Strikmiller, P. K., Ehlinger, S., Cribb, P., & Nader, P. R. (1997). Physical activity in a multiethnic population of third graders in four states. *American Journal of Public Health, 87,* 45–50.

Simons-Morton, B. G., Parcel, G. S., Baranowski, T., Forthofer, R., & O'Hara, N. M. (1991). Promoting physical activity and a healthful diet among children: Results of a school-based intervention study. *American Journal of Public Health, 81,* 986–991.

Simons-Morton, B. G., Taylor, W. C., Snider, S. A., & Huang, I. W. (1993). The physical activity of fifth-grade students during physical education. *American Journal of Public Health, 83,* 262–265.

Simons-Morton, B. G., Taylor, W. C., Snider, S. A., Huang, I., & Fulton, J. E. (1994). Observed levels of elementary and middle school children's physical activity during physical education classes. *Preventive Medicine, 23,* 437–441.

Stucky-Ropp, R. C., & DiLorenzo, T. M. (1993). Determinants of exercise in children. *Preventive Medicine, 22,* 880–889.

Taggart, A. C., Taggart, J., & Siedentop, D. (1986). Effects of a home-based activity program: A study with low fitness elementary school children. *Behavior Modification, 10,* 487–507.

Tappe, M. K., Duda, J. L., & Ehrnwald, P. M. (1989). Perceived barriers to exercise among adolescents. *Journal of School Health, 59,* 153–155.

Taylor, W. C., Baranowski, T., & Sallis, J. F. (1994). Family determinants of childhood physical activity: A social-cognitive model. In R. K. Dishman (Ed.), *Advances in exercise adherence* (pp. 319–342). Champaign, IL: Human Kinetics.

Trost, S. G., Pate, R. R., Dowda, M., Saunders, R., Ward, D. S., & Felton, G. (1996). Gender differences in physical activity and determinants of physical activity in rural fifth grade children. *Journal of School Health, 66,* 145–150.

U.S. Department of Health and Human Services. (1990). *Healthy people 2000: National health promotion and disease prevention objectives.* Washington, DC: U.S. Department of Health and Human Services, U.S. Public Health Service.

U.S. Department of Health and Human Services. (1996). *Physical activity and health: A report of the Surgeon General.* Atlanta, GA: U.S. Department of Health and Human Services, Centers for Disease Control and Prevention, National Center for Chronic Disease Prevention and Health Promotion.

Vallerand, R. J. (1987). Antecedents of self-related affects in sports: Preliminary evidence on the intuitive-reflective appraisal model. *Journal of Sport Psychology, 9,* 61–182.

Wadden, T. A., Foster, G. D., Stunkard, A. J., & Linowitz, J. R. (1989). Dissatisfaction with weight and figure in obese girls: Discontent but not depression. *International Journal of Obesity, 13,* 89–97.

Wardle, J., & Marsland, L. (1990). Adolescent concerns about weight and dieting: A social-developmental perspective. *Journal of Psychosomatic Research, 34,* 377–391.

Zakarian, J. M., Hovell, M. F., Hofstetter, C. R., Sallis, J. F., & Keating, K. J. (1994). Correlates of vigorous exercise in a predominantly low SES and minority high school population. *Preventive Medicine, 23,* 314–321.

Chapter 7

Health Promotion in Old Age

Susan M. Heidrich

School of Nursing

University of Wisconsin—Milwaukee

ABSTRACT

The empirical literature on health promotion in old age was reviewed. A developmental perspective was used to examine 42 studies: studies relating health behaviors to health outcomes, descriptive studies of health promotion in old age, studies of the outcomes of health promotion programs in old age, and studies of factors related to older adults' participation in health promotion activities. In general, elderly adults perceived health promotion activities as beneficial, engaged in health behaviors more frequently than younger adults, and participated in community-based and other health promotion programs. There is little definitive evidence that health promotion activities result in better health outcomes for older adults, however. Identifying appropriate outcomes related to health promotion in old age is a critical need.

Keywords: Health Promotion, Health Behaviors, Health Practices, Health Lifestyle, Old Age, Aging

This chapter includes a review of the empirical literature on health promotion in old age. The focus on old age is important for a number of reasons. First, the aging of the population means that large numbers of people will soon be entering old age, which is the time of life when the majority of health care use, expenditure, and cost occurs. For this reason, efforts at health promotion are seen as potentially of great benefit in reducing the costs of health care. There are two conflicting views in the literature about health promotion in old age, however. One view holds that health promotion efforts in old age are beneficial to both the individual and society because they potentially extend the healthy years of life while compressing the years of disability through disease prevention. They may also increase the quality of life by limiting the impact of disease and illness, allowing older adults to remain independent and able to engage in meaningful pursuits. A number of assumptions underlie the positive view of the efficacy of health promotion and disease prevention in old age. One is that aged persons are able to change their behaviors regarding health. A second is that these behavior changes will result in more positive outcomes, that is, they will have an effect.

An opposing view of health promotion in old age is that such efforts are of limited benefit because the positive effects of health promotion efforts are a result of lifelong health practices, thus to begin health promotion in old age is too late to reap any positive effects. This position is sometimes couched in cost-benefit terms. A related view is that aged persons are resistant to health promotion efforts based on an assumption that learning new behaviors is difficult in old age and that lifelong health practices are resistant to change. Some of the research efforts to date have examined which of these perspectives is closest to the truth.

This review was conducted from a developmental perspective. That is, we considered whether age is an important variable in the study of health promotion. In what ways does age influence health promotion or the precursors, mediators, or outcomes of health promotion efforts? Answers to these questions are important in tailoring nursing interventions that take into account individual and developmental differences in behavior.

For the purposes of this review, health promotion is defined broadly as strategies related to individual lifestyle behaviors that influence health (e.g., physical activity, nutrition), health protection strategies (e.g., fall prevention, oral health), and disease prevention strategies (e.g., health counseling, screening, immunizations). An objective of *Healthy People 2000* (U.S. Department of Health and Human Services [USDHHS], 1991) related to people over 65, focuses on improving functional independence, not just length of life, and increasing the years of healthy life.

This review is organized in four sections. The first section reviews articles relating age and health behaviors to particular outcomes, generally mortality. The second section consists of descriptive studies of health behaviors or health promotion activities in old age. The third section addresses outcomes related to health promotion programs for older adults. The last section is concerned with factors related to older adults' participation in health promotion activities.

CRITERIA FOR REVIEW

This review was limited to research articles published since 1980 in peer-reviewed journals. Articles included examined either health promotion in elderly persons only or age differences in some aspect of health promotion, with at least one age group of the study being elderly persons. Old age was defined as 65 years or older. This cut-off was based on the current convention in gerontological research that "young-old" are those aged 65 to 74, "middle-old" are those aged 75 to 84, and "old-old" are those aged 85 and over. However, some studies were included in which the age range extended somewhat lower (e.g., 55 years). The intent was to exclude primarily middle-aged samples who generally have different health profiles and lower health care usage rates than the elderly.

This review was also limited to research that examined health promotion or health behaviors in a comprehensive manner. The studies were concerned with a range of health behaviors or practices. This is in contrast to numerous studies (not reviewed) that examine one specific health-promoting or disease-preventing behavior or intervention. Typically, the range of health behaviors studied jointly or separately included: exercise, nutrition, immunization, stress management, oral health, smoking cessation, fall prevention, and screening and early diagnosis of cancer, cardiovascular disease, arthritis, osteoporosis, depression, and diabetes. Examining each of these topics independently is beyond the scope of this chapter. It should be noted, however, that much current and important research on health promotion interventions and outcomes in old age focuses on single behaviors. Also, although not planned, all of the studies reviewed were of community-dwelling persons. Despite great need, there is little research involving nursing home residents or the institutionalized elderly.

The literature search used three computer databases: the Cumulative Index of Nursing and Allied Health Literature (CINAHL) from 1982 to 1996, MEDLINE from 1980 to 1996, and PsycLIT from 1980 to 1996. The search concentrated most heavily on studies of the last 10 years, however. These searches were augmented with archival methods. The following terms were searched: "health promotion and aging," "health behaviors and aging," "successful aging," "disease prevention and aging," "health beliefs and aging," "wellness and aging," "self-care and aging," and "quality of life and aging." For each of these, health promotion activities or behaviors had to have been included as a variable. For example, a study examining successful aging would only be reviewed if health promotion activities were linked to successful aging in some way. In addition, searches were conducted by names of authors who are known researchers in the area of health promotion. The search was restricted to English-language articles.

HEALTH BEHAVIORS AND HEALTH OUTCOMES: LONGITUDINAL STUDIES

In the 1970s, an association was found between mortality and seven common health practices: physical activity, cigarette smoking, alcohol consumption, obesity, sleeping habits, daily consumption of breakfast, and snacking between meals (Belloc, 1973; National Center for Health Statistics [NCHS], 1979a, 1979b). This sparked numerous investigations into disease prevention and health promotion efforts. These efforts dovetailed with nursing's commitment to wellness and the enhancement of health, and spurred research in nursing and other disciplines regarding health promotion. It was not clear from the early studies linking health habits to mortality whether this association continued into old age, however. This question is important because it speaks to the efficacy of health promotion activities in old age and to the cost–benefit ratio of spending health care dollars on health promotion in old age.

Four studies were reviewed that examined the relationship between health practices and health outcomes in old age. Two studies examined this relationship for old adults only (Branch & Jette, 1984; Strawbridge, Camacho, Cohen, & Kaplan, 1993), and two compared age groups (Breslow & Enstrom, 1980; Kaplan, Seeman, Cohen, Knudsen, & Guralnik, 1987).

Branch and Jette (1984), using data from the Massachusetts Health Panel Study, examined the relationship between five health practices and mortality in individuals aged 65 and over who were interviewed in 1974, 1976, and 1980. After controlling for age, socioeconomic status, and baseline health status, no significant predictors of mortality in men were found; and only one practice, never smoking, predicted mortality in women. Strawbridge et al. (1993) examined predictors of change in functional health (e.g., ability to perform instrumental and other activities of daily living) over 6 years in 356 adults, aged 65 and over, from the Alameda County study. The Alameda County studies included data on seven health practices as well as demographic, personality, and social support measures. In this study, the number of positive health practices performed was related to increased functional health over 6 years, but the specific predictors differed for men versus women. For men, these were income, education, marital status, never smoking, physical activity, and regular social contact. For women, predictors were never smoking, going out, regular social contact, and internal health locus of control.

Two studies in which age groups were compared suggested that the relationship between health practices and mortality persists in old age (Breslow & Enstrom, 1980; Kaplan et al., 1997). Breslow and Enstrom found that the number of health practices had an inverse relationship with mortality in 6,928 adults in the Alameda Study who were followed from 1965 to 1974. This relationship persisted at older ages, but was weaker. How these analyses were performed was not explicitly described in the article, however. Kaplan et al. examined 17-year mortality in three age cohorts from the Alameda County Study (38–49, 50–59, and 60–74 at baseline). After adjusting for gender, race, and baseline health status, smoking and physical activity were related to mortality in all three age groups.

The majority of these studies support the relationship between health practices and mortality in old age. The strengths of these studies are that they were longitudinal and based on probability samples. Only a few health behaviors have typically been included in these studies, however, and many health behaviors and practices associated with disease prevention and health promotion were not examined (e.g., screening, immunizations, stress reduction). There is also little evidence to suggest which health practice or combination of health practices might be affecting mortality or which individuals might benefit most from positive health practices. It is also unclear whether these results were due to a lifetime of healthy living leading to a selective survival effect in old age or whether changing health practices when one is already old can still affect mortality. Only one study (Strawbridge et al., 1993) examined an outcome other than mortality: functional health. Given the prevalence of chronic illness in old age, outcomes such as functional health, which are typically viewed as important to quality of life in old age, may be even more important than mortality when assessing the impact of health promotion at older ages.

Descriptive Studies of Health Behaviors and Their Correlates, Patterns, and Predictors

A number of studies have examined correlates, patterns, and predictors of health behaviors and health promotion activities. These studies have been grouped into two categories: those examining whether health promotion behaviors and their correlates, patterns, or predictors differ for different age groups and those examining correlates, patterns, and predictors of health promotion activities in samples of older adults only.

Age Differences in Health Behaviors and Their Correlates, Patterns, and Predictors

Before health promotion was studied empirically, conventional wisdom was that older adults would be less likely to engage in health behaviors because by old age it was too late for changes in lifestyle behaviors to make any significant differences in health outcomes. National surveys in the 1970s (Belloc, 1973; Breslow & Enstrom, 1980; NCHS, 1979a, 1979b) demonstrated, however, that health practices were more, rather than less, prevalent at older ages. This led to studies conducted to specifically examine the relationship between age and health behaviors.

Prohaska, Leventhal, Leventhal, and Keller (1985) and Leventhal and Prohaska (1986) examined age differences in the frequency and perceived efficacy of 21 health practices in 396 adults aged 20 to 89. The 21 health practices included 15 health actions and 6 cognitive/affective health strategies, thus increasing the domain of health behaviors from the typical 7 that had been studied in the past. They found that the frequency of 10 of 15 health actions and 4 of 6 cognitive/affective strategies significantly increased from young adulthood to old age. There were no age differences in the perceived efficacy of these behaviors. That is, young adults perceived these activities to be just as important to health as did older adults, but the young adults practiced them less frequently.

Similarly, Bausell (1986) used telephone interviews of 1,254 randomly selected adults, including 177 aged 65 and over, to examine the frequency and efficacy of 20 health behaviors. These included four safety, seven dietary, two health monitoring, and seven general lifestyle behaviors. Compared to young adults, the elderly were more compliant with recommendations for 9 of the 20, particularly for diet, blood pressure monitoring, and home safety. They were less likely to engage in vigorous exercise or visit the dentist. The older adults also perceived health behaviors as more efficacious than younger adults.

Finally, Walker, Volkan, Sechrist, and Pender (1988) examined age differences in a health-promoting lifestyle and its correlates. A convenience sample of 452 adults, aged 18 to 88, responded to questionnaires that included the Health Promoting Lifestyle Profile (HPLP) (Walker, Sechrist, & Pender, 1987). The HPLP is a 48-item scale assessing the frequency of health-promoting behaviors in six areas: self-actualization, health responsibility, exercise, nutrition, interpersonal support, and stress management. Older adults had significantly higher scores (meaning more frequent health-promoting behaviors) for the total HPLP and for the health responsibility, nutrition, and stress-management subscales. HPLP total and subscale scores were also regressed on age, marital status, income, employment status, and gender. Age explained the most variance in health responsibility, nutrition, and stress management and was also a significant predictor of self-actualization.

These studies are consistent with previous surveys indicating that older adults are as likely or more likely to engage in positive health practices as young or middle-aged adults. They also extended the range of health practices and included health-promoting activities related to social, cognitive, and affective strategies that have been implicated in more positive health outcomes. Because they are all cross-sectional, these studies did not answer the question of whether adults are more likely to change to health-promoting lifestyles as they age or whether these findings reflect lifelong differences in health practices that persist into old age. These studies also did not address whether the broader range of health practices examined was related to any health outcomes or mortality. Comparisons across studies are also difficult because of the different kinds of measures used to assess health behaviors, from simple checklists to more comprehensive instruments like the HPLP. In addition, the few studies that examined age difference did not take into account the health status of the respondents and whether changes in health status with age are related to changes in the frequency of or perceptions about health behaviors.

Correlates, patterns, and predictors of health behaviors in old age.
Seventeen descriptive studies were reviewed that examined health behaviors in samples restricted to older adults. Some examined health behaviors in specific samples of older adults (e.g., older women, rural elders), whereas others examined specific variables theoretically related to health promotion practices (e.g., health locus of control). Thus, in contrast to most of the studies previously reviewed, a number of these studies had a theoretical basis. By type of sample or conceptual model there was an insufficient number of studies to come to conclusions about proposed relationships. For this reason, these studies are reviewed together to give an indication of the range of demographic and other variables examined in relation to health behaviors. A number of these studies were also concerned with whether different health behaviors are correlated. That is, are individuals likely to engage in a set of health behaviors or are these behaviors essentially independent?

Jensen, Counte, and Glandon (1992), using data from the first phase of a 3-year longitudinal study, interviewed enrollees in a health maintenance organization (HMO) ($n = 258$) and a random sample of community controls ($n = 144$), aged 62 and over. The majority were White females. This investigation was based on a health belief model in which internal control expectancies were proposed to predict health maintenance behaviors and subsequent health status. Health maintenance behaviors included a number of health practices as well as a preventive health visit to a health care provider within the last 6 months. Differences between HMO enrollees and controls were not reported in this study. Health maintenance behaviors were predicted by higher socioeconomic status and an internal health locus of control, however. Few significant correlations were found among the different health practices, suggesting that health practices are independent.

Martin and Panicucci (1996) also investigated health locus of control in relation to health behaviors in 40 Black female church members. These women had a mean age of 71 and in contrast to many samples found in studies of health, were primarily of low socioeconomic status, with 50% having less than an eighth-grade education. For the 20 health practices examined, adherence to 17 was found; and high importance ratings were given to all 20. High adherence was significantly correlated ($r = .55$) with self-rated health. Lowest adherence was found for preventive dental care, use of smoke detectors, and use of seat belts, suggesting a need for intervention in these areas. Although the small sample size limits the generalizability of the findings, it is important that support for the importance and practice of preventive health behaviors in an older, Black, less educated female population was identified.

At a hypertension clinic, Whetstone and Reid (1991) interviewed 30 rural volunteers aged 55 to 70 regarding barriers to self-care management of hypertension. Respondents completed a health risk appraisal instrument that included lifestyle behaviors related to health. The authors did not present any data regarding responses to this instrument, however. The authors also identified, from open-ended interview responses, that diet and lack of social support were barriers to self-care management. Again, how these barriers were identified was not explicitly stated. The lack of reporting of both data and methods limits the importance or utility of the findings.

Using a very different approach, Quinn, Johnson, and Martin (1996) examined intraindividual differences in older women's health-seeking behaviors. This study used a single-subject design in which the sample was the number of occasions rather than persons. Data from the Georgia Centenarian study (Poon et al., 1992) regarding health-seeking behaviors and diet were examined in a time-series analysis from four women in their 60's and four in their 80's. For the 60–69-year-olds, health-seeking behaviors consisted of both diet and activity items. For 80–89-year-olds, only activity items were related to health-seeking behaviors. For both groups, the health-seeking behaviors were stable over 100 days, suggesting the traitlike nature of these behaviors in old age.

Six studies examined correlates or predictors of a health-promoting lifestyle using the HPLP. Foster (1992) studied 200 Black volunteers (mean age = 73) at a senior center. Significant correlations were found between the HPLP and a measure of life satisfaction, but not with current health, age, or socioeconomic status. The range of these variables may have been restricted, however. There was a significant inverse relationship between HPLP scores and smoking.

Huck and Armer (1996) recruited 50 Roman Catholic nuns, aged 65 to 89, from a blood pressure screening clinic. The majority had been health care professionals and had 16 years of education. Descriptive data on the HPLP were presented. The highest mean subscale scores were found for nutrition and self-actualization and the lowest for exercise. In open-ended descriptions of health-promoting behaviors, the most frequently named were: exercise, nutrition, contact with health care provider, recreation, and sleep. Although health locus of control was also measured, no analysis in relation to health-promoting behaviors was reported.

In contrast, Speake, Cowart, and Pellet (1989) found significant positive correlations between the HPLP and internal health locus of control in a convenience sample of 297 older adults in Florida (mean age = 72, 29% were Black). Predictors of HPLP were examined in a regression analysis in which age, gender, race, marital status, income, and education were controlled. Both internal health locus of control and perceived health were significant predictors of the HPLP subscales of exercise, nutrition, stress management, interpersonal support, health responsibility, and self-actualization. Conceptually, this study differs from many because perceived health was considered a predictor of a health-promoting lifestyle rather than the outcome. Of course the causal direction cannot be determined from this cross-sectional study.

Speake, Cowart, and Stephens (1991) compared HPLP scores of rural (N = 106) and urban (N = 237) elderly. Participants were recruited from senior centers and fairs. Their mean age was 71, and the rural elderly had a higher proportion of female, Black, poor, and less educated persons. The researcher also examined whether an internal locus of control and better perceived health were related to HPLP scores. Regression analyses indicated that the different subscales of the HPLP had different predictors. The most consistent predictors were current health and locus of control. There were no differences between rural and urban elderly. The researchers suggested this was because the rural and urban counties were adjacent so that the environments were more similar than different.

Riffle, Yoho, and Sams (1989) examined the relationships among HPLP, self-reported health, and social support in 113 older (mean age of 74) Appalachian elderly attending nutrition sites. Mailed and on-site surveys were used, but no information was given regarding response rates. The elders were mostly White, female, poor, with an 11th-grade education. Significant but small (r = .22, .30) correlations were found between HPLP, social support, and self-rated health.

Duffy (1993) hypothesized that HPLP scores would be higher for younger, male, White, married, higher income, higher internal locus of control, lower chance and powerful others locus of control, better perceived health, and higher self-esteem. A convenience sample ($N = 471$) of persons associated with retirement communities or centers, with a mean age of 75 years, was interviewed. The hypotheses were tested using canonical correlations. The majority of the hypotheses were supported except that males with higher income and self-esteem but poorer current health were less likely to exercise or use good nutrition. Higher internal locus of control and self-esteem were related to higher HPLP scores.

Frenn (1996) did not use the HPLP, but did examine a health-promoting lifestyle. She used both interviews and participant observation techniques with 31 older adults, aged 62 to 88, to identify patterns of health-promoting behaviors in older adults. Three main patterns were identified from the qualitative data: maintaining relationships, attending to health behaviors, and staying active. In addition, Frenn described patterns that influence health promotion (e.g., learning about health, making choices in the direction of health) and contextual factors influencing health promotion patterns (e.g., life history, financing health care). The purpose of this study was to develop a theory of health promotion for nursing practice and suggest ways in which models of health promotion need to be expanded, rather than to demonstrate empirical evidence for these relationships.

The six studies using the HPLP were carried out with diverse samples, in terms of ethnicity and socioeconomic factors, which adds to the body of knowledge about the HPLP. A number of the studies examined the same correlates and predictors, for example, locus of control, and offer some evidence that an internal locus of control and better perceived health are related to HPLP. On the other hand, some of the samples were small, nonrepresentative of the elder population, and biased in that many were recruited from senior centers, health fairs, or clinics. These persons may be more likely to be interested in lifestyle modification than other elderly. The researchers did not address the possible conceptual overlap between some of the HPLP subscale and some of the hypothesized predictors. For example, there may be some redundancy in the measures of locus of control and the health responsibility subscale, or there may be redundancy between measures of social support and the interpersonal support subscale. These theoretical and measurement issues have not been clearly delineated. Finally, seven studies broadly identified correlates of health behaviors in old age. Rakowski, Julius, Hickey, and Holter (1987) asked whether there were common predictors across numerous different health practices. They grouped health practices into four conceptual areas: health routines, information seeking, medical and self-examinations, and risk avoidance. The correlates examined were demographic characteristics, number of illnesses, health perceptions (locus of control, concerns, and interference), life outlook (morale and future orientation), and social network. They interviewed 172 community-dwelling adults whose mean age was 75 and who were somewhat more educated, White, and Jewish than the general population of elderly. They found that the most consistent correlates across the four health practice groups were gender (female) and a supportive family environment. Each health practice group also had different predictors, however, and health practice groups did not consistently predict each other, suggesting that health practices are somewhat independent. A strength of this study is its comprehensive approach to identifying correlates. One limitation is that the reliabilities of the health practice scales were quite low.

Hickey, Rakowski, and Julius (1988), using the same data, also examined gender differences in health practices in old age. They found few significant relationships between gender and health practices or the correlates identified in the previous study. The authors speculated that it may be more informative to examine the interaction of age and gender over time because of gender differences in morbidity and changing gender-stereotyped behaviors with age.

Johnson (1991) described the health care practices of a randomly selected sample ($N = 250$) of rural (communities of fewer than 4,000 persons) elders (mean age of 84 years). The majority were women who identified at least one chronic health problem. A 24-item personal lifestyle questionnaire was used that measured the frequency of engaging in health practices. Of the 24 health practices, only 7 were engaged in often in this much older group of rural elderly. Fifty percent reported no yearly physical exam; 64% no dental exams; and 73% no self-breast exam ever. The majority also reported never exercising, rarely getting enough sleep, never using a seat belt, and not communicating problems to another. Nutrition was also poor, but few reported smoking. More frequent health practices were associated with younger age, being female, married, and having more education.

The relationship among social support, health-promotive beliefs, and preventive health behaviors was examined for one wave of a longitudinal study of HMO enrollees (Potts, Hurwicz, Goldstein, & Berkanovic, 1992). The sample consisted of 1,099 mostly female elderly (mean age = 73) with a high-school education. Health-promotive beliefs were the extent to which persons endorsed the importance (on a 5-point scale) of five health behaviors. Regression analyses were used to predict health behaviors after controlling for self-rated health and frailty. Social support predicted six of eight behaviors, but after health beliefs were added, this dropped to three behaviors. Health beliefs and gender (being female) explained the most variance in health behaviors, suggesting that interventions should be aimed at bolstering beliefs in the importance of health behaviors.

Brown and McCreedy (1986) surveyed 386 men and women, aged 55 and over, about the extent of their health practices, correlates of health practices (specifically, age, gender, socioeconomic status, and marital status), and their current health status. Respondents were randomly selected from a 7,000-member senior citizen organization. Three age groups were compared: 55 to 64, 65 to 74, and 75 and over. Health status was measured using an index of symptoms, the number of days activities were limited due to illness, physician visits due to illness in the last 2 weeks, and self-rated health. Health protective behaviors were measured by a checklist of 30 behaviors that comprised five subscales: health practices, safety practices, preventive health care, environmental hazard avoidance, and harmful substances. Respondents practiced an average of 17 health behaviors; the most frequent were nutrition, sleep, and smoking behaviors. The least frequent were flossing teeth and using seatbelts. Age was not related to the number of health behaviors, but gender (female) and education (higher) were. Using stepwise multiple-regression procedures, the most variance in health behaviors found was due to gender, with occupation and marital status having small effects. Within gender the strongest predictor of health behaviors for women was socioeconomic status and for men was being married. There were no differences in health status by age (although self-rated health only was lower in the oldest age group), nor was there any significant relationship between health behaviors and health status.

Bergman-Evans and Walker (1996) examined use of clinical preventive services by older women. Using data from the National Health Interview Survey, compliance with recommendations from the U.S. Preventive Services Task Force regarding screening, counseling, and immunizations by health care providers was examined for 5,574 women in three age groups: 65 to 74, 75 to 84, and 85 and over. In stark contrast to studies concerning self-reported individual health behaviors in old age, low compliance across preventive health behaviors and services was found. For instance, fewer than 1% of women received all of the health-history questions, and only 7% received all recommended exams (e.g., height, weight, blood pressure, visual acuity, hearing, and clinical breast exam). The proportion receiving laboratory exams declined with age; pap smears were the exam with the lowest prevalence. Fifty percent of women received health counseling in at least one area (e.g., diet, exercise), but only 5% received all recommended immunizations.

The discrepancy between the results of the Bergman-Evans and Walker study and others points to some of the gaps in the literature and theory concerning health promotion in old age. Although health promotion as a concept is based on what individuals can do to maximize their health related to lifestyle behaviors, disease prevention also is considered an important aspect of health promotion. Many disease prevention and health-screening activities, and perhaps some health promotion activities for some individuals require interaction with and direction from health care providers. This raises the question of the relative efficacy or importance to health of these different activities. If older adults engage in appropriate health behaviors but do not receive recommended disease prevention interventions, are any positive effects of their individual health promotion activities lost? Are efforts better spent educating older adults to advocate for appropriate preventive health services or educating health care professionals to provide them in terms of both health outcomes and costs?

As a group, these studies support the prevalence of health behaviors and a health-promoting lifestyle in old age. These studies also suggest some early attempts at increasing the generalizability of this finding by examining health behaviors in more socially and culturally diverse samples. In general, however, these studies rely on nonrandom samples with few attempts at comparisons among different cultural, socioeconomic, or at-risk groups. Most studies suggest that gender, income, and education are positively correlated with numerous health promotion activities, but again, specific comparative research has rarely been done. A major limitation of the majority of the studies is the reliance on self-report of health behaviors. Whether self-reports of behavior are valid indicators of actual behaviors is an area that deserves the attention of health promotion researchers. Linkages between expanded health behaviors or health-promoting lifestyles and health outcomes have rarely been made.

HEALTH PROMOTION PROGRAMS—OUTCOMES

A number of studies examined the impact of participation in specific health promotion programs on health outcomes. The actual health promotion pro grams differ in substantial ways as do the outcomes examined, making comparisons and conclusions difficult. Some of these studies were reports of demonstration projects, and replication studies have not been done. Studies reviewed in this section have been grouped by method to make comparisons more meaningful. The first group of studies are those in which volunteers were used and control groups were sometimes employed. The second group of studies used randomized trials.

Health Promotion Programs—Volunteer Samples

A number of studies examined the outcomes of community-based health promotion programs for older adults. Barbaro and Noyes (1984) compared attenders and nonattenders at a monthly wellness program held at a congregate living center for older adults. Of the 300 residents, approximately 30% (mean age = 82) attended at least some of the sessions, which were based on health topics identified by residents. Six months postprogram, residents were asked about behavior changes made regarding skin care, bowel habits, memory and learning, nutrition, vision, and exercise. Attenders were more likely to say they had changed their behavior compared to nonattenders in four of the six areas. Actual behavior was not assessed.

"Staying Healthy After Fifty" was a community-based health promotion project studied in 16 communities to assess its effects on participants' satisfaction, perceived benefits, direct effects (health actions, health skills, health care costs), and indirect effects (health status, use of physician services, and health-related quality of life) (Benson et al., 1989; Simmons et al., 1989). The demonstration project, carried out from 1985 to 1987, consisted of eleven 2-hour sessions covering health concerns, emergencies, lifestyle, consumer planning, and instituting a self-change plan. These were presented to groups of 15 to 20 persons. In addition, 26 workshops were held to prepare 38 instructors and 390 educational team members to teach the workshops. Participants in the demonstration project were 2,600 individuals whose mean age was 66. The majority were female, had a high-school education, reported at least one chronic illness, and 70% were American Association of Retired Persons (AARP) members (AARP was one sponsor of the project). Simmons et al. and Benson et al. reported on data from 161 participants and 161 neighbors (comparison group) from 20 of these courses in 16 communities. Preprogram, postprogram, and 6-months-posttest data were compared. Participants scored higher than nonparticipants on their perceived ability to perform self-care tasks (e.g., taking temperature, blood pressures, pulse), use of seat belts, changes in diet, exercise, and stress reduction. There were no differences in health perceptions, health status, or physician usage, or in variables related to quality of life (life satisfaction, social activities) between pre- and postresponses.

A similar community-based health promotion project, the "Self Care for Senior Citizens Program," consisted of 13 2-hour classes on clinical topics and lifestyle behavior changes held in three demographically similar communities (Nelson et al., 1984). Participants were 415 women, aged 60 and over, who generally were high-school educated but low income. Two hundred and four attended the program. The control group ($n = 126$) attended one health education lecture on foot care and hypertension. Pretests and 3- and 12-month posttests were conducted on health skills and health behaviors. Participants reported more confidence than controls in performing health skills (e.g., taking a pulse), more attempts at lifestyle changes (e.g., weight loss, exercise), and more confidence in communicating with physicians. There were no significant group differences in self-reported health status or health care usage.

Similar results were thus found for two different community-based health promotion programs. Although the programs were effective in teaching some positive health behaviors, no significant changes in health outcomes were evident.

In a different vein, Belcher (1990) compared three models of care delivery in a 5-year trial at the Seattle Veterans Affairs Medical Center. The models were: (a) physician oriented, meaning that physicians were educated and motivated to provide preventive services; (b) patient education—patients were given written materials advising them to ask their physicians for certain preventive services; (c) health promotion, in which patients self-referred and were followed by nurse practitioners who practiced health-promotion-based care; and (d) a usual-care control group. The health promotion clinic services included a physical exam and health history, screening laboratory tests, immunizations, and health counseling. Patients were randomized to all but the health promotion clinic. Because of the extra clinic visits required for these activities compared to the other models, veterans had to volunteer to attend. Participants were 1,224 veterans with a mean age of 59; the majority were chronically ill. At baseline, less than 25% of participants had received any health promotion care. At the end of the trial, there was no change in baseline for any of the groups except the health promotion clinic. This group of patients had a three- to fourfold increase in the number of health promotion activities recorded in their charts. There were also higher participation rates and higher satisfaction ratings in this group compared to the other models. This study did not examine whether these differences were related to any changes in health outcomes or costs of care.

Except for one (Belcher, 1990), these studies relied on volunteers' attendance at educational programs. A positive aspect of a number of these studies is their use of control groups to assess the effect of educational health promotion programs. In the Belcher study, the program also consisted of actual health care delivery. A difficulty with all of these studies is that it is not known what aspect of a program might be responsible for changes in health behaviors or perceptions. Is the critical component the actual content of the program, the person delivering the program, the time (e.g., number of classes), or the context of the program in terms of overall health care delivery? These studies also do not explain why some health behaviors are affected and others are not. Again, this is a critical question for health promotion researchers. Finally, these studies, although a number have adequate and somewhat representative samples, again rely mainly on self-report of changes in behaviors or in perceptions and offer little information about actual behavior change or change in health outcomes.

Randomized Trials

Four studies employing randomization with control and experimental groups were reviewed. Vickery, Golaszerski, Wright, and Kalmer (1988) examined the impact of a health promotion program aimed at encouraging self-care on health care use outcomes in 1,294 Medicare Health Maintenance Organization enrollees. Medicare patients in the HMO were randomly assigned to an experimental or control (usual treatment) group. The intervention consisted of written materials including two reference books, a monthly newsletter, lifestyle brochures and self-care education packages, and a telephone intervention service. Service usage was measured 1 year before and 1 year after entry into the program. Eleven risk behaviors (e.g., exercise, smoking, seat belt use, immunization, blood pressure) were measured at 6 and 12 months after the program. No differences in overall use were found; however, there was a decrease in the number of high service users in the experimental compared to the control groups. This resulted in an overall cost savings for the experimental group. The authors suggested that health education programs are feasible for older adults, however, the mechanism by which health education led to changes in behavior needs to be identified.

In a similar study, Mayer et al. (1994) examined the impact of a preventive services program on health behaviors in 1,800 enrollees in a Medicare HMO. Again, participants were randomly assigned to the preventive services or control (usual care) groups. The preventive services package consisted of clinical tests, immunizations, individualized health risk appraisals with individual counseling, and group health promotion sessions covering physical and mental health topics. Mayer et al. reported on a 1-year follow-up of health behaviors. At baseline, the experimental and control groups were comparable in terms of demographic (mean age = 73, the majority were White females with higher education and income) and health risk status ("good" health by self-rating). At 12 months, the experimental group scored significantly higher than the control group in frequency of aerobic exercise, other exercise, decreased dietary fat, and decreased caffeine. There were no differences in blood pressure, sodium intake, general nutrition, and safety. Health care usage or health status was not reported in this article.

Williams et al. (1996), using the same data, attempted to identify specific components of health promotion programs hypothesized to result in improved outcomes. Because previous studies suggested that changes in health attitudes or behaviors did not necessarily result in changes in health status, attention was paid to identifying outcomes for high-risk participants. Three groups of attendees in the prevention group were identified: those attending no health promotion workshops, those attending one or two, and those attending three to four. Smokers and the oldest participants (aged 75 and over) were more likely to be nonattenders, but generally attendance was not associated with any specific health risks, illnesses, or social–psychological factors. Attendance had no effect on measures of physical health status but was associated with an increase in scores on a coping index, suggesting improved coping skills.

Bank of America retirees ($N = 4,712$) participated in a randomized trial of a preventive services program (Fries, Bloch, Harrington, Richardson, & Beck, 1993). In this case, there were two experimental groups. The first group received an individualized health promotion program by mail based on a health-risk assessment. The second experimental group received only the health risk appraisal in year 1, but the full intervention in year 2. The control group received usual care, and only claims data were collected. There was a significant reduction in health risks for both experimental groups after 2 years. This reduction was found in three age groups: 55 to 64, 65 to 74, and 75 and over. There was also a 10% reduction in claims in the experimental groups compared to the control. The risk factors for which there was a significant change at 12 months included systolic blood pressure, seat belt use, weight, salt intake, dietary fat, and total score. No differences were found for dietary cholesterol, smoking, alcohol use, exercise, and stress levels. Although specific physical health parameters were not assessed, the change in claims data suggested better physical health outcomes for the health promotion groups.

Overall, these studies, with more rigorous designs and somewhat similar health promotion interventions, offer some limited support for the impact of health promotion programs. There does appear to be some change in reported health behaviors after participation in structured programs of health promotion. Whether these changes result in better health status is not clear from these studies; however, the time frame is somewhat short (usually 1 or 2 years) for detecting changes in morbidity. Likewise, in terms of the use of preventive services, the data do not clearly indicate a positive impact on health outcomes, although there is some indication of decreased use of health services. Whether decreased usage is an indication of better physical health or some other factor (particularly since most of these samples were drawn from HMOs) is not known, however. Another issue in these studies is the lack of attention to effect size. Although large sample sizes are commendable and necessary when trying to detect small effects, a drawback is that somewhat small effects can achieve statistical significance, but their practical or clinical significance is not clear. These studies, similar to those reviewed in the previous section, also shed little light on which aspects of a health promotion program are of the greatest benefit in terms of outcome. The one study (Williams et al., 1996) that examined the number of sessions attended generally found no differences in outcomes.

What is clear from these studies is that health promotion activities and educational efforts can be used by older adults, and these efforts result in some behavior changes (albeit by self-report) that persist for 1 or 2 years, at least. This is particularly evident from the Medicare studies, which employed random samples more representative of older adults than found in some of the community-based studies.

PARTICIPATION IN HEALTH PROMOTION PROGRAMS

Although the previously reviewed studies suggest that older adults are likely to participate in and benefit from health promotion efforts, a number of studies specifically examined factors related to participation by older adults. Of primary concern is whether those most likely to benefit from health promotion activities actually take part in educational or clinical services. Three studies were reviewed that addressed this question. Buchner and Pearson (1989) investigated factors related to participation in a voluntary 10-week health promotion program offered to all HMO enrollees aged 55 and over in the Group Health Cooperative of Puget Sound. Participants ($n = 103$) from 21 clinics were compared to a random sample ($n = 531$) of nonparticipants. Participants were significantly more likely to be White, better educated, and have higher incomes than nonparticipants, which is similar to previous reports in the literature. Participants were also significantly more likely to report less positive affect and fewer emotional ties than nonparticipants, however. This was true for both men and women.

Durham et al. (1991) examined data from 2,713 members, aged 65 and over, in the same Puget Sound HMO who received health promotion services as part of a demonstration project. Increased participation in health promotion activities was related to younger age and physician involvement, after controlling for chronic illness and proximity to the clinic. Those who were high users of medical services (more than six clinic visits per year) in different age groups were compared to others in terms of participation in health promotion activities. Lower participation was found only for those over the age of 74, particularly if they had multiple chronic illnesses.

Watkins and Kligman (1993) assessed predictors of different attendance patterns at a community-based senior-citizen health promotion program. Lowest attendance was related to lower income, living alone, fewer social contacts, and activity being limited by health problems.

Together these studies suggest that those elders with the most health problems or who may be the most frail or isolated, although not necessarily the oldest, are the least likely to participate in formal health promotion programs. Comparisons are difficult as different studies examined different sets of predictors, however. For instance, some controlled for health status, whereas others did not. Some examined factors like transportation, whereas others did not. It is also not known whether differences among studies may be due to differences in the types of health promotion programs offered; that is, some programs may have been more popular or successful than others due to content, presenters, or the agency involved. Although some studies compared attenders and nonattenders, others examined predictors of high versus low attendance. These differences, again, make conclusions difficult.

SUMMARY AND DIRECTIONS FOR FUTURE RESEARCH

The studies reviewed here indicate that aged adults view health promotion activities as beneficial to their health, engage in numerous health behaviors more frequently than do younger adults, and both participate in and report benefits from health promotion programs. On the other hand, research to date does not provide definitive evidence that health behaviors and health promotion activities result in better health outcomes for older adults. The types of research reviewed here ranged from small, descriptive, cross-sectional studies to large-scale, longitudinal investigations using national probability samples. Given the extremely large number of studies published since 1980 that addressed health behaviors and health promotion, the number concerned with old age is relatively small. Given nursing's long-standing interest in health promotion, the number of studies published in nursing journals seems very small.

A number of important questions and issues should guide further research in this important area. One of the most pressing is identifying appropriate outcomes related to health promotion in old age. Very few of the studies reviewed here examined health status or cost of care outcomes, except in narrowly defined ways (e.g., mortality, self-rated health, physician visits). These are important outcomes but do not take into account important issues of quality of life in old age. Quality of life is an important outcome and may be the most important outcome for aged adults (USDHHS, 1991). Quality-of-life research includes perspectives on successful aging, psychological well-being, and productive aging, as well as physical health status. There is neither a predefined upper limit on quality of health nor on health, however. At what point can one consider life to be of acceptable quality, or that one has successfully or productively aged, or that one is "healthy"? There is no agreed-on reference against which to measure success. Theoretical work examining the links between health promotion activities or a health-promoting lifestyle and important quality of life and other health outcomes is lacking and will be important in guiding future work in this area. Some of the outcomes that should be addressed include functional status, ability to maintain independent living in the community, symptom management, health care utilization, productive activity, and psychological well-being related to mastery, autonomy, control, and positive relations with others (Heidrich & Ryff, 1996).

Few investigators have addressed the important issue of measurement and self-report data, in particular, in the study of health behaviors. No studies were found that examined whether self-reports of behavior or behavior change reflected actual behaviors. Often health behavior measures consisted of checklists with dichotomous format or used Likert scales that have descriptors such as "rarely" and "most of the time." This type of scaling gives little indication of the amount of quality of different health behaviors that may be linked to different types or levels of health outcomes. The validity of these measures remains an open question and needs further research.

Related to scaling problems is the question of whether the relationship between health promotion and health status in old age is linear. Current conceptualizations seem based on the notion that a more healthy lifestyle results in better health. But there may be both lower and upper limits to the effects of health behaviors on health status, particularly in old age.

One way in which these questions, and many others, could be examined is by doing more comparative research and more research on individual differences in health promotion. Older adults are more heterogenous than younger and middle-aged adults in every aspect of behavior. Thus, research from an individual-differences perspective is essential. Although there are some descriptive studies examining health behaviors in different cultural groups, studies using comparison groups are rare. In old age, research comparing frail and healthy elders, individuals with different chronic illnesses that have different profiles of symptoms and functional impairments, and elders living in different environments (e.g., family, neighborhood, and cultural factors) would help in describing the range of health behaviors and factors influencing health behaviors in old age. Theoretical work in this area is also needed to inform hypotheses-testing research and the development of theory-based interventions with older adults. For instance, what interventions or strategies are the most effective and health promoting, and whom do these strategies benefit most?

Further research is also needed to better understand the relationship among different health practices as well as their differential effects on health outcomes. And more thought needs to be given to the question of whether to examine health behaviors individually or together, that is, as a health-promoting lifestyle. The few studies that have examined the relationship among health practices suggest that there is little relationship but are short on explanations as to why. In old age health promotion may mean efforts that can enhance health relative to baseline, and these efforts may be related to specific, individualized behaviors rather than a more global conception of health promotion.

Another important question rarely addressed concerns the developmental profile of health promotion behaviors. Is a health-promoting lifestyle a reflection of lifelong habits or do these behaviors change with age? If health behaviors change with age, what factors influence this change and are these factors related to age or some other characteristics? Identification of these factors could guide interventions tailored to persons of different ages. More attention to developmental theory and research would enrich the study of health promotion.

In summary, there are important theoretical and empirical questions that remain regarding the impact and importance of health promotion in old age. The studies reviewed here provide an important descriptive base to guide future studies that should address the heterogeneity of older adults, the development of health-promoting lifestyles, and the links between health promotion and important health and quality-of-life outcomes in old age. Such research is necessary to inform nursing practice in health promotion and disease prevention over the lifespan.

REFERENCES

Barbaro, E. C., & Noyes, L. E. (1984). A wellness program for a lifecare community. *Gerontologist, 24,* 568–571.

Bausell, R. B. (1986). Health seeking behavior among the elderly. *Gerontologist, 26,* 556–559.

Belcher, D. W. (1990). Implementing preventive services: Success and failure in an outpatient trial. *Archives of Internal Medicine, 150,* 2533–2541.

Belloc, N. B. (1973). Relationship of health practices and mortality. *Preventive Medicine, 2,* 67–81.

Benson, L., Nelson, E. C., Napps, S. E., Roberts, E., Kane-Williams, E., & Salisbury, Z. T. (1989). Self care evaluation of the Staying Healthy After Fifty program. Impact on course participants. *Health Education Quarterly, 16,* 485–508.

Bergman-Evans, D., & Walker, S. N. (1996). The prevalence of clinical preventive services utilization by older women. *Nurse Practitioner, 21,* 88–106.

Branch, L. G., & Jette, A. M. (1984). Personal health practices and mortality among the elderly. *American Journal of Public Health, 74,* 1126–1129.

Breslow, L., & Enstrom, J. E. (1980). Persistence of health habits and their relationship to mortality. *Preventive Medicine, 9,* 469–483.

Brown, J. S., & McCreedy, M. (1986). The hale elderly: Health behavior and its correlates. *Research in Nursing & Health, 9,* 317–329.

Buchner, D. M., & Pearson, D. C. (1989). Factors associated with participation in a community senior health promotion program: A pilot study. *American Journal of Public Health, 79,* 775–777.

Duffy, M. E. (1993). Determinants of health-promoting lifestyles in older persons. *IMAGE: Journal of Nursing Scholarship, 25,* 23–28.

Durham, M. L., Beresford, S., Diehr, P., Grembrowski, D., Hecht, J. A., & Patrick, D. L. (1991). Participation of higher users in a randomized trial of Medicare reimbursement for preventive services. *Gerontologist, 31,* 603–606.

Foster, M. F. (1992). Health promotion and life satisfaction in elderly Black adults. *Western Journal of Nursing Research, 14,* 444–463.

Frenn, M. (1996). Older adults' experience of health promotion: A theory for nursing practice. *Public Health Nursing, 13,* 65–71.

Fries, J. F., Bloch, D. A., Harrington, H., Richardson, N., & Beck, R. (1993). Two year results of a randomized controlled trial of a health promotion program in a retiree population: The Bank of America study. *American Journal of Medicine, 94,* 455–461.

Heidrich, S. M., & Ryff, C. D. (1996). The self in later years of life: Perspectives on psychological well-being. In L. Sperry & H. Prosen (Eds.), *Aging in the 21st century: A developmental perspective* (pp. 73–102). New York: Garland.

Hickey, T., Rakowski, W., & Julius, M. (1988). Preventive health practices among older men and women. *Research on Aging, 10,* 315–328.

Huck, D. G., & Armer, J. M. (1996). Health perceptions and health promoting behaviors among elderly Catholic nuns. *Family and Community Health, 18,* 81–91.

Jensen, J., Counte, M. A., & Glandon, G. L. (1992). Elderly health beliefs, attitudes, and maintenance. *Preventive Medicine, 21,* 483–497.

Johnson, J. (1991). Health-care practices of the rural aged. *Journal of Gerontological Nursing, 17*(8), 15–19.

Kaplan, G. A., Seeman, T. E., Cohen, R. D., Knudsen, L. P., & Guralnik, J. (1987). Mortality among the elderly in the Alameda County Study: Behavioral and demographic risk factors. *American Journal of Public Health, 77,* 307–312.

Leventhal, E. A., & Prohaska, T. R. (1986). Age, symptom interpretation, and health behavior. *Journal of the American Geriatrics Society, 34,* 185–191.

Martin, J. C., & Panicucci, C. L. (1996). Health related practices and priorities: The health behaviors and beliefs of community-living Black older women. *Journal of Gerontological Nursing, 22*(4), 41–48.

Mayer, J. A., Jermanovich, A., Wright, B. L., Adler, J. P., Drew, J. A., & Williams, S. J. (1994). Changes in health behaviors of older adults: The San Diego Medicare Preventive Health Project. *Preventive Medicine, 23,* 127–133.

National Center for Health Statistics. (1979a). *Acute conditions: Incidence and associated disability, United States, July 1977–June 1978.* Series ID-No. 132. Public Health Service. Washington, DC: U.S. Government Printing Office.

National Center for Health Statistics. (1979b). *Physician visits: Volume and interval since last visit, United States—1975.* [Series 10-No. 132.] Public Health Service, Washington, DC: U.S. Government Printing Office.

Nelson, E. C., McHugo, G., Schnurr, P., Devito, C., Roberts, E., Simmons, J., & Zubkoff, W. (1984). Medical self care education for elders: A controlled trial to evaluate impact. *American Journal of Public Health, 74,* 1357–1362.

Poon, L. W., Clayton, G. M., Martin, P., Johnson, M. A., Courtenay, B. C., Sweaney, A. L., Merriam, S. B., Pless, B. S., & Thielman, S. B. (1992). The Georgia centenarian study. *International Journal of Aging and Human Development, 34,* 1–17.

Potts, M. K., Hurwicz, M. L., Goldstein, M. S., & Berkanovic, E. (1992). Social support, health-promotive beliefs and preventive health behaviors among the elderly. *Journal of Applied Gerontology, 11,* 425–440.

Prohaska, T. R., Leventhal, E. A., Leventhal, H., & Keller, M. L. (1985). Health practices and illness cognitions in young, middle aged, and elderly adults. *Journal of Gerontology, 40,* 569–578.

Quinn, M. E., Johnson, M. A., & Martin, P. (1996). Intraindividual and interindividual differences in factors influencing older women's health-seeking behavior. *Health Care for Women International, 17,* 187–196.

Rakowski, W., Julius, M., Hickey, T., & Holter, J. B. (1987). Correlates of preventive health behavior in late life. *Research on Aging, 9,* 331–355.

Riffle, K. J., Yoho, J., & Sams, J. (1989). Health-promoting behaviors, perceived social support, and self-reported health of Appalachian elderly. *Public Health Nursing, 6,* 204–211.

Simmons, T. J., Nelson, E. C., Roberts, E., Salisbury, T. T., Kane-Williams, E., & Denson, P. (1989). A health promotion program: Staying healthy after fifty. *Health Education Quarterly, 16,* 461–472.

Speake, D. L., Cowart, M. E., & Pellet, K. (1989). Health perceptions and lifestyles of the elderly. *Research in Nursing & Health, 12,* 93–100.

Speake, D. L., Cowart, M. E., & Stephens, R. (1991). Healthy lifestyle practices of rural and urban elderly. *Health Values, 15,* 45–51.

Strawbridge, W. J., Camacho, T. C., Cohen, R. D., & Kaplan, G. A. (1993). Gender differences in factors associated with change in physical functioning in old age: A 6 year longitudinal study. *Gerontologist, 33,* 603–609.

U.S. Department of Health and Human Services. (1991). *Healthy people 2000: National health promotion and disease prevention objectives.* [DHHS Publication No. (PHS) 91-50213.] Washington, DC: U.S. Government Printing Office.

Vickery, D. M., Golaszerski, T. J., Wright, E. C., & Kalmer, H. (1988). The effect of self-care interventions on the use of medical services within a Medicare population. *Medical Care, 26,* 580–588.

Walker, S. N., Sechrist, K. R., & Pender, N. J. (1987). The Health-Promoting Lifestyle Profile. Development and psychometric characteristics. *Nursing Research, 36,* 76–81.

Walker, S. N., Volkan, L., Sechrist, K. R., & Pender, N. J. (1988). Health promoting lifestyles of older adults: Comparison with young and middle-aged adults, correlates and patterns. *Advances in Nursing Science, 11,* 76–90.

Watkins, A. J., & Kligman, E. W. (1993). Attendance patterns of older adults in a health promotion program. *Public Health Reports, 108,* 86–90.

Whetstone, W. R., & Reid, J. C. (1991). Health promoting of older adults: Perceived barriers. *Journal of Advanced Nursing, 16,* 1343–1349.

Williams, S. J., Drew, J., Wright, B., Seidman, R., McGan, M., & Boulen, T. C. (1996). Health promotion workshop for seniors: Predictors of attendance and behavioral outcomes. *Journal of Health Education, 27,* 13–20.

Chapter 8

Health Promotion for Family Caregivers of Chronically Ill Elders

BARBARA A. GIVEN
COLLEGE OF NURSING
MICHIGAN STATE UNIVERSITY

CHARLES W. GIVEN
COLLEGE OF HUMAN MEDICINE
MICHIGAN STATE UNIVERSITY

ABSTRACT

Previous research has focused almost exclusively on the burden and the negative effects of caregiving on the primary caregivers of the chronically ill. This prior research has provided a backdrop for understanding the psychological and physical challenges that caregiving incurs. Missing from past research, however, is any focus on the health promotion strategies of this caregiving population. Although some literature focuses on the psychological well-being, few articles deal with the physical health status of caregivers. Fewer yet describe the health promotion strategies that caregivers use to maintain their health.

The chapter reviews existing literature regarding health promotion activities of primary caregivers in the context of articles focused on the psychological and physical health status of caregivers. Health promotion strategies will be discussed, as will recommendations for future research in this topic area.

Keywords: Caregiver, Chronically Ill, Health Promotion, Self-Care, Self-Report, Well-Being

Family caregivers are the key to maintaining the health and well-being of the frail elderly and chronically ill in the community. The role family caregivers play has become critical because of changes in the health care system. Care is becoming more complex external to the acute care setting and, as the aging population grows, the roles of family caregivers will assume even more importance. Given the effects of aging and chronic illness in older adult caregivers, health care providers should become partners with caregivers to assist them in providing care to family members and also to engage in self-care activities to maintain their own health and well-being.

Family caregiving is not a role or activity that individuals typically desire, seek, or expect. The role of the family caregiver is often unexpected and unwanted, but when confronted with a need for care and a sense of family obligations, many wives, husbands, daughters, and sons step forward to become caregivers. Others, however, find themselves providing care because of cultural expectations and obligations rather than out of a personal desire to assist with care. Still other family members become caregivers by default—because they are women, not employed outside of the home, or happen to live close to the care recipient. As caregivers, spouses are the main source of care for the chronically ill elderly; they provide the most extensive and comprehensive care to a disabled spouse; they maintain the caregiver role longer and are more likely to be care providers as well as care managers (Pruchno & Potashnik, 1989). Numerous and various care situations exist (dependent on such factors as race, socioeconomic status, and gender), including those involving patients with severe cognitive deficits (e.g., dementia) and those with serious physical defects (e.g., stroke or cancer). These care situations place varying demands on the caregivers and may influence their health and well-being.

The literature about family caregivers has suggested that due to the role expectations and the chronic stress and strain of caregiving, the deterioration of family caregivers' emotional and physical health can occur (Aneshensel, Pearlin, & Schuler, 1993). Family caregivers struggling with the demands of care and perhaps their own chronic illnesses need to adopt self-care health behaviors to maintain a productive life, to prevent emotional and physical health problems, and to remain in the care provider role. Much scholarly work has been produced in the last 2 decades on caregiver burden and the overall negative effects of caring on the caregiver. This work has broadened the understanding of the problems that occur with caregiving, but a focus on health-promotive behaviors of caregivers for their own health status is absent. It is important to understand the negative effects of the caregiving role and what caregivers do or can do to protect themselves from negative stressors and to maintain their own health.

To facilitate and promote continued family care, health care practitioners must emphasize the caregiver's health status and health behaviors. Social, emotional, physical, financial, and legal changes in a caregiver's life are daily challenges that influence both the care provided to the care recipient and the health status of the caregiver. The caregiving role often demands performance over a long period of time, sometimes years. In order to approach the range of care problems systematically, to modulate the unpleasant effects that problems of care generate, and to postpone personal gratification, the caregiver must develop coping strategies to preserve his or her own health status. Caregivers may, however, fail to engage in self-care and neglect their own health needs because of their focus on the care they provide rather than the care they themselves require. The purpose of this chapter is to examine the state of knowledge of health promotion activities of individuals providing care for the elderly and chronically ill.

Health promotion, as defined for the purposes of this chapter, consists of activities directed toward increasing the level of well-being and actualizing the health potential of individuals, including primary and secondary prevention activities. Primary prevention consists of activities directed toward decreasing dysfunction or disabilities, including active protection against unnecessary stressors. Secondary prevention emphasizes shortening the duration and severity of existing health problems and enabling an individual to function.

LITERATURE-SEARCH PROCESS

When conducting general searches on medical, psychological, social, and family nursing databases, little was found on health promotion or health behaviors of caregivers. English-language publications were searched on the following databases: Cumulative Index to Nursing and Allied Health Literature (CINAHL; 1986 to 1996), MEDLINE (1986 to 1996), Soc Abstracts (1986 to 1996), and Clin Psych (1986 to 1996). Key words used for the computer-based searches included "caregiver," "health promotion," "health," and "health behaviors." A large number of articles on caregiving (1,353) and many nonrelated articles (due to using "health" as a general search term) were found.

Because using "health promotion" and "health behaviors" as key terms did not yield materials appropriate to the scope of this chapter, another search was completed that included paired key terms with specific areas of health behaviors in addition to "family caregivers." This more specific search included "nutrition," "fitness and exercise," "physical activity," "stress reduction," "relaxation," and "drug use" (polypharmacy and psychotropic drugs). A search of the CINAHL database yielded 11 articles, whereas a search of the Clin Psych database provided 62 articles. A MEDLINE search was also completed; some of the articles found were redundant items already found in the CINAHL and Clin Psych searches, but several new articles were found (a total of 147). Abstracts of all 147 articles were reviewed. Only 12 related to nutrition, 9 to exercise and physical fitness, 122 focused on stress and burden, 2 on relaxation, and 2 on psychotropic drugs. Most articles mentioned health promotion and health behavior, but these concepts were not variables under study. From the reviewed abstracts, the following review was completed. All empirical research articles were reviewed without restrictions to research methodology issues. Dissertations were not reviewed.

Those found that were focused on psychological well-being, negative mental health, physical health status, self-care practices, symptom experience, use of sick days, and general life satisfaction were selected for review. For self-care behaviors or intervention studies, articles were reviewed related to sleep, exercise, over-the-counter medications, psychotropic drugs, health practices, and leisure or respite activities.

REVIEW OF THE LITERATURE

Based on this gap in the caregiving literature, articles related to the physical and mental health of family care providers were reviewed to glean any important work related to the health promotion and health behaviors of family caregivers. These caregiver health-and-well-being-related articles were used as the basis of the literature review. The focus is limited to a primary caregiver providing care, usually for an older adult with chronic disease. A review of the state of the science with respect to spousal caregivers by Jackson and Cleary (1995) is a review important to this topic. The review by Clipp and George (1993) of literature related to the health consequences of caregiving is equally important.

The purpose of the review is to summarize what is known from the research literature about the health-related activities of caregivers of adults. Later in the chapter, the implications for future study of health promotion for family caregivers are discussed.

Psychological Health Status of Caregivers

Most studies have shown higher depression levels and negative mental health among caregivers when compared to age- or gender-based population norms (Clipp & George, 1990a; Fischer, Visintainer, & Schulz, 1989; Gallagher, Rose, Rivera, Lovett, & Thompson, 1989; George & Gwyther, 1986; Moritz, Kasl, & Berkman, 1989; Pruchno & Potashnik, 1989). These studies abound and have been reviewed frequently; thus, they will not be reviewed here. Most reviews are focused on the caregivers of dementia patients; for example, the recent work of Schulz, O'Brien, Bookwala, and Fleissner (1995). Readers are also referred to the works of Schulz, Visintainer, and Williamson (1990).

Schulz et al. (1995) reviewed 90 articles to assess the prevalence and magnitude of psychiatric and physical morbidity effects among caregivers and to identify individual and contextual correlates of health-status effects for caregivers of dementia patients. Almost all of the studies in this review reported elevated levels of depressive symptoms among caregivers; those using diagnostic clinical interviews also reported high rates of clinical depression and anxiety. Across these studies, psychiatric morbidity in caregivers was generally linked to patient problem behaviors, income, caregiver self-rated health status, perceived stress, and life satisfaction.

As reported by Schulz et al. (1995), the evidence in these 90 articles, however, was less clear and often contradictory for the association between caregiving and physical morbidity (such as self-rated health, number of medical illnesses, symptoms, health care usage, or preventive health behaviors). Alterations in caregiver health status were generally associated with problem patient behaviors, patient cognitive deficits, and caregiver depression, anxiety, and perceived social support.

A longitudinal design was used by Bull, Maruyama, and Luo (1995) to examine posthospital transitions for family caregivers. Physical function and mental health domains were examined at discharge, 2 weeks postdischarge, and 2 months postdischarge. There was no significant change in physical or functional health during the 2-month period. Although these numbers eventually declined, caregivers did show high scores on anxiety and depression at discharge.

In a study by Neundorfer (1991), the effect of coping patterns on the physical and mental health of caregivers was examined. The gender of caregivers was identified as a significant predictor for physical health status as measured by the OARS (Older Americans Resources and Services) (Fillenbaum & Smyer, 1981). Sick days, physician visits, hospital days, overall health, current health, and the extent to which health limited caregiver activities were also measured. Discussion of these items was limited. Neundorfer acknowledged the stressors of caregiving but concluded that most caregivers of spouses with dementia manage their roles without severe negative effects on their own physical health.

Irvin and Acton (1996) tested a model of caregiver stress mediation based on the modeling and role-modeling theory for caregivers caring for cognitively impaired adults. Perceived support and self-worth were examined to determine if these self-care resources had a mediating effect on stress and well-being. Self-care resources mediated the relationship of stress and well-being for these caregivers.

Physical Health Status of Caregivers

Given the large amount of literature linking physical illness to stress, one would expect that the caregiver literature would include studies focused on physical health status. Instead, few studies could be found that even mentioned physical illness (such as respiratory problems, hypertension, or cardiovascular disease) as associated with the health status of caregivers. The most frequent physical health discussion and analysis of caregivers were self-reports (often single item) of general physical health status and an occasional study that examined physical symptoms, drug or substance use, or health care usage as indicators of health status. Some recent work looked at immune function as an indicator of susceptibility to physical disease. A review of the relevant literature on physical illness follows.

Haley, Levine, Brown, Berry, and Hughes (1987) and Haley, Levine, Brown, and Bartolucci (1987) found that caregivers report alterations in physical health status. Specifically, Haley, Levine, Brown, Berry, and Hughes found that, in a matched group of caregivers, the physical health status of caregivers—as measured by health ratings and number of chronic diseases—was significantly poorer than that of controls. Numbers of common physical symptoms, however, did not differ, but health care usage—as measured by physician visits and the number of prescription medications—was higher among caregivers.

A comparative study by Jutras and Lavoie (1995) consisted of three groups matched by gender and age: one group in which there was a care recipient, one group of subjects who lived with a nonimpaired person over 55 years of age, and one group of subjects who did not live with a person under 54 years of age. Caregivers reported experiencing more stress, more disabilities, and/or more chronic conditions, and also suffered from hay fever, back problems, and diabetes. There were no statistically significant differences found with respect to self-rated perceptions of health, levels of happiness, or satisfaction with health status.

To provide a depression and physical-health-status profile, Bergman-Evans (1994) compared spousal caregivers of Alzheimer's patients living at home and living in a nursing home. Depression was measured using the Center for Epidemiologic Studies—Depression Scale (CES-D; a 20-item, 4-point Likert scale) (Radloff, 1977). Physical health status was assessed via caregiver self-report, reports of nonroutine physician visits, and days when they were unable to do "regular work." Sleep disturbances and arthritis were the two health problems most frequently reported. Few caregivers reported smoking, drinking alcohol, and most exercised more than one time per week. Bergman-Evans (1994) found that both groups reported similar levels of depression and that the majority of caregivers in each group reported their physical health as "good" or "excellent." For home caregivers, depression was found to be closely connected to self-assessed health status and days unable to work; whereas depression was significantly correlated to self-assessed health for nursing home caregivers.

Taylor, Ford, and Dunbar (1995) used a cohort study of individuals 55 years old to compare the health of caregivers to noncaregivers, as well as to examine the changes in caring and health over a 3-year period. Caregivers in this study did not report poorer health as determined by "minor physical symptoms."

From a longitudinal study, McKinlay, Crawford, and Tennstedt (1995) reported that caregiving exerted its greatest impact on the personal life of the caregiver (sleep, leisure, health, and privacy) (61%) in comparison to family life (18%) and employment (15%–20%). All areas of negative impact persisted over time.

Clipp and George (1993) compared spousal caregivers of dementia patients with spousal caregivers of cancer patients. They found that the caregivers of dementia patients had more compromised health than the caregivers of cancer patients. Clipp and George (1990b) found that caregiver characteristics, rather than the severity of patient illness or the care situation, were predictors of antianxiety, antidepressant, or sedative/hypnotic drug use. Overall, 30% of the caregivers used psychotropic drugs on an occasional basis. Levels of satisfaction with leisure and perceived need for support were linked with drug use as were numbers of symptoms, poor self-rated health, and frequent physician visits. Caregivers were reported as being a group at high-risk of exhaustion, depressed appetite, sleeping difficulties, and nervousness.

O'Brien (1993), in a pilot study of caregivers of individuals with multiple sclerosis, examined health-promoting behaviors of spouses. Twenty subjects were included. There was a statistically significant inverse relationship between level of recipient dependence and behaviors of the caregiver. Wives reported higher health-promoting behaviors than did husbands and scored lowest on exercise. Results of the Health Promoting Lifestyle Profile (Walker, Sechrist, & Pender, 1987) used in the study revealed that caregiving wives felt a sense of purpose in their caregiving duties.

Connell, Davis, Gallant, and Sharpe (1994) examined the effect of caring for a demented spouse on caregivers' health behaviors and physical and mental health status. Forty-four spousal caregivers were included in the study. Changes in health behaviors since care provision began were explored in terms of appetite, exercise, smoking, alcohol intake, sleeping, and medication use. Caregivers reported decreased health behaviors, such as a 40% decline in eating nutritious meals and a decline in exercising; caregivers also reported increased alcohol and substance abuse. Half of those who smoked increased their smoking. These caregivers reported that overall their health status was affected negatively.

Fuller-Jonap and Haley (1995), in one of the few studies that was focused on health habits, used a case-control design to study the impact of male spousal caregiving for wives afflicted with Alzheimer's disease. With respect to health habits, caregivers had significantly more difficulty with sleep, were not able to exercise on a regular basis, tended to use over-the-counter medications more frequently, and had more respiratory symptoms than noncaregivers. In contrast with prior studies, caregivers did not show higher rates of cigarette smoking or alcohol consumption. When the caregivers were questioned about using sleeping medication, most of the caregivers responded that they could not take any medication that would keep them from being alert at all times to respond to care-recipient needs.

Pruchno and Potashnik (1989) conducted one of the most relevant studies of the physical health problems of spousal caregivers. Caregivers spent less time sick in bed, reported fewer visits to the physician, and spent fewer days in the hospital than did the general population. Caregivers did, however, rate their own health as "excellent" less frequently than did the general population, yet rated their own health as "good" more often than the general population. Both male and female caregivers reported higher rates of diabetes, arthritis, ulcers, and anemia in the past 12 months than the general population. Female caregivers reported higher rates of hypertension and heart trouble than did women in the general population, whereas men reported higher rates of emphysema. General physical symptoms (e.g., nervousness, perspiration, heart palpitation, dizziness, trembling, headaches, insomnia, bad dreams/nightmares) were also reported at higher rates by caregivers than in the general population. Depression also was higher. There was no report nor any mention by the investigators of any health promotion or self-care activities by caregivers in this study.

In order to study the effects of caregiving on psychological and physical well-being and social support, Haley et al. (1995) performed a four-group comparison study of Black versus White caregivers and Black versus White noncaregivers. With respect to physical health, White participants (caregivers and noncaregivers) had higher numbers of genito-urinary symptoms and digestive tract symptoms. Black participants had a higher frequency of illness and worse self-rated health. When looking at caregivers versus noncaregivers within each ethnic class, however, no significant differences were found. Spousal caregivers reported higher symptoms regarding eyes, ears, cardiovascular system, digestive tract, and musculoskeletal system, as well as using more prescription medications than nonspousal caregivers. Nonspousal caregivers had higher numbers of unhealthy habits. Whereas racial differences in health were apparent, the researchers found no support for an overall negative impact of caregiving on physical health.

In a longitudinal study that sought to develop and evaluate a causal model of the relationship between physical health and depression among a sample of spousal caregivers of individuals with Alzheimer's disease or a related dementia disorder, Pruchno, Kleban, Michaels, and Dempsey (1990) found that strong relationships existed in which depression predicted the self-reported health of caregivers. Depression has been suggested to increase one's vulnerability to physical illness, either through immunological alterations or from failure to care for oneself.

Overall, studies in which investigators examined health care usage (Haley, Levine, Brown, & Bartolucci, 1987; Pruchno & Potashnik, 1989) found that caregivers had fewer physician visits (Moritz, Kasl, & Berkman, 1992), fewer hospital stays and more physician visits (Haley, Levine, Brown, & Bartolucci, 1987), more days in the hospital, more prescription drug use, and fewer sick days (Clipp & George, 1990a). Subjects involved in studies by McKinlay et al. (1995) and Pruchno and Potashnik (1989) reported more psychotropic prescription drug use than general populations (Clipp & George, 1990a). Cattanach and Tebes (1987) found that caregivers of dementia patients did not have more physical symptoms (e.g., headaches, weight change, back pain) than caregivers of functionally impaired patients and did not spend more days in bed or have more physician visits. This contradicts previous research that shows differences among these caregiver groups.

Given the conflicting findings, it is not clear what one should expect as to how caregiving might effect the physical health of caregivers or their use of health care services. In only two studies did investigators report increased substance abuse: the work of Connell et al. (1994) on caregivers of demented spouses and the work of Hall et al. (1994) on caregivers of traumatic brain injury patients.

Moritz, Kasl, and Osfeld (1992), in a study of spousal caregivers of patients with dementia, found increased systolic blood pressure less frequently treated by hypertension medication and more hospitalizations among husbands caring for wives with poor cognitive functioning. Moritz and colleagues did not find an association between caregiving and alcohol use or smoking.

Although there is little information about the influence of stress on caregivers' physical health and the information that exists is confusing and sometimes contradictory, some recent work on the immune system of caregivers would suggest that physical health may be influenced at the immune level due to the stressors related to caregiving.

Kiecolt-Glaser et al. (1987) reported immunosuppression as a result of chronic stress among family caregivers of dementia patients as well as higher levels of depression, lower mental health, and poorer immune responses. In their 1995 work, Kiecolt-Glaser, Marucha, Malarkey, Mercado, and Glaser found that caregivers slept less, had longer illness episodes, and sought more physician visits than did controls. There was no difference in alcohol consumption, smoking, or caffeine use, and subjects had normal albumin levels. Healing took 9 days longer in caregivers than in matched controls. Peripheral blood leukocytes from caregivers produced significantly less Interleukin-2 (IL-2) in response to lipopolysaccharide stimulation. No group differences in health-related behaviors were found among these caregivers.

To determine whether a chronic stressor (i.e., caregiving for a spouse with a progressive dementia) was associated with an impaired immune response to an influenza virus vaccination, Kiecolt-Glaser, Glaser, Gravenstein, Malarkey, and Sheridan (1996) compared the vaccine responses of 32 caregivers with 32 gender-, age-, and socioeconomically matched control subjects. As assessed by two independent methods, caregivers showed a poorer antibody response following vaccination relative to control subjects. These data demonstrated that down-regulation of the immune response to influenza virus vaccination was associated with a chronic stressor in the elderly caregivers. These results have implications for vulnerability to infection that caregivers may have. Long-term implications for the effect of altered immune response are needed.

Vitaliano, Scanlan, Krenz, Schwartz, and Marcovina (1996) examined relationships between chronic stress and insulin/glucose in two groups: nondiabetic men with an average age of about 70 years who were spousal caregivers of persons with Alzheimer's disease and nondiabetic men matched by age and gender who were spouses of nondemented controls. Fasting, insulin/ glucose, and psychological variables were assessed twice over a 15- to 18-month period. Caregivers had significantly higher insulin levels at both assessment points than did controls, even when obesity, exercise, gender, age, consumption of alcohol, hormone replacement therapy (HRT), lipids, and hypertension were considered. Caregivers also generally reported significantly more psychological distress (higher burden, depression, hassles, and lower uplifts) than did controls. These results are important to long-term caregiving because higher insulin and glucose levels are also associated with increased coronary risk and coronary heart disease. In 1995, Vitaliano, Russo, and Niaura also found higher levels of high-density lipoproteins in a group of nonsmoking, nonobese caregivers.

Esterling, Kiecolt-Glaser, Bodnar, and Glaser (1994) found continuing and former caregivers more depressed than controls in a comparison of caregivers of dementia patients with former caregiver and control patients. Current and former caregivers also had a poorer response than controls to cytokines, important in stimulating natural killer cells and suggesting that the consequences of chronic stressors exist beyond the cessation of stressors. Both caregiver groups saw physicians more than two times as often as controls for infectious illness symptoms. Continuing caregivers, bereaved caregivers, and controls did not differ in use of caffeine, cigarettes, alcohol, or sleep. Likewise, no differences were found for use of cardiac drugs, analgesics, or antihistamines.

Critique of Articles Reviewed

Research on the psychological health status of caregivers often uses levels of depression and anxiety to document family members' mental health. These measures are different and because of the variation in duration of caregiving and the point in the caregiving trajectory when the measures were administered, it is difficult to approach and to interpret the findings. Numerous studies on caregiver burden have measures that examine lack of personal time and leisure time for caregivers (C. W. Given, Collins, & Given, 1988). Much work has been done on psychological distress, primarily caregiver burden and depression (Aneshensel et al., 1993; Schulz et al., 1995). Caregivers clearly reported anxiety and depression, but how this relates to overall health practices, self-care, and health-promoting behaviors remains unknown (B. Given, Stommel, Collins, King, & Given, 1990; Kurtz, Kurtz, Given, & Given, 1995; Pruchno et al., 1990).

Caregivers are often recruited from support groups and may have been caregiving for many years. The study by Neundorfer (1991) was one of the few studies that examined use of health care services as an indicator of caregiver health status. Without comparisons to the mental health of other groups or population norms, it is difficult to characterize the influence of caring on the mental health of family members. Also, cross-sectional observations fail to describe changes in caregivers' mental health. More research is needed to describe changes in mental health across the caregiving trajectory and to assess which aspects of patient care (e.g., helping with medications, helping move about the house) and caregiver-related factors (e.g., age, gender, health status) are associated with these changes.

Research on the influence of caring on the physical health status of caregivers indicates that few studies consider physical illness as a variable. If included, physical health status was often reported by a single item. Few longitudinal studies were undertaken and investigators used different caregiver measures to assess "health ratings" or numbers of chronic illnesses. Some researchers included only chronic illnesses, such as diabetes, whereas others include acute problems, such as colds, headaches, and hay fever. Symptom lists were used in two studies, but each list was different. Jutras and Lavoie (1995) used satisfaction with health status, whereas Clipp and George (1990a) used satisfaction with leisure and other family-related dimensions. McKinlay et al. (1995) used "impact" of caregiving on sleep, leisure, family life, and so on.

The three studies that specifically examined health-promoting behaviors were small studies (Connell et al., 1994; Fuller-Jonap & Haley, 1995; O'Brien, 1993). The latter two studies included caregivers of patients with dementia. Again, instruments were dissimilar and various methodologies were used.

Health care usage was not included as a variable in most studies and where it was included, it was in validated self-reports of use of services. Medical record audits were seldom included to validate caregiver reports or usage behavior. Thus, we know little about health promotion strategies or how caregivers are able to sustain such practices.

Among the few studies that employed noncaregiving comparison groups, differences in the physical health between the two groups were modest. Several possibilities might account for this conclusion. First, caregiving really does not have a substantial effect on caregiver physical health. Second, caregivers who have been caregiving have adapted and, so long as there is no significant change in the demand for care, their health remains comparable to that of their noncaregiving counterparts. Third, the stresses imposed at the time of entering the caregiving role or when new demands are imposed are considerable, but following these points in the caregiving trajectory, physical health remains relatively uncompromised. Over the course of the disease, caregiver adaptation occurs and caregiver physical health problems come under remission. These alternative explanations deserve future research and assessment. Each will require caregiving participants who are at known but varying points along the caregiving trajectory and who are facing varying levels of caregiving demands at different points in time. One set of studies that has begun to address these methodologic issues as well as to capture more precise indications of physical health is the recent biomarker studies.

Literature on the immune system and other biomarker studies are in their infancy and both the Kiecolt-Glaser and Vitaliano research teams have focused mostly on caregivers of dementia patients (Kiecolt-Glaser et al., 1987; Kiecolt-Glaser, Dura, Speicher, Trask, & Glaser, 1991; Kiecolt-Glaser et al., 1995, 1996; Vitaliano, Young, Russo, Romano, & Magana-Amato, 1993; Vitaliano et al., 1995, 1996). These studies used case-matched controls and the same blood markers were processed in the same laboratories using identical equipment.

Biological response studies that included health care practices and health care service use offer considerable promise for resolving the understanding of the negative effects that caregiving has on the physical health of family members caring for elderly persons with functional and cognitive deficits. Based on this understanding, health promotion strategies can be suggested.

With the lack of examination of health care activities by the caregiver, there is little knowledge available related to the counteracting or mediating of negative physical effects. Perhaps secondary gain, coping strategies, or other health practices are moderating these effects. What may or may not be occurring, however, remains unexplored in caregiver literature.

Minority and cultural differences in physical health care activities are seldom discussed. Only Haley et al. (1995) compared different racial groups. Much of the research relates to and derives from convenience samples or from those who are already participating in support groups or local agencies and are not from the general population. There are very few controlled studies and no experimental designs (except for the physiological immune studies). Very little attention has been paid by nurse researchers to this area, which is surprising given the focus of nurses on health promotion activities. The health promotive practices of caregivers seem to be a mystery.

IMPACT OF INTERVENTIONS ON THE HEALTH STATUS OF CAREGIVERS

Numerous studies exist that identify strategies leading to positive effects on the caregiver and include coping strategies such as problem-solving skills, information-seeking behavior, and use of social support (Clipp & George, 1990a; Kiecolt-Glaser et al., 1991; Noelker & Bass, 1989). Cognitive strategies to deal with the negative dimensions of caregiving, such as depression and burden, included reappraisal and reframing (Haley et al., 1987; Pratt, Schmall, Wright, & Cleland, 1985; Pruchno & Resch, 1989; Quayhagen & Quayhagen, 1988; Stephens, Norris, Kinney, Ritchie, & Grotz, 1988; Wright, Lund, Pratt, & Caserta, 1987). There is no compelling evidence or indication whether or not these same strategies would work in promoting activities to positively affect caregiver physical health. These interventions might improve physical health if the problem is stress related, as they are based on stress-reduction models. Help-seeking behaviors for self-care health practices have not been addressed in the studies in which researchers examined health and well-being.

Cognitive and behavioral strategies may help the caregiver in regulating his or her behavior during and across stressful situations. Several studies showed that cognitive behavioral strategies like problem solving, positive reappraisal, reframing, learned resourcefulness and secondary skills (e.g., related to time, behavior, or social resource management) are related to caregiver well-being (Pruchno & Resch, 1989; Rosenbaum, 1989; Stephens et al., 1988; Wright et al., 1987).

Rosenbaum (1989) labeled self-controlled skillfulness "learned resourcefulness" and defined it as a way to guide the family caregiver to change ineffective habits, to learn new and more effective behaviors, and to manage the emotional, behavioral, or cognitive disruptions of stressful caregiving behaviors. Self-control behaviors could play an important role in the adjustment of the caregiver to acute and chronic stressors associated with caregiving and may help to explain why some caregivers cope better with the demands of their role than others. Perhaps these strategies could be used by caregivers to adapt their health practices relating to self-care, lifestyle changes, nutrition, physical fitness, stress management, and leisure time. These strategies would be helpful to the caregiver to find the time and resources to enable them to engage in health-promotive practices.

Problem-solving skills aid caregivers in dealing with difficulties that arise and add to feelings of self-control, whether they be directly related to patient care or related to other issues, such as time management (Intrieri & Rapp, 1994). Although there were no articles found that evaluated the effect of self-care in the care situation on health-promoting behaviors, two were found that showed the benefit and inclusion of caregiver self-care in support groups (Greene & Monahan, 1989; Toseland, Blanchard, & McCallion, 1995). These studies did not evaluate if the caregiver actually engaged in self-care and what self-care activities might have been undertaken. Greene and Monahan (1989) reviewed 29 studies of group interventions for caregivers and only two mentioned caregiver self-care.

Social support and respite are mediators of the negative effects of caregiving that have been identified by Baillie, Norbeck, and Barnes (1988) and Clipp and George (1990a). Respite, a time for self-care, leisure, or physical fitness, is often mentioned as a strategy to give caregivers time for themselves. Respite, however, has not been consistently shown to improve burden and mental health, nor is there evidence of a positive effect on physical health (Lawton, Kleban, Moss, Rovine, & Glicksman, 1989). Few studies, however, were focused on the health-promoting activities or health outcomes supported or provided by community agencies. Respite studies do not report that caregivers use this time for leisure, self-care, or health-promoting activities. Little attention has been given to any discussion of strategies that can be used to enable health care practices or self-care practices by caregivers or health promotion interventions for the spousal caregiver. Finally, these models presume a link between perceived stress and mental and physical health. Should this link prove tenuous or nonexistent, then these models would be of little use in improving caregiver health.

RECOMMENDATIONS FOR RESEARCH

Caregivers caring for the chronically ill can live not only longer but better quality lives by following health promotion, self-care, and disease prevention practices. The following recommendations are made to overcome the serious void in the literature related to health promotion among caregivers. Descriptive studies are needed to expand the view of caregiving and to examine the usual health practices of those engaged in caregiving.

Do the negative health effects of caregiving occur differentially among groups? Representative samples of caregivers need to be accrued in future study. Emphasis should be placed on sampling from prevalent chronic diseases and obtaining caregivers of patients who are physically dependent and not just those with dementia. Health promotion behavior studies should be targeted to specific subgroups of caregivers: spouses, adult children, men, or women; by age group; by racial and ethnic groups; and extended to socially marginalized caregivers, such as the poor, as well as those who seem to experience marked distress.

It is important to determine if caregivers maintain usual self-care practices or alter them as the demands for care increase. Factors that influence caregivers' abilities to adopt new health and self-care practices successfully need to be described. Longitudinal studies of caregiver adaptation to the caregiving role over time are needed to explore the complex interactions of caregiver physical health, mental health, and how usual self-care and health promotion and practices are altered given the continuous and constantly changing role of caregiving. One's understanding and perception of caregiving and the role of this perception in reducing stress and promoting physical health deserves further exploration. Baseline health status and health-promotive strategies at the onset of caregiving should be known and assessed so that follow-up and monitoring of changes and overall impact is possible. The self-report, clinical assessment, and biological measures of health status also need to be determined for representative populations and then followed longitudinally.

Factors that interfere with caregivers' ability to maintain their usual self-care and health-promotive practices need to be examined. Analyses of caregivers' usual health-promotive practices will be critical in determining their ability to maintain the caregiving role. Knowledge of which self-care practices (i.e., nutrition, exercise, sleep, stress management) change and which remain stable given increasing care demands is essential. Do hours of care influence the abandonment of usual health care practices? When do the effects of caregiving end—after recovery, death, or institutionalization?

What is the relationship of physical and mental health status? Further study of the actual physical health status of caregivers and the influence of physical and mental health on each other is an important direction for future research. Can health practices such as nutrition, exercise, stress management, and so forth, influence the physical health of the caregiver? What impact, if any, do these activities have on mental health status? Are the negative effects delayed, as would be suggested by the immunology research? Can the health-promotive practices of chronically ill caregivers influence the relationship between caregiver and care-recipient status?

What types of interventions are best suited to inspire caregiver health-promotive behaviors? Controlled intervention studies encouraging health practices and the impact on physical and mental health need to be targeted to specific subgroups of caregivers and those caregivers at high risk for negative health outcomes from the care role. Interventions and clinical trials that assist the caregiver to engage in activities that promote health and build physiological reserve must be explored, including exercise programs, good nutrition, social activation, regular sleep, and monitoring their own physical and emotional health. Clinical interventions that appear promising for improving caregivers' self-care and preventing negative consequences for their health should be explored. Interventions that facilitate behavior change and acquisitions of self-management skills are needed.

How, when, and why do caregivers rely on the health care system to meet their own health care needs? The data on the use of health services are scanty. It is unclear how time spent providing care and how the intensity and duration of caregiving influences the number of visits to physicians, the control of caregivers' existing chronic diseases, the compliance with therapeutic regimens for the caregiver, and the use of prescription medications. Descriptive work is needed in this area. Studies must be undertaken that compare physicians' prescriptive patterns with caregivers' requests for assistance when they seek care for health problems. Are psychotropic drugs often prescribed as a way to try to assist the caregiver with stress? Use of over-the-counter medications and alternative health practices was absent from the literature and needs to be determined.

Measures need to be developed that can be used to systematically determine use of health care practices. The Health Promoting Lifestyle Profile, as developed by Walker, Sechrist, and Pender (1987), would be one such instrument.

How do immunological responses affect caregiver health? Chronic stress has been shown to affect the immune system negatively. It is not known how impaired or how long the immune response occurs before the caregiver becomes physically ill or before chronic diseases appear. Further work is needed to see how quickly in the caregiving process these changes occur. Nurse researchers with an interest in health and welfare are well suited to address this area of research; nurses have an opportunity to make a contribution to the existing knowledge base.

SUMMARY

Attention to health promotion would seem to contribute to the health and well-being of caregivers and be necessary for caregivers to maintain a productive life. Activities that promote good health and build psychologic reserve include regular exercise, good nutrition, stress management, social activity, and sleep. Along with engaging in health-promotive behaviors, caregivers must learn to monitor and evaluate their own physical and emotional health status and make decisions on the basis of symptoms and signs they experience and observe. In partnership with their health care professionals, caregivers should be alert to the impact of their own physical health needs, illnesses, emotions, and self-esteem on their ability to continue to function in caregiving roles. In addition, secondary prevention to control the progression of their own disease processes, such as hypertension, arthritis, and cardiovascular disease, will be important given the projected increase in age of the caregivers in the future.

Health care professionals must provide information, support, and resources to assist caregivers in health promotion. Mental and physical health can at least stabilize if the caregiver's support system is perceived as being adequate and stable (Clipp & George, 1990a).

Unfortunately, the health care system gives priority to the urgent problems of the patient and often takes little time to note or identify the health care needs of the caregiver. Little time or intellectual energy has been devoted to the needs of caregivers. This leads to delays in the detection of caregiver declines in health status due to irregular or incomplete assessments. Very little data are gathered in the multitude of caregiver studies that focus on the physical and mental health of caregivers. Few caregiver burden or depression studies even consider health promotion strategies as mediating factors of the negative effects of providing care. Helping caregivers strengthen self-care resources through time management, nutrition, and exercise may be useful to protect them from the stress of caregiving (Irvin & Acton, 1996).

ACKNOWLEDGMENTS

The authors would like to express their deep gratitude to Danielle DeVoss, M.A., and Sharon Kozachik, R.N.c., B.S.N., M.S.N.c., both Research Assistants for the *Family Care Research Program* at Michigan State University, East Lansing, Michigan, for their assistance in the preparation and revision of this chapter.

REFERENCES

Aneshensel, C. S., Pearlin, L. I., & Schuler, R. H. (1993). Stress, role captivity, and the cessation of caregiving. *Journal of Health and Social Behavior, 34,* 54–70.

Baillie, V., Norbeck, J. S., & Barnes, L. E. (1988). Stress, social support, and psychological distress of family caregivers of the elderly. *Nursing Research, 37,* 217–222.

Bergman-Evans, B. (1994). A health profile of spousal Alzheimer's patients. *Journal of Psychosocial Nursing, 32,* 25–30.

Bull, M., Maruyama, G., & Luo, D. (1995). Testing of a model for post hospital transitions of family caregivers for elderly persons. *Nursing Research, 44,* 132–138.

Cattanach, L., & Tebes, J. (1987). The nature of elder impairment and its impact on family caregivers' health and psychosocial functioning. *Gerontologist, 31,* 246–255.

Clipp, E., & George, L. (1990a). Caregiver needs and patterns of social support. *Journal of Gerontology: Social Sciences, 45,* S102–S111.

Clipp, E., & George, L. (1990b). Psychotropic drug use among caregivers of patients with dementia. *Journal of the American Geriatrics Society, 38,* 227–235.

Clipp, E., & George, L. (1993). Dementia and cancer: A comparison of spouse caregivers. *Gerontologist, 33,* 534–541.

Connell, C. M., Davis, W. K., Gallant, M. P., & Sharpe, P. A. (1994). Impact of social support, social cognitive variables, and perceived threat on depression among adults with diabetes. *Health Psychology, 13,* 263–273.

Esterling, B., Kiecolt-Glaser, J., Bodnar, J., & Glaser, R. (1994). Chronic stress, social support, and persistent alterations in the natural killer cell response to cytokines in older adults. *Health Psychology, 13,* 291–298.

Fillenbaum, G. G., & Smyer, M. A. (1981). The development, validity, and reliability of the OARS Multidimensional Functional Assessment Questionnaire. *Journal of Gerontology, 36,* 428–434.

Fischer, L., Visintainer, P. F., & Schulz, R. (1989). Reliable assessment of cognitive impairment in dementia patients by family caregivers. *Gerontologist, 29,* 333–335.

Fuller-Jonap, F., & Haley, W. E. (1995). Mental and physical health of male caregivers of a spouse with Alzheimer's disease. *Journal of Aging and Health, 7,* 99–118.

Gallagher, D., Rose, J., Rivera, P., Lovett, S., & Thompson, L. W. (1989). Prevalence of depression in family caregivers. *Gerontologist, 29,* 449–456.

George, L. K., & Gwyther, L. P. (1986). Caregiver well-being: A multidimensional examination of family caregivers of demented adults. *Gerontologist, 26,* 253–259.

Given, C. W., Collins, C. E., & Given, B. A. (1988). Sources of stress among families caring for relatives with Alzheimer's disease. *Nursing Clinics of North America, 23,* 69–82.

Given, B., Stommel, M., Collins, C., King, S., & Given, C. W. (1990). Responses of elderly spouse caregivers. *Research in Nursing & Health, 13,* 77–85.

Greene, V. L., & Monahan, D. J. (1989). The effect of a support and education program on stress and burden among family caregivers to frail elderly persons. *Gerontologist, 29,* 472–477.

Haley, W. E., Levine, E., Brown, S. L., & Bartolucci, A. A. (1987). Stress, appraisal, coping, and social support as predictors of adaptational outcome among dementia caregivers. *Psychology and Aging, 2,* 323–330.

Haley, W. E., Levine, E. G., Brown, S. L., Berry, J. L., & Hughes, G. H. (1987). Psychological, social, and health consequences of caring for a relative with senile dementia. *Journal of the American Geriatrics Society, 35,* 405–411.

Haley, W. E., West, C. A. C., Wadley, V. G., Ford, G. R., White, F. A., Barrett, J. J., Harrell, L. E., & Roth, D. L. (1995). Psychological, social, and health impact of caregiving: A comparison of Black and White dementia family caregivers and noncaregivers. *Psychology of Aging, 10,* 540–552.

Hall, K. M., Karzmark, P., Stevens, M., Englander, J., O'Hare, P., & Wright, J. (1994). Family stressors in traumatic brain injury: A two-year follow-up. *Archives of Physical and Medical Rehabilitation, 75,* 876–884.

Intrieri, R. C., & Rapp, S. R. (1994). Self-control skillfulness and caregiver burden among help-seeking elders. *Journal of Gerontology, 49,* P19–P23.

Irvin, B. L., & Acton, G. J. (1996). Stress mediation in caregivers of cognitively impaired adults: Theoretical model testing. *Nursing Research, 45,* 160–166.

Jackson, D. G., & Cleary, B. L. (1995). Health promotion strategies for spousal caregivers of chronically ill elders. *Nursing Practice Forum, 6*(1), 10–18.

Jutras, S., & Lavoie, J. (1995). Living with an impaired elderly person: The informal caregiver's physical and mental health. *Journal of Aging and Health, 7,* 46–73.

Kiecolt-Glaser, J. K., Dura, J. R., Speicher, C. E., Trask, O. J., & Glaser, R. (1991). Spousal caregivers of dementia victims: Longitudinal changes in immunity and health. *Psychosomatic Medicine, 53,* 345–362.

Kiecolt-Glaser, J. K., Glaser, R., Gravenstein, S., Malarkey, W. B., & Sheridan, J. (1996). Chronic stress alters the immune response to influenza virus vaccine in older adults. *Proceedings of the National Academy of Science, 93,* 3043–3047.

Kiecolt-Glaser, J., Glaser, R., Shuttleworth, E. E., Dyer, C. S., Ogrocki, P., & Speicher, C. E. (1987). Chronic stress and immunity in family caregivers of Alzheimer's disease patients. *Psychosomatic Medicine, 49,* 523–535.

Kiecolt-Glaser, J., Marucha, P., Malarkey, W., Mercado, A., Glaser, R. (1995). Slowing of wound healing by psychological stress. *Lancet, 346,* 1194–1196.

Kurtz, M. E., Kurtz, J. C., Given, C. W., & Given, B. (1995). Relationship of caregiver reactions and depression to cancer patients' symptoms, functional states and depression—a longitudinal view. *Social Science and Medicine, 40,* 837–846.

Lawton, M., Kleban, M., Moss, M., Rovine, M., & Glicksman, A. (1989). Measuring caregiving appraisal. *Journal of Gerontology: Psychological Sciences, 44,* P61–P71.

McKinlay, J. B., Crawford, S. L., & Tennstedt, S. L. (1995). The everyday impacts of providing informal care to dependent elders and their consequences for the care recipients. *Journal of Aging and Health, 7,* 497–528.

Moritz, D. J., Kasl, S. V., & Berkman, L. F. (1989). The health impact of living with a cognitively impaired elderly spouse: Depression symptoms and social functioning. *Journal of Gerontology: Social Sciences, 44,* S17–S27.

Moritz, D. J., Kasl, S. V., & Osfeld, A. M. (1992). The health impact of living with a cognitively impaired elderly spouse: Blood pressure, self-rated health, and health behaviors. *Journal of Aging and Health, 4,* 244–267.

Neundorfer, M. M. (1991). Coping and health outcomes in spouse caregivers of persons with dementia. *Nursing Research, 40,* 260–265.

Noelker, L. S., & Bass, D. M. (1989). Home care for elderly persons: Linkages between formal and informal caregivers. *Journal of Gerontology: Social Sciences, 44,* S63–S70.

O'Brien, M. T. (1993). Multiple sclerosis: Stressors and coping strategies in spousal caregivers. *Journal of Community Health Nursing, 10,* 123–135.

Pratt, C., Schmall, V., Wright, S., & Cleland, M. (1985). Burden and coping strategies of caregivers to Alzheimer's patients. *Family Relations, 34,* 27–33.

Pruchno, R. A., Kleban, M. H., Michaels, J. E., & Dempsey, N. P. (1990). Mental and physical health of caregiving spouses: Development of a causal model. *Journal of Gerontology: Psychological Sciences, 45,* P192–P199.

Pruchno, R. A., & Potashnik, S. L. (1989). Caregiving spouses: Physical and mental health in perspective. *Journal of the American Geriatrics Society, 37,* 697–705.

Pruchno, R. A., & Resch, N. L. (1989). Mental health of caregiving spouses: Coping as a mediator, moderator, or main effect? *Psychology and Aging, 4,* 454–463.

Quayhagen, M. P., & Quayhagen, M. (1988). Alzheimer's stress: Coping with the caregiving role. *Gerontologist, 28,* 391–396.

Radloff, L. (1977). The CES-D scale: A new self-report depression scale for research in the general population. *Applied Psychological Measurement, 1,* 385–401.

Rosenbaum, M. (1989). Self-control under stress: The role of learned resourcefulness. *Advances in Behavior Research and Therapy, 11,* 249–258.

Schulz, R., O'Brien, A., Bookwala, J., & Fleissner, K. (1995). Psychiatric and physical morbidity effects of dementia caregivers: Prevalence correlates and causes. *Gerontologist, 35,* 771–791.

Schulz, R., Visintainer, P., & Williamson, G. M. (1990). Psychiatric and physical morbidity effects of caregiving. *Journal of Gerontology: Psychological Sciences, 45,* P181–P191.

Stephens, M. A., Norris, V. K., Kinney, J. M., Ritchie, S. W., & Grotz, R. C. (1988). Stressful situations in caregiving: Relations between caregiver coping and well-being. *Psychology of Aging, 3,* 208–209.

Taylor, R., Ford, G., & Dunbar, M. (1995). The effects of caring on health: A community-based longitudinal study. *Social Science and Medicine, 40,* 1407–1415.

Toseland, R., Blanchard, C., & McCallion, P. (1995). A problem solving intervention for caregivers of cancer patients. *Social Science and Medicine, 40,* 517–528.

Vitaliano, P. P., Russo, J., & Niaura, R. (1995). Plasma lipids and their relationships with psychosocial factors in older adults. *Journal of Gerontology: Psychological Sciences, 50,* P18–P24.

Vitaliano, P. P., Scanlan, J. M., Krenz, C., Schwartz, R. S., & Marcovina, S. M. (1996). Psychological distress, caregiving, and metabolic variables. *Journal of Gerontology: Psychological Sciences, 51,* P290–P299.

Vitaliano, P. P., Young, H. M., Russo, J., Romano, J., & Magana-Amato, A. (1993). Does expressed emotion in spouses predict subsequent problems among care recipients with Alzheimer's disease? *Journal of Gerontology: Psychological Sciences, 48,* P202–P209.

Walker, S. N., Sechrist, K. R., & Pender, N. J. (1987). The Health-Promoting Lifestyle Profile: Development and psychometric characteristics. *Nursing Research, 36,* 76–81.

Wright, S. D., Lund, D. A., Pratt, C., & Caserta, M. S. (1987). *Coping and caregiver well-being: The impact of maladaptive strategies or how not to make a situation worse.* Paper presented at the Annual Scientific Meeting of the Gerontological Society of America, Washington, DC.

PART II

Research on Care Delivery

Chapter 9

Prenatal and Parenting Programs for Adolescent Mothers

Paulette J. Perrone Hoyer
College of Nursing
Wayne State University

ABSTRACT

Adolescence is a time of risk taking and exploration. The adolescent's exploration of the developmental and physical changes taking place often puts the adolescent at greater risk than at any other time in life. The risk-taking behaviors involve sexual activity, experimentation with substances including cigarettes and alcohol, rebellion against paternal norms, suicidal behavior, and violence. This chapter focuses on the potential outcome of one of these risky behaviors: sexual activity. The intent is to summarize the findings of the research community on the pregnancy and parenting programs for adolescents. A summary of some of the recent research and demonstration projects for pregnant and parenting adolescents is provided. Published and unpublished articles from a variety of disciplines are included. These articles vary by method, type of program, location, and outcome measurement. Methodological issues related to the preponderance of quasi-experimental designs with small samples and demonstration projects are addressed. The lack of theoretically driven, longitudinal research that is specific to the developmental level of the population is discussed, and directions are suggested for future research.

Keywords: Adolescent, Teen Pregnancy, Prenatal Care, Pregnancy, Parenting, Adolescent Pregnancy Programs

Adolescence is a time of identity seeking, risk taking, and exploration. It is also a period when the individual perceives the self as immortal. These normal developmental perceptions and actions can put the adolescent at greater health risk than during other life stages (Dryfoos, 1991; Kokotailo & Adger, 1991). Today's adolescents enter puberty sooner and become sexually active at younger ages. In the 1800s the average age of menarche was 16 years. With improvements in health care and better nutrition through the 1980s this age has decreased to 12 years. From 1970 to the mid-1980s the number of 15- to 19-year-old females who ever had premarital intercourse increased from 29% to 52%; the statistics for the same age group in males indicated a rise from 55% to 64% (Moore, Miller, Glei, & Morrison, 1995). In 1993, 32% of females and 43% of males in the 9th grade reported that they had sexual intercourse. By the 12th grade, 66% of females and 70% of males said they had sexual relations (Kann et al., 1995). Data for 1995 (Moore, 1997) indicate that 40% of females and 36% of males, 20 years and under, have had sexual intercourse in the last 3 months. By the time they are between 18 and 21 years, 33% of never-married males and 20% of never-married females have had sex with six or more partners (Adams, Schoenborn, & Moss, 1995). The decreasing age for first sexual intercourse and the increasing number of sexual partners outside of marriage means that more adolescents are at risk for unintended pregnancy and sexually transmitted diseases (STDs) including HIV (human immunodeficiency virus). Eleven percent of 15- to 19-year-olds become pregnant every year; and this same group contracts 25% of the 12 million cases of STDs occurring in the United States each year (Moore, 1996).

A noticeable health-threatening consequence of sexual activity in the adolescent is unwanted or unintended pregnancy, abortions, or babies. The U.S. birth rate for females aged 15 to 19 in 1993 was 60 births per 1,000, which is significantly higher than any other industrialized country. Although teen births among adolescents over 17 years are declining, births to adolescents 17 and younger continue to rise. For 1994, 37.6% of adolescents between 15 and 17 had given birth (Moore, 1997). Further, the number of adolescent girls aged 14 to 17 is projected to increase by 1.2 million between 1995 and 2005. Reflecting this, the number of births to school-age adolescents (14 to 17) is expected to increase linearly, despite an overall slowdown (14 to 20). The never-married teen birth rate has risen to 72%. Among teens 15 to 17 who have babies, 50% of the fathers of these babies are 20 years or older (Moore, 1996).

Bearing a child during adolescence is a stressful life event because it triggers many changes in the physical, emotional, and social life of the teenager. Among the well-documented consequences are dropping out of school, having to care for a child who may have health and developmental problems, depression, and greater chance for a life of poverty (Dryfoos, 1991). Many of these consequences have negative effects on the teenager as well as her offspring.

High pregnancy rates in adolescent girls have led policymakers and program providers to explore the ways that pregnancy can be prevented and teen mothers assisted to achieve better outcomes for themselves and their babies. Many researchers and clinicians have tried to address the multiple needs of the developing adolescent as sexual beings, as pregnant women, and as parents. Intervention programs have been developed throughout the country with varying effects. Unfortunately, many of the programs lack both an evaluative component and a theoretical base.

SCOPE OF THIS REVIEW

In this review prenatal and parenting programs are addressed that have been developed from both a theoretical and atheoretical perspective, as well as those that are demonstration projects or are research based. There are two comprehensive works covering (a) adolescent pregnancy prevention programs, and (b) reviewing recent research on prevention programs available from Child Trends, Inc. (Moore, Miller, Glei, & Morrison, 1995). Therefore, this review does not address pregnancy prevention programs that are covered in the compendium. It is focused on the programs for the adolescent who is pregnant or has delivered a child. In order to accomplish this, the literature was searched manually and through computer databases including Cumulative Index to Nursing and Allied Health Literature (CINAHL) (1980–1996), MEDLINE (1985–1996), SOCIAL SCIENCES (1985–1996), PSYCHINFO (Indexes to psychology journals) (1985–1996), and INDEX MEDICUS (1985–1996). Additional programs were identified through adolescent and child health conference proceedings for the past 5 years and presenters were contacted for information. Statistical information was sought via the Internet and is available online from the federal government, from state governments, and from Alan Guttmacher Institute.

With social awareness of the health consequences of adolescent pregnancy, programs were developed as early as the 1960s. The major focus in this chapter is on the literature and programs developed between 1985 and 1996 with a few selected early programs included. The search identified many programs that were theory-based demonstration projects, clinical trials, intervention research, and natural experiments. The programs that were chosen for this review included those that had something unique to offer or supported a general approach that has been documented as effective. Effective programs were those that had a demonstrated impact on repeat pregnancy, on perinatal outcomes, on infant care, maternal role attainment, or on the contribution of the adolescent in school.

The ideal approach to adolescents should involve a program that is theory driven and guides the development of the study and the interpretations of the findings. This approach should address the health and developmental issues of the adolescent. Additionally, programs should have an evaluative component. Because of the critical nature of the problem, most programs were not developed with consideration of these issues but were rather an attempt to quickly "fix" a societal problem.

PREGNANCY PREVENTION PROGRAMS

Three articles were found that contained programs not covered in the compendium by Moore, Sugarland, et al. (1995). The compendium covers adolescent pregnancy prevention programs and does a thorough job of evaluating the same. Additional work by Moore is also available through the Internet (Moore, Miller, et al., 1995). The Internet also provides a vast storehouse of information that is readily available. The Child Trends group in Washington is on the Internet and tabulates current trends in adolescent pregnancy, pregnancy prevention, and a host of other information related to the family and the child.

In reviewing the literature regarding pregnancy prevention few programs were not identified by Moore et al. (1995). The high-school-based experimental work by Bayne-Smith (1994) used a holistic health-promoting approach and incorporated the "Teen Incentives" model developed by Schinke (1981). Her work combined concepts of self-perception and external locus of control and involved an evaluative component. Experimental teens attended a 6-month, 3-phase program. Those in the control group received written information covering sexual activity, contraception, and access to health care. Significant findings included a decrease in sexual activity and an increase in contraceptive use in the experimental group. The control group also had a reduction in sexual activity. The research has many potential sources of bias. Because teens were from the same class, potential cross-contamination could occur leading one to suspect that results are not due to the intervention. Further bias existed in the identified sample, only teens from an inner city freshman class were included. Although the results were intriguing and suggestive, they cannot be generalized beyond the sample involved.

Frost and Forrest (1995) describe another comprehensive approach. These researchers used comparison groups to evaluate five pregnancy prevention programs that incorporated decision-making and negotiation skills, education on sexuality and contraception, as well as an emphasis on delay or abstinence of sexual activity. Four of the five programs were school based and included access to contraceptive services. "Postponing Sexual Involvement" in Atlanta used a mentoring method in a school-based educational curriculum aimed at eighth graders. "Reducing the Risk" targeted 10th graders in California classes who were randomly assigned to control or experimental groups and followed for 1 1/2 years. The "School/Community Program" in rural South Carolina targeted 14- to 17-year-olds who were matched and followed for 3 to 6 years. "Self-Center" in Baltimore linked school-based sexuality and reproductive health education with access to contraception and provision of medical services at a nearby clinic. Schools were matched and adolescents within the groups were followed for 3 years. "Teen Talk" in both Texas and California targeted 13- to 19-year-olds and randomly assigned classes and individuals to a condition. There is no indication of length of follow-up.

Frost and Forrest (1995), using meta-analytic techniques, concluded that programs are most effective in reducing sexual activity and increasing contraceptive use when they targeted the sexually inexperienced younger teenagers, and that pregnancy prevention was enhanced when contraceptive services were easily accessed. Effect size was calculated for all studies using the same measures (proportions of sexually active, proportions using contraceptives, and proportions becoming pregnant). The behavior of adolescents who participated was compared to behavior of similar adolescents. Control students received some variation of the alternative or a traditional program. Four of the programs used posttests but administered them at different times. These researchers identified some major issues prevalent in existing literature on prevention programs. Samples tend to be limited to Black or African American adolescents from low-income areas. Issues that need to be addressed include the effects of environment (i.e., media, poverty, parent or sibling teenage pregnancy) on early sexual activity. Programs need to be implemented with different ethnic and racial groups in areas with higher socioeconomic (SES) status. Program reports need to be more detailed to allow for replication. Because the authors of most existing programs did not report the value and standard deviation for each outcome measure as well as the p value for significant as well as nonsignificant results, the meta-analysis was limited to the five programs. This meta-analysis clearly identified one of the major problems with the current literature on adolescent pregnancy programs. The methodology was not sufficiently described to replicate the study nor are there sufficient data for meta-analytic techniques.

Jones and Mondy (1994) compared outcomes of two Texas programs: "Special School" program and the "Lifespan Program" with a comparison group. The authors compared short-term perinatal outcomes and birth patterns over a 5-year period. Differences between the groups disappeared over the 5 years. Age at first pregnancy was a significant predictor of number of subsequent pregnancies and high-school graduation. They argue that effectiveness of programs depends on long-term community involvement. In this article, the authors used a quasi-experimental design to compare a school-based program with a clinic-based program and with general care for adolescents. Groups were compared on the following variables: number of births, mean age at target births, number of prenatal visits, gestational age, and birth weight. Major limitations of the work are based on sampling technique and data collection method. Samples were not comparable. Comparisons were based on nonequivalent, unequal samples (Lifespan, $N = 37$; Special School, $N = 71$; and Comparison, $N = 108$). Groups within the programs had prenatal care on site, biasing entry into prenatal care. As with other programs, samples were limited by including only low-income groups from inner-city neighborhoods. Data were collected retrospectively from chart review over a 5-year period.

Despite limitations, some consistent findings relative to prevention programs do recur. Effective strategies that reduce the incidence of pregnancy include (a) use of a holistic approach that incorporates knowledge about sexuality, (b) mentoring by older teens, (c) life strategies to identify and avoid risk behavior, (d) access to contraceptives, and (e) decision-making skills and strategies. Interventions that are school- or community-based appear to have the best chance for success in reducing teen pregnancy.

PRENATAL AND PARENTING PROGRAMS

As so few experimental studies were found (Bayne-Smith, 1994; Field, Widmayer, Stringer, & Ignatoff, 1980; Hoyer, Jacobson, Ford, & Walsh, 1994; Jones & Mondy, 1994; O'Sullivan & Jacobsen, 1992; Porter, 1984), both prenatal and parenting programs were combined in this discussion. Programs were found that are based in clinics (Covington et al., 1991; Fullar et al., 1991; Hardy, King, & Repke, 1987; Hoyer et al., 1994; Morris, Berenson, Lawson, & Wiemann, 1993; Neeson, Patterson, Mercer, & May, 1983; O'Sullivan & Jacobsen, 1992; Roye & Balk, 1996), hospitals (Porter, 1984; Smith & Gingiss, 1996; Smoke & Grace, 1988; P. Thompson, Powell, Patterson, & Ellerbee, 1995), schools (Bachman, 1993; Bayne-Smith, 1994; Chen, Telleen, & Chen, 1995; Jones & Mondy, 1994; Kleinfeld & Young, 1989; McAfee & Geesey, 1984), and communities (East, Matthews, & Felice, 1994; Garcia-Coll, Hoffman, & Oh, 1987; Lapierre, Perreault, & Goulet, 1995; Musick, 1993; Polit & Kahn, 1985; J. Thompson, 1993). Some unique settings included homeless shelters (Borgford-Parnell, Hope, & Keisher, 1994; Sheaff & Talashek, 1995) and maternity homes (Koniak-Griffin, 1994; Koniak-Griffin & Verzemnieks, 1991). Programs offered a multitude of intervention strategies and evaluative techniques.

Limitations were consistent across studies. It is very difficult to randomly assign subjects to groups, as these are very costly to conduct and providers often resist "denying services" to clients. Therefore, most of the work was quasi-experimental (Bachman, 1993; Covington et al., 1991; Field et al., 1980; Fullar et al., 1991; Garcia-Coll et al., 1987; Hardy et al., 1987; Kleinfeld & Young, 1989; Koniak-Griffin, 1994; Koniak-Griffin & Verzemnieks, 1991; Lavery, Chaffee, Marcell, Martin, & Reece, 1988; Mikanowicz, Nicholson, Olsen, & Wang, 1992; Morris et al., 1993; Musick, 1993; Neeson et al., 1983; Opuni, Smith, Avery, & Solomon, 1994; Polit et al., 1984; Roye & Balk, 1996; Smith & Gingiss, 1996; Smoke & Grace, 1988; Stevens-Simon, Fullar, & McAnarney, 1992; Stevens-Simon, Kaplan, & McAnarney, 1993; Talashek, 1992; Warrick, Christianson, Walruff, & Cook, 1993) with comparisons of a treatment group with a similar, nontreatment population. Without random assignment, it is difficult to be certain that the effects result from the treatment rather than preexisting differences between the groups. Many programs were found that simply did a posttest assessment of the groups (Bayne-Smith, 1994; Covington et al., 1991; Mercer, 1980; Morris et al., 1993; Neeson et al., 1983); some included both pre- and posttest (Hoyer et al., 1994; Koniak-Griffin & Verzemnieks, 1991). Additionally, natural experiments or demonstration projects were simply described in the literature (Grogger & Bronars, 1993; Hall et al., 1987; Mikanowicz et al., 1992; Musick, 1993; National Adolescent Health Resource Center, 1993). Comparison groups often used data from previous years leading to questions of historical validity (Anderson & Dahlberg, 1992; Borgford-Parnell et al., 1994; Chen et al., 1995; Diener, Mangelsdorf, Contreras, Hazelwood, & Rhodes, 1995; East et al., 1994; Garcia-Coll et al., 1987; Koo, Dunteman, George, Green, & Murray, 1994; Lapierre et al., 1995; McAfee & Geesey, 1984; Records, 1994; J. Thompson, 1993; P. Thompson et al., 1995). A few studies combined qualitative and quantitative methodology (Bayne-Smith, 1994; Field et al., 1980). A few qualitative studies were found (Lee & Grubbs, 1993; Mercer, 1980). Sampling problems were consistent across studies. Most samples included only lower socioeconomic groups (Bayne-Smith, 1994; Covington et al., 1991; Diener et al., 1995; East et al., 1994; Field et al., 1980; Fullar et al., 1991; Hardy & Duggan, 1988; Hoyer et al., 1994; Lapierre et al., 1995; McAfee & Geesey, 1984; Morris et al., 1993; Nelson, Key, Fletcher, Kirkpatrick, & Feinstein, 1982; Opuni et al., 1994; O'Sullivan & Jacobsen, 1992; Polit & Kahn, 1985; Records, 1994; Roye & Balk, 1996; Stevens-Simon et al., 1992) and predominantly inner-city, minority adolescents with nonequivalent comparison groups (Mercer, 1985). Many sample sizes were 60 or less (Diener et al., 1995; Garcia-Coll et al., 1987; Koniak-Griffin & Verzemnieks, 1991; McAfee & Geesey, 1984; Porter, 1984; Thompson et al., 1995; Williams-Burgess, Vines, & Ditulio,

1995). Extraneous variables were not taken into account. Many studies used researcher-developed instruments without established psychometrics (Bachman, 1993; Kelen, Hunt, Sibeko-Stones, & Varga, 1991; Koniak-Griffin & Verzemnieks, 1991; Records, 1994); instruments developed for the adult population without norms for adolescents (Diener et al., 1995; Garcia-Coll et al., 1987; Koniak-Griffin & Verzemnieks, 1991; Records, 1994); and retrospective chart review, school records, or birth certificate data (Covington et al., 1991; Hardy et al., 1987; Jones & Mondy, 1994; Kleinfeld & Young, 1989; Koo et al., 1994; Lavery et al., 1988; Mikanowicz et al., 1992; Neeson et al., 1983; Opuni et al., 1994; Setzer & Smith, 1992). Long-term follow-up was limited to less than a year in most studies (Bachman, 1993; Chen et al., 1995; Diener et al., 1995; Kleinfeld & Young, 1989; McAfee & Geesey, 1984; Morris et al., 1993; Nelson et al., 1982; O'Sullivan & Jacobsen, 1992; Porter, 1984; Records, 1994; Smith & Gingiss, 1996; Smoke & Grace, 1988; J. Thompson, 1993; P. Thompson et al., 1995). Without controlling extraneous variables and accounting for changes over time, and with the other methodological limitations, it is difficult, if not impossible to truly evaluate these programs.

There is a plethora of exploratory/descriptive work and a large number of demonstration projects. All of the work indicated the urgency felt by society to deal with this major problem.

TYPES OF PROGRAMS

The following programs are those that were deemed most effective at changing maternal or fetal outcomes, regardless of sample size. Programs in which the investigator offered a unique approach or contributing factor to adolescent pregnancy were included. Comprehensive programs that covered reproductive health services in total or in part are community, school, or hospital based; involved mentoring or role modeling; and had both short- and long-term follow-up were viewed as essential.

Comprehensive Programs

Comprehensive programs used a school- or community-based approach and addressed total lifestyle. Most were quasi-experimental in design and used a matched sample that did not receive the treatment for comparison. In this discussion, programs are organized relative to time, with the earliest program addressed first.

Johns Hopkins Center for Teenage Mothers and Their Infants program is one of the longest running programs for adolescents (Hardy & Duggan, 1988; Hardy et al., 1987). This highly successful program is a blueprint for the comprehensive approach. The program used a team approach with individual case management; included health, nutrition, pregnancy, and parenting programs; linked adolescents and their parents to community resources; and included an evaluative component. Targeted adolescents were 18 and under, unmarried, of low socioeconomic status, and predominantly African American. Program participants were compared with adolescents in standard prenatal care programs at the same institution. Program adolescents were different from controls in almost all aspects of perinatal and long-term health outcomes (Duffy & Coates, 1989). This program is quasi-experimental and at the time of the latest report had enrolled over 1,500 adolescents. As previously stated, the sample has been limited in that it included predominately low socioeconomic status, minority adolescents, with a comparison group from a nonequivalent population.

The Project Redirection (Polit, 1989; Polit & Kahn, 1985) is a community-based model funded by the Ford Foundation and the U.S. Department of Labor. Sites included communities in Boston, New York City, Phoenix, and Riverside, CA. The targeted population was disadvantaged adolescents 17 and under who were parents or currently pregnant. Comparison groups were nonequivalent. The program was unique in the use of both peer groups and role models. Sampling programs affected the ability to truly understand the differences that appeared. The groups were unequal, with no attempts made to control extraneous variables.

The Rochester Adolescent Maternity Program (RAMP) is an ongoing program that provides comprehensive care to the adolescent (Fullar et al., 1991; Stevens-Simon et al., 1992; Stevens-Simon et al., 1993). The program was designed with ongoing evaluation, thus allowing multiple quasi-experimental studies to be undertaken. Outcomes continuously measured include prenatal data: demographic, pregnancy, family structure and support, housing arrangements, school attendance or special programs; involvement of the father, risk problems in the adolescent; and data collected postnatally: birth outcomes, support systems, referrals, insurance. The advantage of this program lies in the tremendous data collected on an ongoing basis. The major disadvantage lies in the lack of randomness, the predominantly minority sample, and little attempt to account for extraneous influences.

Ounce of Prevention Fund—Parents Too Soon (OPF) (Mosena & Ruch-Ross, 1996a, 1996b; Musick, 1993) is a public/private partnership including private philanthropists and the Illinois Department of Children and Family Services. This natural experimental program is now a "state-wide system for research, training and technical assistance working with community based organizations to address high risk adolescents' needs" (Musick, 1993, p. 2) and has been in existence since 1981. Included are both prevention and health promotion services. Pregnancy outcomes were compared favorably with a national sample of adolescents (Ruch-Ross, Jones, & Musick, 1992). As is typical of state initiatives, however, most of the reported results are either descriptive or qualitative in nature. Comparison groups are nonequivalent and from a different historical period. The major advantage of the state initiatives lies in the large data set that is relatively untapped.

Another school-based model is the TAPP program or The Teenage Pregnancy and Parenting Project (Warrick et al., 1993). Seven sites in Phoenix and Tucson were used. Investigators used five different educational approaches to compare services and to evaluate outcomes. Pregnant students were followed longitudinally. The major outcome variable was the success of the adolescent in school. By using many sources of support, the multiple comprehensive programs were successful in encouraging at least a high-school completion. Methodological issues lie in the unequal, nonequivalent, predominantly minority sample as well as reliance on retrospective record review.

One notable pilot project was school and community based, and involved both a governing board and a community advisory board. The Northeast Adolescent Project (NEAP) in Houston (Opuni et al., 1994) is described by the authors as a collaborative effort that included a school district, a county commissioner, a hospital district, and Baylor College of Medicine's Teen Health Clinic. NEAP adolescents, compared to controls, had consistently better performance on outcome measures including premature birth, maternal health, postpartum compliance, low-birth weight (LBW) babies, and continued school attendance. Ten schools participated in the program with a potential pregnant adolescent sample of 63. Thirty-one pregnant teens were randomly selected for follow-up. Matching on demographic variables created a comparison group. Although the limited sample affects interpretation of the results, this pilot work is promising and does support the overall effectiveness of supportive comprehensive programs.

Hoyer et al. (1994) piloted a theoretically driven, peer-centered model for adolescent care. Adolescents in an HMO (health maintenance organization) clinic were randomly assigned to either experimental groups or the control condition. Those in the experimental groups were paired with a pregnant peer for prenatal care. The program was designed to empower the adolescent and encourage healthy behavior. Adolescents in the experimental groups consistently attended prenatal care classes, had good perinatal outcomes, and had less repeat pregnancies when compared to the control group. Although the sample was limited to lower socioeconomic minority adolescents, the theory-

driven, longitudinal pre–posttest experimental design allows for broader interpretation of the results.

Other Programs

There are a number of programs that are described in the literature. These
programs contain many elements that are the hallmark of successful programs,
but because of a lack of evaluative strategies and random assignment, they
are difficult to evaluate. Most authors used convenience samples and described
the work. These programs date from the mid-1980s. Those listed below are
organized with the earliest program listed first.

The Ealing Teen Mums' Club is one such program (J. Thompson, 1993).
Set up in a London borough by a nurse midwife, the program was intended
as a health education and social resource for the adolescent mother. All
teenagers who were pregnant were booked into the club for care. No attempt
was made to compare teenagers who were pregnant with any type of comparison group. The group was multiethnic, used community resources, but limited
follow-up to 6 weeks. Evaluation was anecdotal responses from the teenagers.

Changing Roles, an educational curriculum, was described by McAfee
and Geesey (1994). The authors found that adolescents dropped out of school
as they became pregnant. The intent of this program was to keep the adolescent
in school and reduce truancy. The authors contend that the program was
effective. The sample was limited to 52 multiethnic, low socioeconomic teens,
however. There was no comparison group and evaluation is based on anecdotal
information from teachers.

Canadian work by Lapierre et al. (1995) describes shared governance in
peer-counseling groups. This is community based and involves mothers in a
given community called "godmothers" and health care workers who supervise
them. "Godmothers" have two defined areas of responsibility: individually
they promote well-being in the mother by making home visits and bringing
food supplements; collectively they educate and inform the mother by organizing social, informational, and recreational activities. This program is theory
based and uses the developmental dependence of adolescents on their peers.
Another seldom seen feature is the use of a mentor in the community. The
sample is limited to low socioeconomic adolescents and had no comparison
group.

The descriptive programs seldom included a comparison group and are
limited to small samples of predominantly low socioeconomic minority adolescents. Long-term follow-up seldom occurred beyond a year and was often
limited to the first postpartum visit. These programs do suggest alternatives

to traditional programs and give insights into the types of interventions and supports that might best be incorporated into successful programs. The use of peer-group support as well as mentors to model parenting behaviors are methods that need further evaluation.

Parenting Among Ethnic or Racial Groups

Some authors looked at differences in parenting among ethnic or racial groups. Multiple measures were used and data were collected on behaviors, anxiety, depression, competence, and infant involvement. Caucasian adolescent mothers and early parenting supports were examined by Garcia-Coll et al. (1987). Fifty low- to middle-class Caucasian adolescent and nonadolescent mothers with their 4-month-old infants were interviewed and videotaped in their homes. When compared to adults, adolescents were less verbal with their infants and scored lower on responsiveness and involvement scales. Support from adolescent peers and maternal support were found to be more important than other types of support in mediating the effect. Small sample size is at issue here ($n = 25$ adolescent mothers, $n = 25$ adult mothers) as well as the limited subject pool (one site used). Further sample issues are those of nonequivalence, as the use of predominantly lower socioeconomic, lower educational adolescents compared to a middle-class, educated adult sample. Because socioeconomic status has been found to be a powerful predictor variable in both maternal behavior and perinatal outcomes (Sameroff & Chandler, 1975; Tulkin, 1977) findings need to be interpreted cautiously. The authors did attempt to match on socioeconomic status, further limiting their sample to 34 (17 in each group).

East et al. (1994) examined the interrelations among adolescent mothers' parenting attitudes, confidence, and stress levels; and differences in those relationships across race, age and parity. The sample was comprised of 119 former-adolescent mothers. The authors concluded that the younger the adolescent is when giving birth, the more at risk she is for poor acceptance of her child. White adolescents had significantly more positive values than the other two groups. African American mothers had more confidence in their ability than did Hispanic mothers. For all adolescents, the authors found high stress associated with low confidence in mothering, low acceptance of the child, and low empathy for the child's needs. Mothers with low confidence in their role and low confidence in future relationships with their child valued physical punishment, tended to view the child as nurturer, and had little empathy for the child's needs. The authors identified relationships between low confidence, high stress, and inappropriate values. Younger mothers were less accepting of their child, independent of the age of the child. Sample issues occur in this study. The relatively small subsamples may have prevented detection of some differences and allowed questionable interpretation to significant differences. Additionally, mothers self-selected into the study, limiting generalizability of the findings. Concepts such as maternal confidence were used interchangeably with competence. This is one of the few studies found that examined multiple racial or ethnic groups, however. Its value lies in the fact that it points to the need for different assessments when examining racial and ethnic groups.

P. Thompson et al. (1995) also described adolescent parenting. A small sample ($N = 19$) was obtained from a randomly selected chart audit of mothers ($N = 92$) who were part of the university hospital-based, multidisciplinary program. Variables of interest were subsequent pregnancies, child development, parenting attitudes, school completion, and family support. All adolescents tended toward nonnurturing attitudes. The sample of 19 included only those adolescents who could be located from the original 92, however. Assumptions about adolescent parenting were made based on very small numbers. There was no attention to racial or ethnic differences in the adolescents nor to the multiple variables that influence parenting.

In an attempt to understand differences between adult models of parenting competence and parenting of Latina adolescent mothers, Diener et al. (1995) recruited 50 Latina adolescents from high schools and community agencies. The sample included Puerto Rican, South American, and Mexican Latinas. Data were collected on depression, anxiety, social support, life events, economic strain, maternal behaviors, and competing time demands. Relationships were posited between social support and parenting competence. Support from mother and peers was most important in reducing the demand of the child felt by the adolescent. The authors combined the Puerto Rican and Mexican mothers for analyses stating that the only difference was marital status. They also eliminated the 6% South American group from the sample. The final sample included the 47 remaining mothers. Assumptions were made regarding maturity of the mothers based on marital status, however, only six mothers were married. The report discussed results in terms of the original sample of 50 as well as the final sample of 47. The sample size was not large enough to detect effects. Tools were used that did not have normative data for the adolescent population, let alone for different ethnic groups. Although there are problems with this study, the attention to different populations within the adolescent parenting community is a vital issue in the study of adolescent mothers.

Adolescents are different from adults, they are both different from and similar to each other. Sample size and use of tools that do not have normative data for the adolescent population limit these studies. Assumptions are made based on very small subsamples of the population. Although methodological issues exist, the value of this type of research is immeasurable. The limited attention to ethnic and racial differences in the literature on adolescent parenting identifies a need to design programs specific to different populations and to develop instruments specific to adolescents.

Location of the Program

Some researchers examined the location of the program in an attempt to identify the best place to address adolescent needs. Sites included schools, hospitals, prisons, and homeless shelters. Each had unique problems and positive aspects.

Pregnancy outcomes from a Kentucky program initiated by the Board of Education were described by Lavery et al. (1988). Data were collected from 2,293 students enrolled in the Teenage Parent Program. Comparisons were made based on location of primary antenatal care (TAPP, University Clinic, Health Department, and private physician). Results indicated that these comprehensive programs improved health, increased use of contraception and improved school attendance. This study used retrospective chart review as well as school and hospital records to obtain data and then comparisons were made across locations. Socioeconomic status becomes a factor in the results reported, however. Private physician clients were more likely to be of higher socioeconomic status than the adolescent clinic patient, thus biasing interpretation of these results.

The San Diego Adolescent Pregnancy and Parenting Program (SAN-DRAPP) described by Kleinfeld and Young (1989) examined the temporal relationship between dropping out of school and teen-age pregnancy, and whether or not teens in special education programs were at greater risk for dropping out than students not in these programs. A random numbers table was used to select a final sample of 135 cases from an 800-caseload database. Findings supported their hypothesized relationships and also identified an unexpected result. Teenagers in special education appeared to be at higher risk for pregnancy and dropping out of school than their counterparts in regular classes. Data were collected retrospectively from records. There was no attempt to identify other reasons that these teenagers dropped out of school. The other special education teens may drop out at the same rate, leading one to question the conclusions of the study. The finding of increased risk of pregnancy for special education students needs to be further explored.

The Rural Approach to Pregnancy and Parenting: Outreach Resources to Teens (RAPPORT) compared outcomes from birth certificates of adolescents from four counties with those of teenagers in a voluntary adolescent program for rural Pennsylvania (Mikanowicz et al., 1992). RAPPORT, funded federally and locally, provided a school and home program to teenagers and their families. The intent was to improve perinatal outcomes, support educational aspirations and encourage independence. There was a significant difference in timing of onset into prenatal care, birth-related complications, timing of repeat births for the two cohorts, and completion of education. Sampling issues continue as adolescents self-select into the programs and data are collected at different time points for comparison groups. For this analysis, data were collected prospectively from RAPPORT teenagers and retrospectively from state health department birth certificates and annual statistics for all teenagers. All analyses were based on these data.

Bachman (1993) investigated the effect of a structured learning program designed to provide health education to high-school students over a 7-year period. The self-described learning needs of pregnant 7th- to 12th-grade students in an alternative educational setting were examined. Multiple teaching methods were assessed and needs identified. The researcher concluded that a need exists in both grade and high schools for pregnant teens to have perinatal education. The use of investigator-designed tools without established psychometrics limits the use of this study. The value of the study lies in the identification of multiple modes of teaching that appeal to adolescents.

In a collaborative effort, the Delaware Division of Public Health, the University of Minnesota's National Adolescent Health Resource Center (1993), and the University of Delaware collected baseline and survey data to compare the effect of Delaware's school-based Wellness Centers for adolescents on access to care, help-seeking, and risk-taking behaviors. Comparisons were made between self-identified users and nonusers of the Centers (National Adolescent Health Resource Center, 1993). Based on the findings of the survey, the researchers recommended that the use of school-linked clinics is critical and they should be strategically located based on needs assessment. Community health programs should be integrated and evaluation plans established with the start-up of any new programs. In general, comprehensive programs, linked to community and school, are effective methods of providing health care to adolescents. These findings cannot be generalized beyond the small group of individuals within the wellness center programs. Perceptions reported are those of a limited sample who were present at one of three schools on the day that the survey was administered.

Another neglected population, the homeless, was addressed in descriptive work by Borgford-Parnell et al. (1994). The Out-of Home Teen Pregnancy Project is a collaborative effort that mobilized the community to address pregnancy and infant outcomes in the increasing numbers of pregnant and parenting homeless or runaway adolescents. An intensive case management team consisting of a public health nurse and a social worker provided services. All services were in nontraditional settings, including shelters, city and county parks, detention centers, and youth drop-in centers. The team was not restricted by district and thus able to develop many alternative interventions to engage and maintain relationships with the ever-changing needs of the teens. Study findings can only be applied to this self-selected population; however, the authors do identify a population that needs to be addressed in future research.

Breuner and Farrow (1995) identified a major deficit in health care to adolescents by survey research. These researchers sent surveys to 430 prisons across the United States. From the responses of 261 institutions, they identified a population of 2,000 pregnant teenagers and 1,200 teenage mothers. Nearly half of the agencies continued incarceration despite the pregnancy and of those, 70% did not have parenting classes and 31% provided no prenatal care. This population represents a "captive" population that deserves health care and is ripe for research. Little is known about the pregnant or parenting convict. Would the knowledge of pregnancy prevent the crime? Methods should be established to identify pregnant or parenting teenagers and multidisciplinary research conducted to establish the most effective method of intervening with this population.

Smith and Gingiss (1996) used a random quota sample to compare differences between teenagers who used programs that were either hospital or school based. Their intent was to profile the client characteristics of teenagers who used the two types of clinics. Hospital-based programs drew teens who had dropped out of school and were predominately Hispanic. The school-based clinics reflected the racial and ethnic composition of the city. African American teens used the school clinics. The teens in the school clinics had higher educational goals. They saw their mothers as role models and also the major source of support. These teens were more likely to use alcohol and other substances, however. This study emphasizes the need to look at service delivery setting when designing programs for adolescents. Attending to the preferences can lead to a structure that would improve the perinatal outcome.

The literature identified multiple sites that can be used to intervene in the pregnancy and parenting of the adolescent. Alternative settings can provide positive support to the adolescent.

Models for Practice

There have been some attempts to develop models for practice that are usually based in health promotion. The Parent Enhancement Program (PEP) (Porter, 1984) was a hospital-based model started in southwestern Pennsylvania and expanded to northern West Virginia. A study was conducted to test the feasibility of the program. Adolescents were randomly assignment to either PEP or usual care. This model included three phases: prenatal, perinatal, and postnatal components and used a holistic approach that emphasized nursing roles of teaching, practice, and research. Materials were presented over 6 months, in 2 1/2-hour sessions. One of the goals of the program was to develop the adolescent as a family health resource. This is the only work found that suggested using the teen as a community resource following completion of the program. The work has much potential, however, no further evidence extending the work was found.

Sheaff and Talashek (1995) used Talashek's (1992) Nursing Model for Teen Pregnancy in a retrospective descriptive design to compare teens in temporary housing who had been pregnant with those who had never been pregnant. Data were collected through chart review of 136 adolescents who were admitted to a 12-bed housing shelter during a 1-year period. The teenagers who had been pregnant were more likely to be older, both chronologically and gynecologically, to be at a higher grade level, and to report significant histories of sexual activity and sexual abuse. The authors stated that these adolescents reported twice as many pregnancies as those in the general population and had fewer resources available to them. This study identifies a major unaddressed population of adolescents in temporary housing. Further, the issue of sexual abuse as a major factor in unintended teenage pregnancy needs to be addressed.

A descriptive correlational design along with causal modeling was used to test an Adolescent Family Assessment Model (Records, 1994). Using a convenient sample from teen-parent programs and an obstetrician's office, an attempt was made to describe relationships between caregiving behaviors, knowledge, peer and family approval, and family functioning. A combination of White or Native American ethnicity and age of the first child explained variance in caregiver activity. A notable finding was the strong feeling of burden felt by the adolescent mothers. The use of a convenience sample is at issue here. There is attention to another understudied population, however, the Native American. As previously suggested, the attention to other racial and ethnic groups needs attention from researchers.

These studies highlight a major problem in adolescent pregnancy research. There exist few theoretically driven studies of pregnant or parenting teens. Convenience samples compared to nonequivalent controls continue to be an issue.

Intervention Studies

Intervention studies have focused on one of two areas (a) maternal and newborn outcomes, or (b) maternal role attainment. The intervention studies usually involved a small sample size. They were more likely to include either random assignment or a comparison group. Programs that address perinatal outcomes are listed first, followed by those that address maternal role attainment.

Some nicely designed studies were conducted in the 1980s and 1990s in which researchers examined the effects of programs on various maternal or neonatal outcomes. An excellent example is the work by Field et al. (1980). These researchers had two major foci: (a) to assess the risks of being born preterm or preterm to a teenage mother, and (b) to evaluate the effects of an early intervention program on infants born to lower-class, Black teen mothers. Mothers were randomly selected into one of five groups. Teen mothers and their preterm infants who agreed to participate were randomly assigned to intervention or control. These teens were then compared to teens that had full-term infants, and to adult mothers who had either preterm or full-term infants. Biweekly home visits were made after school hours to the intervention group, by two-person teams, a trained interventionist and a teenage Black female work/study student. Infant developmental outcomes were superior for the intervention group on standardized infant development measurements. The measures do not have normative data for the adolescent population, however. This study is unique in that it uses both random assignment to an intervention or control group as well as comparison groups. The use of blocking variables, (a) term versus preterm infants, and (b) adult versus teenage mother, lend sophistication to the study. The study would have been strengthened by random assignment of both teenage and adult mothers.

Mercer's seminal work was reported in 1980. Mercer used qualitative methodology including semi-structured interviews and naturalistic field observations to examine the teenage mother's view of motherhood and to look at how their infants fared (Mercer, 1980). Data were also collected retrospectively from records. This work by Mercer is classic and highlights the beginning of an illustrious program of research.

In another group of studies, researchers examined the effects of more comprehensive intervention programs on adolescents using quasi-experimental designs. Nelson et al. (1982) conducted an evaluation of the Teen Tot clinic in Alabama. Despite using a convenient sample with matched controls some favorable short-term outcomes were evident when compared with the general clinic experience. In another comprehensive program, investigators used random assignment of 243 mothers and their infants to "special care" or routine well-baby care (O'Sullivan & Jacobsen, 1992). The focus of the special health care program was on (a) prevention of repeat pregnancy, (b) return to school by the mother, (c) up-to-date immunizations for the infant, and (d) reduced use of the emergency room. In the program, investigators used a multidisciplinary team including a social worker, a pediatrician, and a nurse practitioner.

Major differences were found in the repeat pregnancy rate and the immunization rate. Neeson and colleagues (1983) described a comprehensive program
using a retrospective, quasi-experimental design to compare outcomes of mothers in three groups: (a) teens receiving care from nurse practitioners in the
Young Women's clinic ($n = 261$); (b) teens receiving care from the resident
clinic ($n = 318$); and (c) adult women receiving care from residents in the
University clinic ($n = 2,655$). Outcomes were notably different for the teens
receiving care from the nurse practitioners. Infant weight, gestational age
assessments, APGAR scores, and hospital stays were better than the general
clinic population. These studies (Neeson et al., 1982; Neeson et al., 1983;
O'Sullivan & Jacobsen, 1992) have the same issues, convenience samples,
nonequivalent comparison groups, and the use of retrospective chart review.
The value of these programs cannot be assessed without random assignment
or matched comparison groups.

Smoke and Grace (1988) used a quasi-experimental design to examine
the differences between two groups, one group received prenatal education
through a team approach in the Adolescent Obstetrical Service (AOS) at a
university hospital, and a comparison group who received care from health
department clinics. Nine classes were designed as an education program for
the experimental group. A management team was set up that included a
registered nurse, nutritionist, and social worker coordinated by a nurse midwife. Researchers found a significant difference in knowledge gained as well
as fewer maternal and fetal complications for the intervention group. This
study has similar problems to those above, the use of a self-selected convenience sample ($n = 70$) compared to a combined sample from four health
departments across the country ($n = 46$). Unequal samples and lack of equiva-
lence is an obvious issue. Regional differences exist as well as significantly
different racial compositions of the comparison group.

A retrospective initiative described by Morris et al. (1993) compared
outcomes of three different groups of adolescents. The multiethnic adolescent
sample of 1,080 included 660 (61%) from a comprehensive teen-pregnancy
clinic, 143 (13%) who had no prenatal care, and 277 (26%) who had traditional
care. Outcomes were similar for adolescents who received prenatal care when
compared with those who had no prenatal care. Unlike other comprehensive
programs, the authors found little difference between the groups in the comprehensive program and those in the regular program with the exception of
numbers of visits and trimester of onset of prenatal care. Despite different
findings regarding comprehensive programs, the authors did not recommend
eliminating comprehensive programs for adolescents. The authors indicated
that outcomes not measured may be more significant than the ones they
examined including repeat pregnancy, completion of education, and long-term

child outcomes. The groups were different on many of the baseline variables including marital status, parity, abortion history, and gynecologic age. The lack of group equivalency may have biased the findings as reported.

Koniak-Griffin (1994) devised a 6-week aerobic exercise program (AEP) for pregnant adolescents in an attempt to have a positive effect on depression, self-esteem, and physical discomforts of pregnancy. Fifty-eight pregnant adolescent residents of a maternity home agreed to participate in the study. The adolescents were ethnically diverse, including Hispanic, Black, and White teens. Adolescents self-selected into one of two groups, those who exercised ($n = 35$) and those who did not ($n = 23$). Comparisons between the groups indicated measured outcomes significantly enhanced for the treatment group. One interesting ethnic note—the AEP group included mostly Hispanics, whereas the control group included most of the White group. The ethnic finding regarding exercise would need to be verified with a much larger sample. Although having the typical problems of quasi-experimental research (nonequivalent, unequal comparison groups), the findings do suggest that aerobic exercise would be a psychologically beneficial addition to any program for pregnant adolescents.

Unique work by Roye and Balk (1996) compared outcomes of two different programs. Young Black or Hispanic mothers attended a teen mother program (TAM) or a teen mother–grandmother group (TAM-GM). Teens whose mothers participated in the program were significantly less likely to drop out of school and had significantly better self-esteem than the TAM mothers had. The uniqueness of this program lies in the incorporation of the grandmother. The grandmothers were able to meet separately from the teens and were able to confront their own feelings about the pregnancy in a nonjudgmental environment and were more able to support their adolescent daughters and new grandchildren. Measures used were researcher developed or lacked normative information for the adolescent population. As with most comparison studies, the self-selection, nonequivalent groups, and lack of random assignment affects the generalizability of the results.

A number of studies were focused on aspects of maternal role attainment as the primary outcome. Koniak-Griffin and Verzemnieks (1991) evaluated the effects of a nursing intervention on behavioral and affective dimensions of maternal role attainment in pregnant adolescents. Using a predominantly Black and Hispanic convenience sample from a residential maternity home, the researchers randomly assigned adolescents to an experimental or control group. Intervention adolescents met in four 1 1/2-hour classes at weekly intervals that focused on fetal awareness, interactive activities, and maintaining a maternal diary. The results suggested that this type of program has the potential to significantly improved maternal–fetal attachment and early mother–infant interactions. A suggestive finding was the fact that maternal self-confidence and attitudes toward themselves as mothers did not relate to mothering behaviors. Maternal confidence was not adequately described, measures do not have normative data for the adolescent population, and the sample was small ($N = 20$), thus findings need to be interpreted carefully.

The impact of an educational intervention program on rapid repeat pregnancies was described by Covington et al. (1991). The target population was young, poorly educated, and of low socioeconomic status. A retrospective review of all hospital and clinic records was used to identify teens having a first birth between 1985 and 1987. Medical records of these same teens were used to identify those who had a repeat pregnancy within 2 years of the first birth and prior to age 20. Forty-one percent had a repeat pregnancy within 2 years despite the use of oral contraceptives as a method of birth control. The Teens in Transition Through Education program was designed to address multiple repeat pregnancies as well as to improve the outcomes of the current pregnancy and to address parenting skills. The pregnant teens attended 9 to 10 group educational sessions in their regularly scheduled adolescent prenatal clinic. Significant others and parents attended and participated. After delivery, participants returned to share their experiences with the group. Although the authors stated that the program is too new to evaluate, they believe that their program will have a significant effect. The use of gifts to encourage attendance, the low socioeconomic status, and the use of one site limit the generalizability of the results. This program identifies the use of peer support and family members as a valuable addition to pregnancy intervention programs for adolescents.

The Parent–Baby (Ad)Venture Program (PBA), an innovative community-based program (Williams-Burgess et al., 1995) was designed to support high-risk adolescents in the early postpartal period and to prevent child abuse. The program offered meetings 3 days a week during the first 12 weeks postpartum and then weekly involvement for the first year of the infants' life. The focus of the program was on three areas: (a) performance of basic parenting skills, (b) management of parental stress, and (c) networking with community resources. Additionally, the program was intended to increase self-esteem through maternal role attainment. The program actively involved adolescents and community members by using them as volunteer helpers for the later groups. Community program volunteers included foster grandmothers, students from nearby colleges, and community members. Evaluation was conducted through interviews with a small number ($N = 15$) of participants and measures were not identified. Despite its methodological problems, the Parent–Baby (Ad)venture program offered a promising short-term approach to maternal role attainment and parenting behaviors.

The programs that addressed either maternal role attainment or infant outcomes suffered from the same type of methodological problems. Programs were insufficiently described to allow interpretation. Sample sizes were unequal and nonequivalent and therefore insufficient to draw conclusions. Instruments were developed for the project or did not have normative data for the adolescent population.

The Adolescent Father

The adolescent father is neglected in most programs. Work by Sachs, Poland, and Giblin (1990) addresses an ongoing initiative that involves the adolescent father more fully in pregnancy and childbearing. The father is seen as a support system for the adolescent mother. The Adolescent Prenatal Clinic was used to assess resources and to involve both partners. Fathers had limited involvement despite every effort to address their needs. This program suggests a need to include and support adolescent fathers in pregnancy and parenting care.

Social support was explored in a school-based descriptive study. Chen et al. (1995) used a convenient sample of African American unmarried, pregnant teenagers to examine relationships between support, age of the father of the baby, and prenatal care. Data from birth certificates indicate that the younger father who was also in school was more likely to be involved with the pregnancy and to encourage attendance at prenatal care appointments.

Adolescent fathers are a neglected member of the adolescent pregnancy experience. The lack of literature addressing the needs of the father is a clear gap in the research. The two studies identified fathers only insofar as they were supports for the mother. There were no studies identified that addressed the adolescent father as a unique individual.

SUMMARY AND FUTURE DIRECTIONS
FOR RESEARCH

As the reader can see, there are multiple programs for adolescents. Programs are run in many sites including schools, communities, hospitals, and clinics. Most states have some type of initiative. Providers include all types of health care professionals. Those who direct the programs believe that they will effect teen reproductive health in some way. Management teams and interdisciplinary groups provide care in the more effective programs. Most research on programs used quasi-experimental designs. Very few programs are culturally or ethnically specific. Ongoing evaluations are built into the longer running programs.

Mentoring exists in many programs. The mentoring takes the form of role models or women who connect the pregnant or parenting adolescent with another in the community. Some programs use a peer or peer group to support the pregnant adolescent.

Theory testing has occurred for models developed for adolescent care. The models that are based on existing theory are driven by social learning theory (Bandura, 1977) or a health belief/health promotion model. Interventions have been designed to effect perinatal outcomes as well as maternal role attainment. Programs offered many evaluative techniques.

There are many methodological issues. It is very difficult to randomly assign subjects to groups as these are very costly to conduct and providers often resist denying services to clients. Most of the work that was found included quasi-experimental designs with comparisons of a treatment or experimental group with a group from the general population. Comparison groups were nonequivalent and unequal. Comparisons were made based on population statistics, retrospective data from different time periods, and from other areas of the country. Low socioeconomic minority teenagers were overrepresented. Small samples were further subdivided into racial or ethnic groups, reducing the possibility to interpret the results. Sample sizes were often insufficient to detect effects. Teenagers self-selected into programs. Convenience samples were the main sampling technique. No attention was given to developmental level of the adolescent. Without random assignment and attention to these issues, it is difficult to be certain that the effects are due to the treatment rather than preexisting differences between the groups. Concepts such as maternal confidence and competence, self-esteem, and self-concept are not defined and used interchangeably. Investigator-designed instruments were used for many studies and established tools do not have normative data for adolescents. There was no attempt to control extraneous variables and account for changes over time. All of these methodological limitations reduce the ability to assess true effects.

The future direction for researchers is clear. Research with adolescents has suffered from a shotgun approach. A more rigorous and systematic approach to the conduct of research with adolescent populations is needed to build a body of knowledge with a strong theoretical base and conceptual clarity.

This will require communication between researchers and shared knowledge and experience. The explosion of information available on the Internet allows researchers to be more creative and to simultaneously examine the same programs across the country with different ethnic and racial groups. Innovative designs that address the extraneous variables including developmental level, program location, ethnicity, culture, age at first birth, and support systems can be developed through electronic communication. Although it is difficult to randomly assign adolescents to care, this rigor is necessary if health professionals and researchers are to understand the multiple factors and relationships involved in successful outcomes. Alternative approaches to sampling could include stratifying or blocking on the extraneous variables. Shared resources across the country would allow results from this type of sampling to be interpreted more generally.

Data indicated that the first pregnancy is often unplanned and not voluntary. Motivational factors that enter into the decision to become sexually active and to carry a baby to term are yet to be explored. The motivational factors may be different for different ethnic groups. Samples are necessary that examine issues in all adolescents, not only the low socioeconomic, minority, inner-city youth. Additionally, the emotional developmental level of the adolescents influences their interpretation of events. The adolescent who is developmentally dependent on peers is different from the one who listens to parents or has moved on to a significant other. Mentors and peer groups appear to be effective in supporting the adolescent mother. Conduct of research and development of programs for the adolescent should explore these supports and attend to these differences.

Though fragmented, the research conducted indicated that comprehensive programs appear more effective in changing outcomes. The comprehensive programs would benefit greatly from a concerted effort across the country. If this is the most effective and efficient approach to adolescent health care, then this needs to be documented and evaluated in multiple sites, with multiethnic, multiracial, multi-socioeconomic adolescents. With the anticipated increase in number of young adolescents under 17 years of age, it will be necessary to examine adolescent pregnancy and parenting much more carefully. Answers to these issues depend on the innovative designs and methodological rigor in adolescent research. More careful attention to design, sample and measurement better suited to the adolescent is necessary to determine the long-term effect of adolescent pregnancy and parenting on the adolescent and her child. Interdisciplinary, cross-country, clinical-trial research is the future of effective adolescent research initiatives.

ACKNOWLEDGMENT

The preparation of this chapter was supported in part by the National Institutes of Health, National Institute of Nursing Research under grant R01 NR04123 Health Promotion of the Pregnant Adolescent.

REFERENCES

Adams, P. F., Schoenborn, C. A., & Moss, A. J. (1995). *Health risk behaviors among our nation's youth: United States*, 1992. Vital and Health Statistics, Series 10, 192. DHHS Publication No. (PHS) 95-1520. Hyattsville, MD: National Center for Health Statistics.

Anderson, J. E., & Dahlberg, L. L. (1992). High-risk sexual behavior in the general population: Results from a national survey, 1988–1990. *Sexually Transmitted Diseases, 19,* 320–325.

Bachman, J. (1993). Self-described learning needs of pregnant teen participants in an innovative university/community partnership. *Maternal–Child Nursing Journal, 21,* 65–71.

Bandura, A. (1977). Self-efficacy: Toward a unifying theory of behavior change. *Psychological Review, 84,* 191–215.

Bayne Smith, M. (1994). Teen incentives program: Evaluation of a health promotion model for adolescent pregnancy prevention. *Journal of Health Education, 25,* 24–29.

Borgford-Parnell, D., Hope, K., & Keisher, R. (1994). A homeless teen pregnancy project: An intensive team case management model. *American Journal of Public Health, 84,* 1029–1030.

Breuner, C., & Farrow, J. A. (1995). Pregnant teens in prison—Prevalence, management and consequences. *Western Journal of Medicine, 162,* 328–330.

Chen, S. C., Telleen, S., & Chen, E. (1995). Adequacy of prenatal care of urban high school students. *Public Health Nursing, 12,* 47–52.

Covington, D. L., Churchill, P., Wright, B., Plummer, J., Cushing, D., & McCorkle, B. J. (1991). Adolescent rapid repeat pregnancy: Problem and intervention in a North Carolina hospital. *Health Values, 15*(5), 43–48.

Diener, M., Mangelsdorf, S., Contreras, J., Hazelwood, L., & Rhodes, J. (1995, March). *Correlates of parenting competence among Latina adolescent mothers.* Paper presented at the biennial meeting of the Society for Research in Child Development. Indianapolis, IN.

Dryfoos, J. G. (1990). *Adolescents at risk* (pp. 61–78). New York: Oxford University Press.

Dryfoos, J. G. (1991). Adolescents at risk: A summation of work in the field—Programs and policies. *Journal of Adolescent Health, 12,* 630–637.

Duffy, J., & Coates, T. J. (1989). Reducing smoking among pregnant adolescents. *Adolescents, 24,* 28–37.

East, P., Matthews, K., & Felice, M. (1994). Qualities of adolescent mothers' parenting. *Journal of Adolescent Health, 15,* 163–168.

Field, T., Widmayer, S., Stringer, S., & Ignatoff, E. (1980). Teenage, lower class, black mothers and their preterm infants: An intervention and developmental follow-up. *Child Development, 51,* 426–436.

Frost, J. J., & Forrest, J. D. (1995). Understanding the impact of effective teenage pregnancy prevention programs. *Family Planning Perspectives, 27*(5), 188–195.

Fullar, S., Eisinger, S., Engerman, J., Jefferson, J., Sprik, M., Martin, S., & Thompson-Scott, (1991). Information on a shoestring: A practical database at an adolescent pregnancy program. *Pediatric Nursing, 17,* 540–557.

Garcia-Coll, C., Hoffman, J., & Oh, W. (1987). The social ecology and early parenting of Caucasian adolescent mothers. *Child Development, 58,* 955–963.

Grogger, J., & Bronars, S. (1993). The socioeconomic consequences of teenage childbearing: Findings from a natural experiment. *Family Planning Perspectives, 25,* 156–174.

Hall, B., Dip, A., Lamont, L., App, B., Mackintosh, J., & St. John, W. (1987). Adolescent parenting education: The WA experience. *Australian Nurses Journal, 17,* 52–55.

Hardy, J., & Duggan, A. (1988). Teenage fathers and the fathers of infants of urban, teenage mothers. *American Journal of Public Health, 78,* 919–922.

Hardy, J., King, T., & Repke, J. (1987). The Johns Hopkins Adolescent Pregnancy Program: An evaluation. *Obstetrics & Gynecology, 69,* 300–306.

Hoyer, P., Jacobson, M., Ford, K., & Walsh, E. (1994). Pregnancy care for the adolescent. *Nurse Practitioner, 19,* 27–32.

Jones, M. E., & Mondy, L. W. (1994). Lessons for prevention and intervention in adolescent pregnancy: A five-year comparison of outcomes of two programs for school-aged pregnant adolescents. *Journal of Pediatric Health Care, 8,* 152–159.

Kann, L., Warren, C. W., Harris, W. A., Collins, J. L., Douglas, K. A., Collins, M. E., Williams, B. I., Ross, J. G., & Kolbe, L. J. (1995). Youth risk behavior surveillance—United States, 1993. *Morbidity and Mortality Weekly Report, 44,* 1–56.

Kelen, W., Hunt, W., Sibeko-Stones, L., & Varga, E. (1991). The special delivery club. *Canadian Nurse, 4,* 21–23.

Kleinfeld, L., & Young, R. (1989). Risk of pregnancy and dropping out of school among special education adolescents. *Journal of School Health, 59,* 359–361.

Kokotailo, P., & Adger, H. (1991). Substance use by pregnant adolescents. *Clinics in Perinatology, 18,* 113–138.

Koniak-Griffin, D. (1994). Aerobic exercise, psychological well-being, and physical discomforts during adolescent pregnancy. *Research in Nursing and Health, 17,* 253–263.

Koniak-Griffin, D., & Verzemnieks, I. (1991). Effects of nursing intervention on adolescent's maternal role attainment. *Issues in Comprehensive Pediatric Nursing, 14,* 121–138.

Koo, H., Dunteman, G., George, C., Green, Y., & Murray, V. (1994). Reducing adolescent pregnancy through a school- and community-based intervention: Denmark, South Carolina, revisited. *Family Planning Perspectives, 26,* 206–217.

Lapierre, J., Perreault, M., & Goulet, C. (1995). Prenatal peer counseling: An answer to the persistent difficulties with prenatal care for low-income women. *Public Health Nursing, 112,* 53–60.

Lavery, J. P., Chaffee, G., Marcell, C. C., Martin, S., & Reece, K. (1988). Pregnancy outcome in a comprehensive teenage-parent program. *Journal of Adolescent and Pediatric Gynecology, 1,* 34–38.

Lee, S., & Grubbs, L. (1993). A comparison of self-reported self-care practices of pregnant adolescents. *Nurse Practitioner, 18,* 25–29.

McAfee, M., & Geesey, M. (1984). Meeting the needs of the teen-age pregnant study: An in-school program that works. *Journal of School Health, 54,* 350–352.

Mercer, R. (1980). Teenage motherhood: The first year. *Journal of Obstetric and Gynecologic Nursing, 9,* 16–26.

Mercer, R. (1985). The process of maternal role attainment over the first year. *Nursing Research, 34,* 198–204.

Mikanowicz, C., Nicholson, M., Olsen, L., & Wang, M. (1992). Adolescent pregnancy outcomes from a rural Pennsylvania program. *Health Values, 16,* 23–30.

Morris, D. L., Berenson, A., Lawson, J., & Wiemann, C. (1993). Comparison of adolescent pregnancy outcomes by prenatal care source. *Journal of Reproductive Medicine, 38,* 375–380.

Moore, K. (January, 1996). *Child Trends: Facts at a glance.* Washington, DC: Child Trends.

Moore, K. (June, 1997). *Child Trends: Facts at a glance.* Washington, DC: Child Trends.

Moore, K., Miller, B. C., Glei, D., & Morrison, D. R. (1995). *Adolescent sex: Contraception, and childbearing: A review of recent research.* Washington, DC: Child Trends.

Moore, K., Sugarland, B. W., Blumenthal, C., Glei, D., & Snyder, N. (1995). *Adolescent pregnancy prevention programs: Interventions and evaluations.* Washington, DC: Child Trends.

Mosena, P., & Ruch-Ross, H. S. (1996a, December). *Multisite implementation of a community based model for delaying second pregnancies among adolescent mothers.* Annual meeting of the American Public Health Association, Session 1163.

Mosena, P., & Ruch-Ross, H. S. (1996b, December). *CBD in the inner city: A strategy for delaying second birth among adolescent mothers.* Annual meeting of the American Public Health Association, Session 3109.

Musick, J. S. (1993). *Young, poor, and pregnant.* New Haven, CT: Yale University Press.

National Adolescent Health Resource Center. (1993). *Final report—Evaluative review: Findings from a study of selected high school Wellness Centers in Delaware* (pp. 1–10). Division of General Pediatrics and Adolescent Health, University of Minnesota.

Neeson, J. D., Patterson, K., Mercer, R., & May, K. (1983). Pregnancy outcome for adolescents receiving prenatal care by nurse practitioners in extended roles. *Journal of Adolescent Health Care, 4,* 94–99.

Nelson, K., Key, D., Fletcher, J., Kirkpatrick, E., & Feinstein, R. (1982). The Teen-Tot clinic: An alternative to traditional care for infants of teenage mothers. *Journal of Adolescent Health Care, 3,* 19–23.

Opuni, K. W., Smith, P. B., Arvey, H., & Solomon, C. (1994). The Northeast Adolescent Project: A collaborative effort to address teen-age pregnancy in Houston, Texas. *Journal of School Health, 64,* 212–214.

O'Sullivan, A., & Jacobsen, B. (1992). A randomized trial of a health care program for first-time adolescent mothers and their infants. *Nursing Research, 41,* 210–215.

Polit, D. F. (1989). Effects of a comprehensive program for teenage parents: Five years after Project Redirection. *Family Planning Perspectives, 21,* 164–169.

Polit, D. F., & Kahn, J. R. (1985). Project Redirection: Evaluation of a comprehensive program for disadvantaged teenage mothers. *Family Planning Perspectives, 17,* 150–155.

Porter, L. (1984). Parenting enhancement among high-risk adolescents: Testing a holistic patient-centered nursing practice mode. *Nursing Clinics of North America, 19,* 89–102.

Records, K. (1994). Adolescent mothers: Caregiving, approval, and family functioning. *Journal of Obstetric, Gynecologic and Neonatal Nursing, 23,* 791–797.

Roye, C., & Balk, S. (1996). Evaluation of an intergenerational program for pregnant and parenting adolescents. *Maternal–Child Nursing Journal, 24,* 32–40.

Ruch-Ross, H., Jones, E., & Musick, J. (1992). Comparing outcomes in a statewide program for adolescent mothers with outcomes in a national sample. *Family Planning Perspectives, 24,* 66–71, 96.

Sachs, B., Poland, M., & Giblin, P. (1990). Enhancing the adolescent reproductive process: Efforts to implement a program for black adolescent fathers. *Health Care for Women International, 11,* 447–460.

Sameroff, A., & Chandler, M. (1975). Reproductive risk and the continuum of caretaking casualty. In F. D. Horowitz (Ed.), *Review of child development research* (Vol. 4, pp. 187–244). Chicago: University of Chicago Press.

Schinke, S. P. (1981). Primary prevention of adolescent pregnancy. *Social Work with Groups, 4,* 1–2.

Setzer, J., & Smith, D. (1992). Comprehensive school-based services for pregnant and parenting adolescents in West Dallas, Texas. *Journal of School Health, 62,* 97–102.

Sheaff, L., & Talashek, M. (1995). Ever-pregnant and never-pregnant teens in a temporary housing shelter. *Journal of Community Health Nursing, 12,* 33–45.

Smith, P. B., & Gingiss, P. L. (1996). Characteristics of pregnant adolescents receiving prenatal care at school-based or hospital-based clinics. *Journal of Health Education, 27,* 30–37.

Smoke, J., & Grace, M. (1988). Effectiveness of prenatal care and education for pregnant adolescents: Nurse-midwifery intervention and team approach. *Journal of Nurse Midwifery, 33,* 178–184.

Stevens-Simon, C., Fullar, S., & McAnarney, C. (1992). Tangible differences between adolescent-oriented and adult-oriented prenatal care. *Journal of Adolescent Health, 13,* 298–302.

Stevens-Simon, C., Kaplan, D., & McAnarney, C. (1993). Factors associated with preterm delivery among pregnant adolescents. *Journal of Adolescent Health, 14,* 340–342.

Talashek, M. (1992). *Nursing model of adolescent maturity and pregnancy* (Grant no. NR02512). Bethesda, MD: National Institutes of Health, Division of Research Grants.

Thompson, J. (1993). Supporting young mothers: Midwifery, teenage pregnancies. *Nursing Times, 89,* 64–67.

Thompson, P., Powell, M. J., Patterson, R., & Ellerbee, S. (1995). Adolescent parenting: Outcomes and maternal perceptions. *Journal of Obstetric, Gynecologic and Neonatal Nursing, 24,* 713–718.

Tulkin, S. (1977). Social class differences in maternal and infant behavior. In P. H. Leiderman, S. R. Tulkin, & A. Rosenthal (Eds.), *Culture and infancy* (pp. 495–538). New York: Academic Press.

Warrick, L., Christianson, J. B., Walruff, J., & Cook, P. C. (1993). Educational outcomes in teenage pregnancy and parenting programs: Results from a demonstration. *Family Planning Perspectives, 25,* 148–155.

Williams-Burgess, C., Vines, S., & Ditulio, M. (1995). The Parent-Baby Venture program: Prevention of child abuse. *Journal of Child and Adolescent Psychiatric Nursing, 8,* 15–23.

PART III

Other Research

Chapter 10

Chronic Obstructive Pulmonary Disease: Strategies to Improve Functional Status

Janet L. Larson
College of Nursing
University of Illinois at Chicago

Nancy Kline Leidy
Health Outcomes Research
MEDTAP International, Inc.

ABSTRACT

People with chronic obstructive pulmonary disease (COPD) experience deterioration in functional status, therefore improving functional status is a major goal of treatment. We reviewed interventions to improve functional status in people with COPD published from 1980 through September 1996. Randomized controlled clinical trials were reviewed to document outcomes in terms of functional capacity and functional performance for the following interventions: pharmacologic therapy including theophylline, inhaled bronchodilators, steroids, antianxiolytics and antidepressants; general exercise strategies including exercise training, exercise and comprehensive pulmonary rehabilitation, and upper extremity training; inspiratory muscle therapy including inspiratory muscle training and inspiratory muscle rest; nutritional therapy; oxygen therapy; and specialized nursing care. Improvements for functional capacity were documented in terms of strength of the inspiratory muscles and upper extremities, walking tests, and peak oxygen uptake. Most interventions were targeted to enhance functional capacity, and few were aimed at enhancing functional performance. Further research is needed to examine the relationship between functional capacity and functional performance and to design and test interventions to improve functional performance.

Keywords: Chronic Obstructive Pulmonary Disease, Functional Status, Pulmonary Rehabilitation, Clinical Outcomes

FUNCTIONAL STATUS

People with chronic obstructive pulmonary disease (COPD) experience a gradual deterioration in functional status. The underlying lung disease is characterized by airflow obstruction, air trapping, and impaired gas exchange associated with a decrease in exercise tolerance and physical symptoms such as cough, dyspnea, and fatigue. These people have fixed airflow obstruction that is not reversible with bronchodilators. There is no cure for this illness. Rather, most intervention strategies, such as pharmacologic therapy, exercise, strength training, nutritional supplementation, oxygen therapy, and home care, are designed to improve functional status. Improving functional status will optimize lung function, minimize symptoms, enhance or maintain day-to-day performance and ultimately, improve quality of life. The imperative in today's health care climate is to demonstrate not only the efficacy of such programs, but their cost-effectiveness as well.

This review addresses the outcome of functional status by synthesizing information derived from randomized controlled trials of people with fixed airflow obstruction, that is, those with a medical diagnosis of chronic bronchitis, emphysema, or COPD. Leidy's (1994b) analytical approach serves as the framework for selecting and evaluating trials designed to improve functional status in people with this debilitating pulmonary disease.

This review is based on a model that defines functional status as a multidimensional concept characterizing the ability to perform activities people generally do in the normal course of their lives to meet basic needs, fulfill usual roles, and maintain their health and well-being (Leidy, 1994b). According to this model, four dimensions of functional status should be distinguished in assessing outcomes: capacity, performance, reserve, and capacity utilization (Leidy, 1994a). Briefly, functional capacity is an individual's maximum potential to perform activities. Performance refers to the day-to-day corporeal activities people do in the normal course of their lives, subject to limits imposed by capacity; reserve is the difference between capacity and performance and refers to latent abilities that can be called on in times of need; and capacity utilization is the extent to which capacity is called on in the selected level of performance (Leidy, 1994a). This review is focused on interventions designed to improve two of these dimensions: capacity and performance.

Functional Capacity

Functional capacity is defined within the context of one's maximum potential to perform daily activities (Leidy, 1994b). The term is used in exercise physiology to delineate the maximum metabolic rate (peak oxygen uptake) achieved during exercise. Within the context of functional status, however, functional capacity goes much further and can include factors such as skeletal muscle strength or oxygen delivery (Leidy, 1994b). Although functional capacity can involve cognitive, psychological, social, and sociodemographic potential, this review will be limited to the physiologic dimension of capacity.

In COPD, physiologic capacity is limited by a combination of ventilatory impairment and physical deconditioning. Limitations of ventilatory capacity are related to increased airway resistance and impaired function of inspiratory muscles. Increased airway resistance increases the work of breathing, and hyperinflation of the chest places the inspiratory muscles at a mechanical disadvantage, reducing their force-generating capacity. Symptomatically, people with COPD experience progressive exertional dyspnea, evidence that they are impinging on reserve. They gradually reduce their physical activities to avoid experiencing dyspnea. The sedentary lifestyle, in turn, contributes to physical deconditioning, characterized by generalized muscle weakness and a reduction in exercise tolerance.

Capacity-targeted strategies are designed to halt or slow this downward spiral. Specifically strategies are aimed at improving capacity for walking and inspiratory muscle function. Thus, the most frequently used outcome measures in clinical trials designed to improve physiologic capacity are symptom-limited exercise tests, exercise tests for endurance at a submaximal workload, timed walking tests such as the 6- or 12-minute–distance walk tests, as well as strength and endurance of the inspiratory muscles and peripheral muscles. The maximal inspiratory pressure (PI_{max}) was frequently used as a measure of inspiratory muscle strength.

Functional Performance

The performance dimension of functional status is defined as the extent to which people actually execute various activities on a daily basis (Leidy, 1994b). These activities reflect individual choice, operating within the constraints imposed by capacity (Leidy, 1994a). Relatively little is known about the factors contributing to variations in performance in people with COPD (Leidy & Haase, 1996). Reduced pulmonary capacity, reflected in forced expiratory volume in second (FEV_1) percentage predicted, accounts for less than 10% of the variance in self-reported functional performance scores. A stronger relationship has been found between walking tests, generally the 6- or 12-minute–distance walk test, and functional performance (Leidy, 1995). Psychosocial factors appear to influence functional performance, independent of the physiologic effects, with anxiety, depression, and psychosocial resources among the significant predictors (Leidy & Traver, 1995). Cross-sectional, multivariate studies suggest a combination of physiological and psychosocial factors account for 27% to 62% of the performance variations seen in this population, leaving a significant portion unexplained (Leidy, 1995).

Self-report is the most frequently used approach for evaluating performance outcomes, with the Sickness Impact Profile (SIP) (Bergner, Bobbitt, Carter, & Gilson, 1981) among the most common measures. Unfortunately, the inclusion of symptoms and the merging of physical and psychosocial performance into an "overall" score make this instrument less than ideal for this purpose (Leidy, 1994a, 1995). Other self-report measures include the Barthel Index (Mahoney & Barthel, 1965), Katz Activities of Daily Living questionnaire (Katz, Ford, Moskowitz, Jackson, & Jaffe, 1963), and various subscales of the Medical Outcomes Study Short Form-36 (Ware & Sherbourne, 1992), Nottingham Health Profile (Katz et al., 1963), and the St. George's Respiratory Questionnaire (P. W. Jones, Quirk, Baveystock, & Littlejohns, 1992). Of these, the Barthel Index and the Katz Activities of Daily Living questionnaires come closest to true performance as defined here (Bloom et al., 1989). Two disease-specific measures to assess functional performance have appeared in the nursing literature: The Pulmonary Functional Status and Dyspnea Questionnaire (Lareau, Carrieri-Kohlman, Janson-Bjerklie, & Roos, 1994) and the Pulmonary Functional Status Scale (Weaver & Narsavage, 1992). Finally, there is emerging evidence that actigraphy, an instrument for counting and tracking movement over time, and calimetry, an instrument for tracking caloric expenditure, may be useful methods for objectively evaluating functional performance and documenting outcomes (Leidy, Abbott, & Fedenko, 1997). Most of the above instruments have been used to test interventions for people with COPD.

REVIEW PROCESS AND CONSTRAINTS

The purpose of this review is to synthesize the empirical evidence related to the efficacy of interventions designed to improve functional status in people with COPD. The review focuses on randomized controlled clinical trials with the following functional capacity outcomes: walking and related variables and inspiratory muscle function. These outcomes were emphasized because they were commonly measured across interventions. Other outcomes were discussed when directly relevant to functional capacity, and cost-effectiveness was discussed when that information was available. The review does not address the efficacy of interventions specifically targeted at pulmonary impairment (pulmonary function) and dyspnea.

Trials employing functional performance outcomes were included in the review if the intent of the study and the outcome indicators were consistent with the conceptual definition of performance. That is, a study was included if it evaluated corporeal day-to-day activities, independent of symptoms, such as dyspnea. Performance measures could be objective, self-report, or simulation. It is important to note that the terms "functional status," "health status," "quality of life," and "health-related quality of life" have been used interchangeably in the literature (Leidy, 1995). Studies represented by these terms were included only if performance outcomes could be evaluated through the presentation of results. Several studies presented results from the Sickness Impact and Nottingham Health Profiles, for example, and are included in this review.

Randomized controlled clinical trials, from 1980 through November 1995, that examined interventions to improve functional status in people with COPD were reviewed. Studies were identified through multiple searches of the MED-LINE database, searching for all studies published in English and using chronic obstructive lung disease as one key word in combination with each of the following: functional status, rehabilitation, quality of life, health status, activities of daily living, and functional ability. To increase the likelihood of obtaining all relevant studies, the results of the initial search were verified by a second series of MEDLINE searches with the addition of exercise, oxygen, nutrition, rehabilitation, and randomized controlled clinical trials. Additionally some studies were identified from the reference lists of published studies.

The search yielded a large number of studies addressing the efficacy of pharmacologic therapy, exercise training, comprehensive pulmonary rehabilitation, and inspiratory muscle training (IMT). Fewer studies were located that examined the effects of resting the inspiratory muscles, nutritional therapy, oxygen therapy, and specialized nursing care. This review addresses the following therapies designed to improve functional status in people with COPD: pharmacologic therapy, exercise therapy, inspiratory muscle therapy, nutritional supplementation, oxygen therapy, and specialized nursing care.

PHARMACOLOGIC THERAPY

Pharmacologic therapy is the traditional mainstay for the treatment of people with COPD, specifically methylzanthines, inhaled anticholinergics, inhaled beta-adrenergic agonists, and inhaled and oral steroids. The primary goal of pharmacologic therapy is to decrease airway resistance and reduce pulmonary impairment as measured by pulmonary function tests. But pharmacologic therapy has the potential to enhance functional capacity and functional perfor-mance, directly through effects on skeletal muscles or indirectly through the amelioration of symptoms. Most studies tested the effect of pharmacologic agents on functional capacity on exercise testing and inspiratory muscle strength. Functional performance outcomes were evaluated in trials testing the therapeutic effects of bronchodilators, steroids, and antidepressants (Borson et al., 1992; van Schayck et al., 1995; van Schayck, Rutten-van Molken, van Doorslaer, Folgering, & van Weel, 1992).

Theophylline

Although theophylline is regularly prescribed for people with COPD, all of its effects are not known. It is reported to improve respiratory muscle function and stimulate respiratory centers of the brain, but it has a narrow therapeutic range and potentially serious side effects result when serum levels exceed upper limits. Eight controlled clinical trials (double-blind cross-over studies) examined the efficacy of theophylline in terms of functional capacity, either for bicycling or walking (Dullinger, Kronenberg, & Niewoehner, 1986; Eaton, MacDonald, Church, & Niewoehner, 1982; Fink, Kaye, Sulkes, Gabbay, & Spitzer, 1994; Guyatt et al., 1987; Mahler, Matthay, Snyder, Wells, & Loke, 1985; McKay, Howie, Thomson, Whiting, & Addis, 1993; Mulloy & McNi-cholas, 1993; Newman, Tamir, Speedy, Newman, & Ben-Dov, 1994). Studies were included in this review if theophylline treatment was administered for 1 week or longer.

Results from these eight studies were conflicting. Four (Fink et al., 1994; Guyatt et al., 1987; McKay et al., 1993; Newman et al., 1994) suggested that theophylline improves capacity for walking and/or bicycling, whereas the remainder did not. All of these studies included people with moderate to severe COPD, most with irreversible airway disease, and few with oxygen dependence. Improvements in functional capacity were typically very modest in magnitude. Guyatt et al. (1987) studied people with fixed airway disease and compared performance on the 6-minute–distance walk test after 2 weeks of each of the following: placebo, theophylline, salbutamol, salbutamol, and theophylline. Results demonstrated that people walked more than 40 meters further after either drug alone, compared to placebo, but there was no additive benefit to the combination of both drugs. McKay et al. (1993) compared the effects of 5 weeks of treatment with placebo, low-dose theophylline

(10 mg/L), and high-dose theophylline (17 mg/L). People walked significantly further on a submaximal treadmill test after the high-dose theophylline compared to placebo and low-dose theophylline, with a 95% confidence interval for the differences between the two groups of 7 to 126 meters. Newman and colleagues (1994) compared the effects of 4 weeks of theophylline to 4 weeks of placebo and found a 14% increase in peak oxygen uptake and a 17% increase in maximal ventilation. Fink and associates (1994) examined the effects of 1 month of theophylline compared to placebo. People in the treatment group experienced a modest improvement in peak oxygen uptake (12%) and maximal ventilation (12%) compared to placebo. In contrast the remaining four studies (Dullinger et al., 1986; Eaton et al., 1982; Mahler et al., 1985; Mulloy & McNicholas, 1993) reported no improvement in exercise performance after treatment with theophylline, despite comparable samples and sample sizes.

Inconsistencies in results can be explained by differences in sample characteristics and in research design. Issues related to sample characteristics include differences in airway response to bronchodilators and severity of airflow obstruction. People with fixed airway disease may be less likely to benefit from inhaled bronchodilators. The two studies (Mahler et al., 1985; Mulloy & McNicholas, 1993) with the most stringent inclusion criteria excluded people with >15% improvement in the FEV_1 after the administration of inhaled bronchodilators. Both of these studies reported no improvement in either FEV_1 or exercise performance with theophylline. Additionally, people with moderate airflow obstruction may be more likely to respond to theophylline than people with severe airflow obstruction because of differences in functional reserve. The mean FEV_1 was slightly higher for three of the four studies (Fink et al., 1994; Guyatt et al., 1987; Newman et al., 1994) that demonstrated an improvement in exercise performance after theophylline, ranging from 38% to 41% of predicted normal values. Most of the above studies used relatively small sample sizes, however, making it difficult to sort out the effects for subgroups. From a research-design perspective one would expect people to respond differently depending on the dose of theophylline and concurrent medications. But differences across studies cannot be explained based on the differences in the serum level of theophylline or the dose of theophylline, possibly because of the confounding effects of concurrent medications.

The effects of theophylline on respiratory muscle strength were examined in three studies (Jaeschke, Guyatt, Singer, Keller, & Newhouse, 1991; Murciano, Aubier, Lecocguic, & Pariente, 1984; Murciano, Auclair, Pariente, & Aubier, 1989). All three studies demonstrated an increase in respiratory muscle strength, ranging from 8% to 24%. The underlying mechanism for increased functional strength was not clear, however. In all three studies theophylline treatment produced concurrent improvements in airflow obstruction, which could improve inspiratory muscle mechanics if accompanied by a reduction in hyperinflation of the chest. Decreased hyperinflation and improved muscle mechanics would increase functional strength of the inspiratory muscles. Murciano and coworkers (1984, 1989) argued that the changes in airflow obstruction were not accompanied by changes in hyperinflation as measured by functional residual capacity, making it unlikely that there was a substantial change in muscle mechanics. In the final analysis the effects of theophylline on respiratory muscles are not well understood, but from a functional perspective the improvement in functional strength of the inspiratory muscles appears to be consistent across controlled studies of people with COPD.

Inhaled Bronchodilators

The effects of inhaled bronchodilators, adrenergic beta agonists, and anticholinergics in terms of functional capacity were tested in three clinical trials. Two weeks of treatment with salbutamol (British name for albuterol) alone produced an improvement in the 6-minute–distance walk test (Guyatt et al., 1987) and no change in PI_{max} (Jaeschke et al., 1991). One week of treatment with metaproterenol alone did not increase the 12-minute–distance walk, but a week of combined therapy, metaproterenol and theophylline, produced an increase in the 12-minute–distance walk (Dullinger et al., 1986). Concurrent improvements in FEV_1 were noted in all three of these studies and could account for the observed improvements in functional capacity. Three additional trials were reported, one examining the dose–response relationship for terbutaline and two comparing an inhaled beta agonist to inhaled anticholinergic therapy. Jaeschke and colleagues (1994) found no differences in the 6-minute–distance walk test or PI_{max} after a 1-week treatment with each of three doses of inhaled terbutaline, 500, 1,000, and 1,500 μg four times a day. Blosser, Maxwell, Reeves-Hoche, Localio, and Zwillich (1995) found that inhaled albuterol and inhaled ipratropium (an anticholinergic drug) produced similar responses with a mean increase in the 12-minute–distance walk over baseline of 59.9 and 64.6 m, respectively. Van Schayck and coworkers (1992) found that inhaled salbutamol and inhaled ipratropium produced similar responses in terms of functional performance as measured by the Nottingham Health Profile (Katz et al., 1963). Across studies the observed inconsistencies with respect to functional capacity could be accounted for by the differences in the specific drugs studied. Although results are promising, they are preliminary as a relatively small number of people were studied.

Steroids

The effects of steroids were examined in terms of functional capacity and functional performance in persons with severe but clinically stable COPD. Grove, Lipworth, Ingram, Clark, and Dhillon (1995) demonstrated that treatment with 3 weeks of oral prednisolone was associated with a significant increase in peak oxygen uptake (10%), but no change in 6-minute–distance walk and no change in functional performance as measured by an activity questionnaire.

Antianxiolytic and Antidepressant Drugs

People with COPD are thought to have elevated levels of anxiety that may contribute to reduced functional capacity, hence the effects of buspirone, an antianxiolytic drug, were examined in two studies. Singh, Despars, Stansbury, Avalos, and Light (1993) found that buspirone produced no effect on the 12-minute–distance (12 MD) walk and peak performance on a graded exercise test, specifically peak work rate, peak oxygen uptake, and peak ventilation. In contrast Argyropoulou, Patakas, Koukou, Vasiliadis, and Georgopoulos (1993) observed no change in peak oxygen uptake and peak ventilation but did report significant improvements in peak work load (13%) and the 6-minute–distance walk (6 MD) (4%). Improvements in exercise performance found in the latter study could be attributed to increased efficiency rather than an actual increase in capacity. This would be consistent with an overall reduction in muscle tension that one would expect to accompany a decrease in anxiety. These findings are preliminary because they involve only two studies and the actual usefulness of antianxiolytic drugs is unclear.

The effects of antidepressants on capacity and performance were examined in one randomized, double-blind trial. Borson et al. (1992) studied 30 people with moderate to severe COPD and coexisting depressive disorder, evaluating functional status before and after 12 weeks of treatment with nortriptyline. No change was observed in capacity as measured by the 12MD. Functional performance improved in both groups, according to the Pulmonary Functional Status Instrument (Lareau et al., 1994) and the Sickness Impact Profile (Bergner et al., 1981) scores, however, only the treatment group experienced statistically significant changes. The Nortriptyline group reported a significant reduction in the number of activities rated "markedly affected" and a decrease in the degree to which activity in general was affected by the disease, according to the Pulmonary Functional Status Instrument. Significant nortriptyline effects were also seen in the SIP overall, physical, and psychosocial scores, although the differential treatment effect was significant only for the overall score.

From this group of drug studies it can generally be concluded that pharmacologic therapy has the potential to produce subtle improvements in functional capacity and possibly functional performance. The expected outcomes have not been clearly defined for individual drugs, however, and continued work is needed to determine which subgroups of people are most likely to benefit from specific drugs.

GENERAL EXERCISE THERAPY

Studies of exercise training can be organized into three groups: general exercise training for endurance, the combination of exercise training for endurance and comprehensive pulmonary rehabilitation, and upper extremity training for strength and endurance. The largest number of studies examined general exercise training and the combination of general exercise training and comprehensive pulmonary rehabilitation.

Exercise Training

The methods of general exercise training included bicycle training, walking, stair climbing, and methods that incorporate multiple exercises. The functional capacity outcomes of exercise training in the outpatient and/or home setting were reported in six randomized controlled clinical trials. Four (Busch & McClements, 1988; Degre et al., 1974; Lake, Henderson, Briffa, Openshaw, & Musk, 1990; McGavin, Gupta, Lloyd, & McHardy, 1977) of the six studies reported evidence of improved functional capacity, but the strength of the evidence was very modest. Two studies (Lake et al., 1990; McGavin et al., 1977) demonstrated a significant improvement in functional capacity for walking as reflected by either the 12MD or the 6MD. In these studies subjects trained for 3 months with stair climbing (McGavin et al., 1977) and for 2 months with stair climbing (Lake et al., 1990). In both studies significant improvements were reported within the treatment group, accompanied by no improvement in the control group and no report of between-group differences and interaction effects. In two other studies no change was found in functional capacity for walking: in one case after 9 weeks of stair climbing (Booker, 1984) and in the other after 10 weeks of multiple exercises including walking, step-ups, and stand-ups (D. T. Jones, Thomson, & Sears, 1985). In all of the exercise studies, however, subjects increased the intensity of training over the course of the intervention, either by increasing the training load or by increasing the duration of training sessions; and this is strong evidence for an increase in functional capacity to perform work.

The bulk of the evidence suggested that observed improvements in functional outcomes were not related to an aerobic training effect of the skeletal muscles in people with COPD. Two of the above studies (Lake et al., 1990; McGavin et al., 1977) demonstrated no change in functional capacity as reflected by the peak oxygen uptake after exercise training. One (Degre et al., 1974) demonstrated a significant improvement in peak oxygen uptake after training (mean increase of 10%) compared to baseline and no significant change in the control group (mean increase of 5%), but did not examine between-group treatment effects. Alternatively, improvements in functional outcomes could be accounted for by one of the following: improved coordination of skeletal muscles that reduced the effort required for a given level of activity, decreased sensitivity to dyspnea that reduced fear of exertional dyspnea, and enhanced motivation to perform.

The effects of workload were examined by Patessio, Carone, Ioli, and Donner (1992). People trained on bicycles 5 days a week for 8 weeks at either a low work rate, below the anaerobic threshold, or a high work rate, above the anaerobic threshold. A significant difference was found between the groups with respect to endurance time for cycling at a fixed work rate, increasing by 71% and 8% for people who trained at the high and low work rates, respectively.

Long-term follow-up after exercise training was examined in two studies. Swerts, Kretzers, Terpstra-Linderman, Verstappen, and Wouters (1990) examined the effects of 12 weeks of follow-up with weekly supervised exercise in the outpatient setting compared to written instructions for home exercise. The two conditions were imposed after an 8-week program of supervised exercise training in the outpatient setting. The group with supervised follow-up retained their improved performance on the 12-minute–distance walk, whereas the group without supervised follow-up decreased performance on the 12-minute–distance walk at 26 weeks and at 52 weeks ($p < .05$). In contrast Tydeman, Chandler, Graveling, Culot, and Harrison (1984) demonstrated no treatment-group differences after 6 months of supervised follow-up compared to unsupervised exercises at home. Improvements in the 12-minute–distance walk were retained for both groups over a period of 6 months. This was accompanied by an improved ability to carry out activities of daily living for 75% of subjects in the group with supervised follow-up and in 50% of the group with no supervised follow-up.

Functional performance outcomes were reported in one study. Booker (1984) observed an increase in self-reported activities of daily living after 9 weeks of stair-climbing exercises as compared to a no-treatment control group. The perceived increase in activities of daily living occurred without a concurrent improvement in the 6-minute–distance walk.

Toevs, Kaplan, and Atkins (1984) examined the efficacy and cost-effectiveness of behavioral interventions to improve compliance with exercise and to ultimately improve functional performance. They studied 90 people with COPD, randomly assigned to one of five groups, three experimental groups participating in behavioral programs to improve compliance and two control groups. All participants were given an individualized exercise prescription, with the Health Status Index (HSI) (Bush, Chen, & Patrick, 1973) used as the outcome measure in determining cost-effectiveness. Briefly, the HSI involves the classification of participants into one of 43 states of functioning that are weighted from 0 (death) to 1 (optimum functioning) according to social preference or utility. Although utilities are often equated with quality of life and used to compare treatment groups and to estimate quality-adjusted life years, the health states of the HSI were described in terms of performance variations. These scores are used to compare treatment groups and estimate the well-year, or quality-adjusted life years, associated with the intervention. In this study, differences between the experimental and control groups were statistically significant ($p < .002$) at 3 months, improvements in health status were greater in the treatment groups, becoming only marginally significant over time as a result of increased variability in the two groups. Dividing this number by cost yields a cost-effectiveness or cost-utility ratio for the program, a common metric that can then be compared across different intervention programs. Costs were calculated by combining direct costs of treatment, indirect costs, and averted hospitalization charges. Using this method, Toevs, Kaplan, and Atkins (1984) estimated the cost per well-year of the treatment (experimental) program to be between $10,834 and $36,897. To put this in perspective, they provided the following guidelines proposed earlier by Kaplan and Bush (1982): Less than $20,000, cost-effective; $20,000 to $100,000 possibly controversial but justifiable; greater than $100,000 per well-year, questionable when compared with other health care expenditures.

Exercise and Comprehensive Pulmonary Rehabilitation

Comprehensive pulmonary rehabilitation includes a range of therapeutic modalities designed to decrease respiratory symptoms, improve functional status, and ultimately to improve quality of life (American Thoracic Society, 1995). Components of pulmonary rehabilitation that are directly aimed at improving functional capacity include exercise training and inspiratory muscle training.

Other elements such as education and psychosocial support are specifically aimed at reducing symptoms, psychosocial morbidity, and improving functional performance. Comprehensive pulmonary rehabilitation has been widely used since the 1970s in the treatment of COPD and multiple uncontrolled studies were conducted to examine its effects. The first clinical trial of comprehensive pulmonary rehabilitation was reported by Toshima, Kaplan, and Ries (1990), and since that time an additional four trials have been reported (Goldstein, Gort, Stubbing, Avendano, & Guyatt, 1994; Reardon et al., 1994; Ries, Kaplan, Limberg, & Prewitt, 1995; Wijkstra et al., 1995). The results of these studies suggest that comprehensive pulmonary rehabilitation programs can improve functional capacity in people with COPD if adequate exercise training is a major component of the rehabilitation program. Because only one study (Toshima et al., 1990) addressed performance outcomes, the extent to which these improvements translate into greater day-to-day performance is not yet known.

Two (Reardon et al., 1994; Ries et al., 1995) of the studies measured peak oxygen uptake during a symptom-limited incremental exercise test, the traditional measure of functional capacity for clinical studies of exercise training. In all four studies functional capacity was measured with a skill test, either a walking test or the endurance time for exercising at a fixed workload on a treadmill or cycle ergometer.

Significant increase in peak oxygen uptake was observed in the larger study ($N = 119$) (Ries et al., 1995); but not in the smaller study ($N = 20$) (Reardon et al., 1994), suggesting the latter result was due to insufficient power. An increase of 9% in peak oxygen uptake was observed in a group of people with moderate to severe COPD after a pulmonary rehabilitation program that included 12 4-hour sessions over 8 weeks with supplemental walking two times a day at home (Ries et al., 1995). The improvements in peak oxygen uptake were no longer present 10 months after the end of the pulmonary rehabilitation program.

In three (Goldstein et al., 1994; Reardon et al., 1994; Ries et al., 1995) of the studies significant improvements were observed in the skill tests. Endurance time for walking on the treadmill at a submaximal workload increased by 85% (10.5 minutes) after 8 weeks of pulmonary rehabilitation with a persistent increase of 40% (5 minutes) at 18 months, though measurable improvements were no longer apparent at 24 months (Ries et al., 1995). Smaller but significant improvements were noted for endurance time in two other studies. After 2 months of inpatient pulmonary rehabilitation with 4 months of outpatient follow-up, an increase of 4.7 minutes was documented on the cycler ergometer (Goldstein et al., 1994). After 6 weeks of pulmonary rehabilitation an increase of 2.1 minutes was observed on the treadmill (Reardon et al., 1994). Similar improvements were noted for the walking tests. People with COPD increased the 6-minute–distance walk by a mean of 37.9 meters after 2 months of inpatient pulmonary rehabilitation and 4 months of outpatient follow-up (Goldstein et al., 1994). In contrast no change was observed in the 6-minute–distance walk after 6 weeks of pulmonary rehabilitation that included progressive muscle relaxation, breathing retraining, pacing, self-talk, and panic control, but no exercise training (Sassi-Dambron, Eakin, Ries, & Kaplan, 1995). This illustrates the importance of exercise as a component of pulmonary rehabilitation when considering functional outcomes.

For some people pulmonary rehabilitation may delay deterioration in functional outcomes, even when no initial improvements resulted from the rehabilitation program. One study (Wijkstra et al., 1995, 1996) demonstrated no significant change in the 6-minute–distance walk and peak work load on a bicycle after 12 weeks of home-based pulmonary rehabilitation. The pulmonary rehabilitation sessions were limited to 30-minute visits twice a week, substantially less than most of the other programs. This could account for the lack of improvement in walking. After the initial training subjects were followed with weekly or monthly pulmonary rehabilitation sessions. At 12- and 18-month follow-up the control group demonstrated a significant decrease in the 6-minute–distance walk and peak work load on a bicycle, whereas the pulmonary rehabilitation treatment groups experienced no change from baseline (Wijkstra et al., 1995, 1996). This suggests that the pulmonary rehabilitation program produced a positive outcome in terms of functional capacity by preventing deterioration.

Strijbos, Postma, van Altena, Gimeno, and Koeter (1996) compared the duration of effect for outpatient hospital-based and home-care pulmonary rehabilitation programs both of which were of 12 weeks' duration. Both groups significantly increased functional capacity as demonstrated by an increase in peak workload on a bicycle and a 4-minute–distance walk as compared to a control group. But the home-care pulmonary rehabilitation group retained their benefits longer, suggesting the possibility of an increase in the level of exercise and/or physical activity on a daily basis at home. To retain the benefits of exercise one must continue exercising, hence it is likely that the home-care pulmonary rehabilitation group increased their functional performance, but functional performance was not measured.

The bulk of the evidence supports the notion that the functional capacity of people with COPD can be improved by a comprehensive pulmonary rehabilitation program that includes exercise as one of its major components. The magnitude of improvement varied and further research is needed to determine the optimal intensity and duration of exercise training combined with educational and psychosocial support. It is generally thought that the combination of exercise training, education, and psychosocial support is more effective than training alone, because of its potential to assist people in modifying their lifestyle, but there is no empirical evidence to support this view. Moreover the efficacy of individual components of pulmonary rehabilitation and the strategies for sustaining prolonged benefits are not well established.

Although an improvement in performance outcomes is clearly a goal of pulmonary rehabilitation and general exercise training, only one trial evaluated this outcome (Ries, Ellis, & Hawkins, 1988). Ries and colleagues (1988) found that the time needed to complete a series of simulated activities of daily living did not change for people after participating in a pulmonary rehabilitation program. Many subjects reported anecdotal evidence of subjective improvements in the performance of activities of daily living after participating in the pulmonary rehabilitation program.

Upper Extremity Training

People with COPD experience difficulty in performing physical work with their arms, especially activities that require physical work with unsupported arms, such as lifting objects and combing hair. This leads to avoidance of upper arm work and loss of strength in the major muscles of the arms and shoulders. Functional outcomes were examined in four (Lake et al., 1990; Martinez et al., 1993; Ries et al., 1988; Simpson, Killian, McCartney, Stubbing, & Jones, 1992) studies of upper extremity training, with three studies including a no-treatment or sham treatment control group. Two (Martinez et al., 1993; Ries et al., 1988) of the four studies added upper extremity training to a comprehensive pulmonary rehabilitation program that included other forms of exercise training. All four studies examined functional capacity in terms of upper extremity strength and none of them examined outcomes in terms of functional performance.

Simpson and colleagues (1992) examined the effects of weight lifting that included single arm curls. They observed a significant increase in dynamic strength as measured by the maximal weight lifted one time with a one-repetition maximum. Lake and coworkers (1990) examined the effect of arm-cycle ergometry and functional unsupported arm exercises. Their results demonstrated a significant treatment effect as reflected by an increase in the maximal workload on an arm ergometer (Lake et al., 1990). In both studies subjects in the training group increased functional capacity by increasing the intensity of training.

Methods used for arm training were compared in two studies (Martinez et al., 1993; Ries et al., 1988) with subjects participating in comprehensive pulmonary rehabilitation. Martinez and coworkers compared supported- and unsupported-arm exercise training. Improvements in endurance for supported and unsupported arm exercises were detected with significantly greater improvements in the group that trained with unsupported arm exercises. Ries and coworkers compared the effects of upper extremity training, upper extremity training with gravity resistance, and upper extremity training with proprioceptive neuromuscular facilitation techniques, all superimposed on a pulmonary rehabilitation program. Both upper extremity training groups improved endurance time on the isokinetic arm cycle and the total number of upper extremity lifts.

Results of these studies demonstrate that it is possible to increase strength and endurance of the upper extremities, but it is not known if this will be associated with improvements in the ability to perform unsupported work with the arms. Additionally it is not known how this will affect functional performance on a day-to-day basis.

INSPIRATORY MUSCLE THERAPY

Respiratory muscle dysfunction is recognized to be a major problem for people with COPD. They develop a functional weakness of the inspiratory muscles that places them at risk for the development of respiratory muscle fatigue and ventilatory failure and contributes to sensations of dyspnea (Younes, 1990), ultimately leading to a decline in functional capacity and functional performance. Interventions have been designed to directly or indirectly improve inspiratory muscle function including inspiratory muscle training and resting the respiratory muscle.

Inspiratory Muscle Training

Inspiratory muscle training is designed to improve inspiratory muscle function by increasing strength and endurance of the inspiratory muscles. It is reasoned that the increased strength of the inspiratory muscles will delay the onset of inspiratory muscle fatigue with exertion and thereby allow people to perform submaximal levels of activity for longer periods of time. The effects of inspiratory muscle training have been studied in terms of functional status outcomes, reflecting both functional capacity and functional performance.

Two general types of training have been developed and studied: isocapnic hyperventilation and inspiratory resistance. With isocapnic hyperventilation the inspiratory muscles are trained with a protocol that incorporates many repetitions and light loads to increase endurance of the inspiratory muscles during hyperventilation. The equipment used for isocapnic hyperventilation is relatively complex and typically includes a pneumotachometer, rebreathing system, carbon dioxide analyzer, and carbon dioxide source to maintain isocapnia (Ries & Moser, 1986). With resistance training the inspiratory muscles are trained with a protocol that incorporates fewer repetitions and heavier loads to improve both strength and endurance of the inspiratory muscles. In early studies of inspiratory muscle training with resistance, people with COPD were trained by inhaling through a small inspiratory orifice to increase the airway pressures required to generate inspiratory flow. With this type of device the training load is unreliable because it depends on the rate of inspiratory airflow. The results of these studies were inconsistent and will not be reviewed in this chapter because of the unreliable nature of the training stimulus.

In recent studies the intensity of the inspiratory muscle training load has been controlled in one of two ways. One method of inspiratory muscle training uses the original style of resistive breathing device with a small inspiratory orifice and controls the training load by providing feedback when the targeted inspiratory flow is achieved, referred to as targeted inspiratory flow. Alternatively, inspiratory muscle training is performed with a threshold inspiratory pressure load. These devices have a large inspiratory orifice and inspiratory pressure loads are independent of inspiratory airflow. The inspiratory orifice is occluded by a valve and a given amount of negative pressure must be generated by the individual to open the valve and allow inspiratory airflow.

The effects of isocapnic hyperventilation training were reported in two studies and the results were inconsistent with respect to dimensions of functional capacity: respiratory muscle endurance and walking. In the first study the effects of isocapnic hyperventilation training were compared to the effects of a placebo treatment of intermittent positive pressure breathing in 32 people with COPD (Levine, Weiser, & Gillen, 1986). The isocapnic hyperventilation training group demonstrated a significant increase in respiratory muscle endurance as measured by the maximal sustained ventilatory capacity. There was no significant improvement in the 12-minute–distance walk and a symptom-limited bicycle test, but both groups reported improvements in activities of daily living on a single item instrument. In the second study isocapnic hyperventilation training was compared to a walking program in 11 people with COPD (Ries & Moser, 1986). No change was observed in the maximal sustained ventilatory capacity, though the isocapnic hyperventilation training group demonstrated a significant increase in the 12MD (mean increase = 77 m) and a significant increase in performance on a symptom-limited exercise test (peak ventilation and peak oxygen uptake) (Ries & Moser, 1986). The training intensity appeared to be similar for both studies, but in the latter study

(Ries & Moser, 1986) both groups of people were also participating in a pulmonary rehabilitation program and this could have confounded results. Further research will be required to clarify these apparent inconsistencies. However, there has been little interest in this type of training in recent years, possibly because the equipment is more complex and costly than other types of inspiratory muscle training.

The effects of inspiratory muscle training with resistance were reported in 13 studies, with treatment duration of 1 to 6 months. Four (Berry, Adair, Sevensky, Quinby, & Lever, 1996; Goldstein, De Rosie, Long, Dolmage, & Avendano, 1989; Wanke et al., 1994; Weiner, Azgad, & Ganam, 1992) of the studies added inspiratory muscle fatigue to an existing pulmonary rehabilitation program that included exercise training. The results of the 13 studies supported the notion that inspiratory muscle training improves inspiratory muscle strength if the intensity of training is adequate. Four (Goldstein et al., 1989; Harver, Mahler, & Daubenspeck, 1989; Kim et al., 1993; Larson, Kim, Sharp, & Larson, 1988) of the studies trained people with relatively moderate loads, and nine trained people with relatively heavy loads. People demonstrated a significant increase in PI_{max} in seven studies that trained people with heavy loads (Alex, Berry, Larson, Covey, & Wirtz, 1997; Belman & Shadmehr, 1988; Dekhuijzen, Folgering, & van Herwaarden, 1991; Heijdra, Dekhuijzen, van Herwaarden, & Folgering, 1996; Larson et al., 1997; Wanke et al., 1994; Weiner et al., 1992) and in one of the studies that trained people with moderate loads (Larson et al., 1988). The magnitude of the increase in PI_{max} ranged from -10 cm of water to -21 cm of water (Belman & Shadmehr, 1988; Weiner et al., 1992). After 10 weeks of targeted flow inspiratory muscle training, the maximal transdiaphragmatic pressure (an indicator of diaphragm strength) increased by 48% in the group trained with a relatively heavy inspiratory load, equal to 60% of PI_{max}, and by 3% in the group trained with a very light load, equal to 10% of PI_{max} (Heijdra et al., 1996). Similarly Preusser, Winningham, and Clanton (1994) compared the effects of training with heavy versus lighter loads and demonstrated a significant increase in PI_{max} over time for both groups, but no differences related to the training load, possibly because the sample size was too small. Three studies failed to detect a treatment effect with respect to PI_{max}, two of which trained people at relatively modest inspiratory loads (Harver, Mahler, & Daubenspeck, 1989; Kim et al., 1993). In the third study (Goldstein et al., 1989), people were followed for only 1 month of inspiratory muscle training, and this is probably too short a training period to fully demonstrate effects.

The results of these studies suggest that inspiratory muscle training improves selected elements of capacity, that is, inspiratory muscle strength but not for other activities such as walking. Walking was measured in seven of the above studies with either the 6- or 12-minute–distance walk tests. Four studies (Dekhuijzen et al., 1991; Goldstein et al., 1989; Preusser et al., 1994; Wanke et al., 1994) reported a significant increase in walk distance in both the treatment group and the control group, but in three of those studies the control group also received pulmonary rehabilitation. Two of the studies (Larson et al., 1988; Weiner et al., 1992) reported an increase in the 12-minute–distance walk only in the inspiratory muscle training group, and one study reported no increase in the 12-minute–distance walk for the treatment or control group after 6 months of training with moderate loads (Kim et al., 1993).

Three studies (Berry et al., 1996; Dekhuijzen et al., 1991; Wanke et al., 1994) examined functional capacity in terms of symptom-limited maximal exercise testing and found no evidence that inspiratory muscle training improves functional capacity over and above the effects of aerobic exercise training alone. All three studies compared whole-body aerobic exercise training to the combination of whole-body aerobic exercise training plus inspiratory muscle training. In two of the studies (Dekhuijzen et al., 1991; Wanke et al., 1994) peak oxygen uptake and peak ventilation increased for both groups, but with no differences between the groups. Peak oxygen uptake did not improve for either group in the third study (Berry et al., 1996).

Two studies evaluated the effectiveness of the inspiratory muscle training intervention on functional performance outcomes and the results suggest that an improvement in the functional strength of the inspiratory muscles is not associated with improvements in functional performance (Kim et al., 1993; Larson et al., 1988). Functional performance was measured in both studies with the Sickness Impact Profile (Bergner et al., 1981). These results may represent reality that inspiratory muscle training has no effect on performance. Alternatively these negative results may be attributed to the sensitivity of this instrument. The Sickness Impact Profile measures a wide range of functional impairment and is generally considered to be relatively insensitive to the small changes in functional status that could potentially result from inspiratory muscle training.

Inspiratory Muscle Rest

The inspiratory muscles are rested at scheduled intervals using noninvasive mechanical ventilation with either negative pressure ventilation or positive pressure ventilation administered by mask or nasal techniques. The rationale for respiratory muscle rest stems from an assumption that the inspiratory muscles are functioning in a perpetual state of fatigue; and resting them on a regular basis will improve respiratory muscle function and reduce dyspnea on exertion, ultimately leading to an improved functional status (Shapiro et al., 1992). This intervention is targeted at people with severe and very severe COPD with hypercapnia and/or hypoxemia. The potential benefits of resting the inspiratory muscles were first explored in a number of uncontrolled clinical studies in the late 1980s, and results were somewhat promising but inconsistent. Since then functional capacity outcomes have been examined in controlled clinical trials, but functional performance outcomes have not been studied. Seven controlled studies (Celli et al., 1989; Gay, Hubmayr, & Stroetz, 1996; Gigliotti et al., 1994; D. J. M. Jones, Paul, Jones, & Wedzicha, 1995; Renston, DiMarco, & Supinski, 1994; Shapiro et al., 1991, 1992; Zibrak, Hill, Federman, Kwa, O'Donnell, 1988) were published to examine the effects of intermittently resting the inspiratory muscles. Three examined the effects of negative pressure ventilation, and four examined the effects of noninvasive positive pressure ventilation.

The results were negative for all three studies of negative pressure ventilation. In one study the effects of 3 weeks of negative pressure ventilation were examined in 14 people with COPD admitted to the hospital for the purpose of the study (Celli et al., 1989). In another study the effects of 6 months of negative pressure ventilation were examined in nine people with COPD in the home setting (Zibrak et al., 1988). In the largest study the effects of 12 weeks of negative pressure ventilation in the home setting was compared to sham treatment in 184 people with COPD (Shapiro et al., 1991, 1992). Many problems were identified with the application of the intervention. In general, subjects did not like the intervention, found it to be uncomfortable and cumbersome, and were not willing to use it on a regular basis.

Since then four small clinical trials have been conducted using noninvasive positive pressure as the method of noninvasive mechanical ventilation. Although the positive pressure techniques appear to be easier for people to tolerate they have not demonstrated consistent benefits with respect to inspiratory muscle strength or walk distance. Jones and colleagues (1995) and Gay and associates (1996) observed no change in 6-minute–distance walk after 3 months treatment with nocturnal nasal pressure support ventilation. Renston and colleagues (1994) found a significant increase in the 6-minute–distance walk after 5 days of positive pressure ventilation administered nasally for 2 hours a day, but they observed no change in PI_{max}. In contrast Gigliotti and colleagues (1994) observed a significant increase in PI_{max} after 4 weeks of treatment with negative pressure ventilation combined with an inpatient rehabilitation program. Negative pressure ventilation was administered 5 hours a day for 5 consecutive days a week, divided in two sessions a day. The control group received 4 weeks of inpatient exercise rehabilitation and both the treatment and the control groups demonstrated a significant increase in the 6-minute–distance walk and a significant decrease in dyspnea, indicating that the improvement in the 6-minute–distance walk and dyspnea were most likely a result of the exercise rehabilitation (Gigliotti et al., 1994).

NUTRITIONAL THERAPY

The functional outcomes of nutritional support were examined in six controlled clinical trials. In general it was acknowledged that nutritional repletion was difficult to accomplish as people had a tendency to reduce their dietary source of calories when nutritional supplements were introduced (Knowles, Fairbarn, Wiggs, Chan-Yan, & Pardy, 1988; Lewis, Belman, & Dorr-Uyemura, 1987). This made it necessary to closely monitor intake, and in three studies all or part of the nutritional intervention was conducted in an inpatient setting (Rogers, Donahoe, & Costantino, 1992; Schols, Soeter, Mostert, Pluymers, & Wouters, 1995; Whittaker, Ryan, Buckley, & Road, 1990). Even with these extreme efforts the average weight gain was less than 2.5 kg in all but one study where people gained an average of 4.2 kg after 3 months of oral supplementation (Efthimiou, Fleming, Gomes, & Spiro, 1988). Two studies monitored nutritional status after nutritional supplementation was discontinued, and in both cases nutritional status deteriorated within 4 weeks (Efthimiou et al., 1988; Knowles et al., 1988). All six studies examined the functional outcomes of nutritional repletion with respect to respiratory muscle strength, and three (Efthimiou et al., 1988; Rogers et al., 1992; Schols et al., 1995) examined functional outcomes in terms of walk distance.

Some of the studies produced borderline improvements in nutritional status, but when nutritional status was clearly improved, it was accompanied by improvements in functional strength of the respiratory muscles (Efthimiou et al., 1988; Rogers et al., 1992; Whittaker et al., 1990). Two studies demonstrated an improvement in maximal expiratory pressure (PE_{max}), but not in PI_{max} (Rogers et al., 1992; Whittaker et al., 1990). Schols and coworkers (1995) demonstrated a significant increase in PI_{max} with the combination of nutritional support plus anabolic steroids as compared to placebo, with a mean increase of $-.9.2$ cm of water and -1 cm of water, respectively. The treatment effects were significant for depleted people but not for nondepleted people. Moreover, no significant improvements were observed in PI_{max} with nutritional support alone, compared to placebo in both nutritionally depleted and nondepleted people (Schols et al., 1995). All people in this study were concurrently participating in an intensive inpatient exercise program, which may have influenced the results.

In general the magnitude of the improvement in respiratory muscle strength was modest, and the clinical significance of these relatively modest improvements is not clearly established. Efthimiou and coworkers (1988) demonstrated a mean increase of −7.3 cm of water for PI_{max}. Whittaker and coworkers (1990) and Rogers and coworkers (1992) observed a mean increase in PE_{max} of 34 and 14.9 cm of water, respectively.

Two studies provide evidence for an improvement in walk distance following nutritional supplementation. Rogers et al. (1992) observed a mean increase of 429 feet versus 1 foot for the treatment versus control group. Efthimiou (1988) observed a mean increase of 53 m in the 6-minute–distance walk after 3 months of oral supplementation and no change in the control group. The treatment effects deteriorated after discontinuation of supplementation and 3 months after discontinuation the 6-minute–distance walk had declined to a mean of 16 m above baseline. Schols et al. (1995) found no additional improvements in the 12-minute–distance walk when anabolic steroids were given with nutritional supplementation versus nutritional supplementation alone.

Only one study (Rogers et al., 1992) examined the effect of nutritional repletion on performance. They found no significant effect on SIP score, which was described as a quality-of-life outcome. These studies demonstrated potential benefits of nutritional repletion in terms of respiratory muscle strength and walking. But extreme measures were required to accomplish modest improvements in nutritional status, and the effects were short-lived after discontinuation of the intervention.

OXYGEN THERAPY

The beneficial therapeutic effects of oxygen therapy are well documented for people with hypoxemic COPD. The nocturnal oxygen therapy trial was one of the first randomized controlled trials to evaluate the effectiveness of this intervention in terms of functional capacity and performance in people with COPD (Heaton, Grant, McSweeny, Adams, & Petty, 1983). Performance outcomes were evaluated through the SIP. No change was noted in functional capacity or functional performance after 6 months' treatment with either nocturnal oxygen therapy or continuous oxygen therapy.

The effects of supplemental oxygen taken during exercise over a 6-week period were examined in people with COPD and mild hypoxemia (McDonald, Blyth, Lazarus, Marschner, & Barter, 1995). With the acute administration of oxygen, small but significant improvements were observed in the 6-minute–distance walk (mean increase of 21 m). After 6 weeks of supplemental oxygen there was a small but significant increase in the 6-minute–distance walk measured while breathing room air (mean increase of 16 m), but there was no change in the 6-minute–distance walk while breathing supplemental oxygen. These small improvements in functional capacity are of little clinical value.

Given the therapeutic benefits of oxygen therapy, the impact of delivery systems on functional performance becomes important. Bloom et al. (1989) found significantly better performance outcomes in people randomly assigned to a transtracheal oxygen delivery system ($n = 22$) compared with nasal cannula or face mask ($n = 21$) according to scores on the Barthel Index and Katz Activities of Daily Living questionnaire. Improvements were noted in both independence and frequency of activity at the 6-month follow-up. Depression levels decreased and morale improved among experimental subjects, whereas the control group experienced no change in depression and a decline in morale. Although the experimental group experienced fewer hospital days than the control group, conclusions regarding cost-effectiveness of the intervention could not be made due to the small sample size.

Vergeret, Brambilla, and Mounier (1989) compared performance levels of people randomly assigned to portable or fixed oxygen delivery systems, using a monthly activity recording system over 1 year. They found that for those on oxygen therapy more than 18 hours per day, people on portable systems spent more time outside and walked further than people with fixed delivery systems. There was no difference in activity for those using their oxygen less than the prescribed 15 hours a day.

These results suggested that the mode of oxygen delivery does have an effect on functional performance. The extent to which the alternatives are cost-effective, in terms of performance outcomes, has not been determined.

SPECIALIZED NURSING CARE

Specialized nursing care is designed to stabilize the disease and improve or maintain performance. Interventions generally include education, support, adjustment or fine-tuning of pharmacologic or respiratory therapy, and modification in the household or family environment. Bergner et al. (1988) conducted a controlled trial of home nursing care in the treatment of people with COPD. Three-hundred-one people were randomly assigned to one of three treatment groups: routine office care, standard home care, and respiratory home care with trained respiratory nurses. Upon completion of the 1-year study, there were no differences in survival, pulmonary function, or SIP score among the three treatment groups. The per-person cost of respiratory home care was

$1,710 more than standard home care and $4,717 more than routine office care. "Special needs," home nursing service, and inpatient costs were significantly higher in the routine-home-care group. The authors concluded that home care services for people not at risk of institutionalization did not improve functional performance and did not yield cost saving. The study did not address differential outcomes for the subgroup of high-risk people who would generally be targeted for home care.

The Cockcroft and coworkers' (1987) clinical trial involved 75 people randomly assigned to monthly visits by a respiratory nurse or a control group, with randomization stratified by hospital admissions during the previous 3 years. Nursing intervention involved a monthly visit for education and support focused on the needs of the individual. The model involved the identification of problems in activities of daily living and goal setting to increase independence. People were encouraged to recognize indications of exacerbations or deterioration in their condition and contact the physician if necessary. Mobility and degree of disability were among the outcomes. Although no differences were found in disability ratings, the treatment group had fewer deaths. Results also suggested that more of the less severely ill people in the control group were admitted to the hospital unnecessarily. In addition, more of the control subjects died at home, suggesting that had their problem been detected earlier and followed up in hospital, they might have been saved. These results suggested that the performance outcomes may have been insensitive to change or that the group differences in morbidity and mortality were not controlled in the analysis of performance outcomes.

More recently, Littlejohns, Baveystock, Parnell, and Jones (1991) studied 152 people and found that respiratory health nurses in England had a positive impact on functional performance (SIP), with the treatment group showing significantly ($p < .01$) more improvement in physical dimension scores of the SIP (mean change of 5.53 of impairment in treatment group versus a change of 1.65 of impairment in the control group). Outcomes for the treatment and control group were not significantly different with respect to pulmonary function tests, the 6-minute–distance walk test, and the paced-step test; however, the treatment group had fewer deaths and loss to follow-up.

In general the results of the specialized nursing care were disappointing, but the lack of a measurable effect could be related to the study designs. Nursing may actually make a difference in the trajectory of functional status, that is, the rate of decline, but the effects are difficult to detect by measuring outcomes over a short period of time. It may be necessary to monitor outcomes at more frequent intervals over a prolonged period of time and compare the slope of decline. Failure to detect a treatment effect could be a function of study design, however. The people enrolled in these studies were severely ill, making improvement difficult if not impossible to achieve. Further, two (Cockcroft et al., 1987; Littlejohns et al., 1991) of the studies found lower mortality rate in the treatment group; it is possible that the severity of the survivors masked a treatment effect. Finally, nursing interventions may actually have an effect on the trajectory of functional status, that is, reduce the rate of decline. Such effects are difficult to detect over short time periods. It may be necessary to monitor outcomes at more frequent intervals over a prolonged period of time, comparing slopes and controlling for differential mortality.

SUMMARY AND FUTURE RESEARCH DIRECTIONS

The purpose of this review was to synthesize the results of randomized controlled trials testing the efficacy of interventions designed to improve functional status in people with COPD. Most of the studies reviewed examined capacity-targeted interventions and measured capacity outcomes with few measuring performance outcomes. To interpret this body of research and to improve future research the following issues must be addressed: statistical significance versus clinical significance of changes in functional status, severity of illness in the target group, specificity of the intervention, and sensitivity of the outcome measures.

Many of the studies demonstrated statistically significant improvements in functional outcome, but statistical significance cannot be equated with clinical significance, as it does not necessarily reflect a clinically meaningful change. Consequently it is important to determine if the observed outcomes were clinically significant.

There are no published guidelines for determining a clinically meaningful change in walking tests, but it would be reasonable to consider a 20% improvement as clinically meaningful if subjects were given adequate practice to learn the test prior to the baseline measurement. It has been demonstrated that the walking tests have a substantial learning effect with improvements ranging from 13% to 33%, depending on the number of tests taken within a short period of time (Knox, Morrison, & Muers, 1988; Larson et al., 1996). Most of the studies reviewed here provided practice sessions prior to conducting walking tests. Clinically meaningful improvements in walking were demonstrated in exercise studies that incorporated walking in combined programs of exercise and rehabilitation and in the two nutritional studies that measured walking. Borderline improvements were observed after the use of inhaled bronchodilators.

To interpret changes in inspiratory muscle strength one must recognize that measurements of PI_{max} will fluctuate from day to day, and the technical error of measurement is estimated to be 10 cm of water for people with moderate to very severe COPD (Larson et al., 1993). Thus the clinical significance of smaller improvements in PI_{max} is questionable. Nutritional therapy resulted in very small increases in PI_{max} of less than −10 cm of water, whereas inspiratory muscle training with heavy loads was associated with greater increases in PI_{max} from −10 to −21 cm of water. The combined effects of nutritional repletion and inspiratory muscle training have not been examined.

The efficacy of treatment should be viewed within the context of severity of illness. The effects of pharmacologic and exercise training were seen primarily in people with mild to moderate disease. It is possible that people with severe and very severe COPD are limited in their ability to improve functional capacity because they have less reserve. Within the body of research greater emphasis has been placed on improving the functional status of persons with moderate and severe airflow obstruction, leaving a gap in knowledge related to improving functional status in people with very severe airflow obstruction.

Interventions to improve functional status should be specifically targeted to capacity or performance outcomes. It is unlikely that a significant change in capacity can be directly or linearly translated into significant changes in functional performance. Strategies to improve functional capacity may or may not be accompanied by improvements in day-to-day performance. Between capacity and performance lies a host of influential moderating variables, factors that influence a person's choice to perform up to observed levels. Psychosocial strategies or individualized, relevance-targeted interventions may enhance motivation to increase performance (Leidy & Haase, 1996; Leidy & Traver, 1995). These issues have not been addressed for people with COPD, and research is needed to develop and test interventions for improving performance outcomes. Moreover, interventions designed to improve functional capacity, such as inspiratory muscle training and exercise training, should be accompanied by supportive interventions directed toward performance if they are to be effective in improving performance (Leidy, 1994b, 1995).

Functional capacity and performance as elements of functional status are important outcomes in today's health care environment. Capacity is potentially related to trajectory of illness and is probably a major contributor to health care resource usage. Interventions that are successful in improving or stabilizing capacity have the potential to reduce the number of emergent care visits and hospitalizations. These effects can translate into direct cost savings as well as improved quality of life. Improvements in performance can reduce caregiver burden, increase the work capabilities of younger people with COPD, and improve people's ability to contribute to the family as in caring for grandchildren. These effects reduce the indirect costs of illness and contribute to improved quality of life.

In the studies reviewed here the poor functional performance outcomes suggest that either interventions did not affect people's day-to-day functioning or the instruments were not sensitive to the change. The SIP was used as an outcome measure in nine of the studies reviewed; seven reported no treatment effects. Most did not report effect size, making it difficult to determine whether the studies had insufficient power to detect changes in SIP score. It may be that the SIP did change, but the changes were so small that a large sample is required to detect the difference statistically. To move forward in this area the use of an instrument that specifically addresses functional performance with evidence of clinically meaningful change is recommended.

Few studies evaluated the long-term effects of pulmonary rehabilitation or specialized nursing care, in terms of either capacity or performance. This may be due to the fact that these interventions are multi-faceted, making it difficult to sort out effects in evaluating outcomes. As the health care environment changes, however, the efficacy and cost-effectiveness of these traditional interventions are being called into question. Carefully designed controlled trials are needed that evaluate outcomes in terms of capacity as well as performance. The work of Wijkstra and colleagues (1995, 1996) offered evidence that rehabilitation programs serve to stabilize, rather than reverse, the physical deconditioning process in people with COPD; this may be true of nursing care as well. It seems prudent, therefore, to power trials accordingly and include frequent, long-term, postintervention follow-up.

For people with COPD, the ultimate goal is to improve functional performance. But it is difficult to interpret the observed improvements in functional capacity until more is known about the relationship between specific dimensions of functional capacity and functional performance in people with COPD. Most of the research has been directed toward improving functional outcomes for capacity, and little is known about strategies to improve functional outcomes for performance of day-to-day activities. In future research, emphasis should be placed on clarifying the relationship between capacity and performance and on developing and testing performance-targeted strategies.

REFERENCES

Alex, C. G., Berry, J., Larson, J. L., Covey, M. K., & Wirtz, S. (1997). High intensity inspiratory muscle training (IMT) in patients with chronic obstructive pulmonary disease and severely reduced function [Abstract]. *American Journal of Respiratory and Critical Care Medicine, 155,* A451.

American Thoracic Society. (1995). Standards for the diagnosis and care of patients with chronic obstructive pulmonary disease. *American Journal of Respiratory and Critical Care Medicine, 152,* S77–S120.

Argyropoulou, P., Patakas, D., Koukou, A., Vasiliadis, P., & Georgopoulos, D. (1993). Buspirone effect on breathlessness and exercise performance in patients with chronic obstructive pulmonary disease. *Respiration, 60,* 216–220.

Belman, M. J., & Shadmehr, R. (1988). Targeted resistive ventilatory muscle training in chronic obstructive pulmonary disease. *Journal of Applied Physiology, 65,* 2726–2745.

Bergner, M., Bobbitt, R. A., Carter, W. B., & Gilson, B. S. (1981). The Sickness Impact Profile: Development and final revision of a health status measure. *Medical Care, 19,* 787–805.

Bergner, M., Hudson, L. D., Conrad, D. A., Patmont, C. M., McDonald, G. J., Perrin, E. B., & Gilson, B. S. (1988). The cost and efficacy of home care for patients with chronic lung disease. *Medical Care, 26,* 566–579.

Berry, M. J., Adair, N. E., Sevensky, K. S., Quinby, A., & Lever, H. M. (1996). Inspiratory muscle training and whole-body reconditioning in chronic obstructive pulmonary disease—controlled randomized trial. *American Journal of Respiratory and Critical Care Medicine, 153,* 1812–1816.

Bloom, B. S., Daniel, J. M., Wiseman, M., Knorr, R. S., Cebul, R., & Kissick, W. L. (1989). Transtracheal oxygen delivery and patients with chronic obstructive pulmonary disease. *Respiratory Medicine, 83,* 281–288.

Blosser, S. A., Maxwell, S. L., Reeves-Hoche, M. K., Localio, A. R., & Zwillich, C. W. (1995). Is an anticholinergic agent superior to a B_2-agonist in improving dyspnea and exercise limitation in COPD? *Chest, 108,* 730–735.

Booker, H. A. (1984). Exercise training and breathing control in patients with chronic airflow limitation. *Physiotherapy, 70,* 258–260.

Borson, S., McDonald, G. J., Gayle, T., Deffebach, M., Lakshminarayan, S., & Van Tuinen, C. (1992). Improvement in mood, physical symptoms, and function with nortriptyline for depression in patients with chronic obstructive pulmonary disease. *Psychosomatics, 33,* 190–201.

Busch, A. J., & McClements, J. D. (1988). Effects of a supervised home exercise program on patients with severe chronic obstructive pulmonary disease. *Physical Therapy, 68,* 469–474.

Bush, J. W., Chen, M., & Patrick, D. L. (1973). Cost-effectiveness using a health status index: Analysis of the New York State PKU screening program. In R. Berg (Ed.), *Health status indexes* (pp. 171–208). Chicago: Hospital Research and Educational Trust.

Celli, B., Lee, H., Criner, G., Bermudez, M., Rassulo, J., Gilmartin, M., Miller, G., & Make, B. (1989). Controlled trial of external negative pressure ventilation in patients with severe chronic airflow obstruction. *American Review of Respiratory Disease, 140,* 1251–1256.

Cockcroft, A., Bagnall, P., Heslop, A., Andersson, N., Heaton, R., Batstone, J., Allen, J., Spencer, P., & Guz, A. (1987). Controlled trial of respiratory health worker visiting patients with chronic respiratory disability. *British Medical Journal,* *294,* 225–228.

Degre, S., Sergysels, R., Messin, R., Vandermoten, P., Salhadin, P., Denolin, H., & de Coster, A. (1974). Hemodynamic responses to physical training in patients with chronic lung disease. *American Review of Respiratory Disease, 110,* 395–402.

Dekhuijzen, P. N. R., Folgering, H. T. M., & van Herwaarden, C. L. A. (1991). Target-flow inspiratory muscle training during pulmonary rehabilitation in patients with COPD. *Chest, 99,* 128–133.

Dullinger, D., Kronenberg, R., & Niewoehner, D. E. (1986). Efficacy of inhaled metaproterenol and orally-administered theophylline in patients with chronic airflow obstruction. *Chest, 89,* 171–173.

Eaton, M. L., MacDonald, F. M., Church, T. R., & Niewoehner, D. E. (1982). Effects of theophylline on breathlessness and exercise tolerance in patients with chronic airflow obstruction. *Chest, 82,* 538–542.

Efthimiou, J., Fleming, J., Gomes, C., & Spiro, S. G. (1988). The effect of supplementary oral nutrition in poorly nourished patients with chronic obstructive pulmonary disease. *American Review of Respiratory Disease, 137,* 1075–1082.

Fink, G., Kaye, C., Sulkes, J., Gabbay, U., & Spitzer, S. A. (1994). Effect of theophylline on exercise performance in patients with severe chronic obstructive pulmonary disease. *Thorax, 49,* 332–334.

Gay, P. C., Hubmayr, R. D., & Stroetz, R. W. (1996). Efficacy of nocturnal nasal ventilation in stable, severe chronic obstructive pulmonary disease during a 3-month controlled trial. *Mayo Clinic Proceedings, 71,* 533–542.

Gigliotti, F., Spinelli, A., Duranti, R., Gorini, M., Goti, P., & Scano, G. (1994). Four-week negative pressure ventilation improves respiratory function in severe hypercapnic COPD patients. *Chest, 105,* 87–94.

Goldstein, R., De Rosie, J., Long, S., Dolmage, T., & Avendano, M. A. (1989). Applicability of a threshold loading device for inspiratory muscle testing and training in patients with COPD. *Chest, 96,* 564–571.

Goldstein, R. S., Gort, E. H., Stubbing, D., Avendano, M. A., & Guyatt, G. H. (1994). Randomised controlled trial of respiratory rehabilitation. *Lancet, 344,* 1394–1397.

Grove, A., Lipworth, B. J., Ingram, C. G., Clark, R. A., & Dhillon, D. P. (1995). A comparison of the effects of prednisolone and mianserin on ventilatory, exercise and psychometric parameters in patients with chronic obstructive pulmonary disease. *Journal of Clinical Pharmacology, 48,* 13–18.

Guyatt, G. H., Townsend, M., Pugsley, S. O., Keller, J. L., Short, H. D., Taylor, D. W., & Newhouse, M. T. (1987). Bronchodilators in chronic air-flow limitation. *American Review of Respiratory Disease, 135,* 1069–1074.

Harver, A., Mahler, D. A., & Daubenspeck, J. A. (1989). Targeted inspiratory muscle training improves respiratory muscle function and reduces dyspnea in patients with chronic obstructive pulmonary disease. *Annals of Internal Medicine, 111,* 117–134.

Heaton, R. K., Grant, I., McSweeny, A. J., Adams, K. M., & Petty, T. L. (1983). Psychologic effects of continuous and nocturnal oxygen therapy in hypoxemic chronic obstructive pulmonary disease. *Archives of Internal Medicine, 143,* 1941–1947.

Heijdra, Y. F., Dekhuijzen, P. N. R., van Herwaarden, C. L. A., & Folgering, H. T. M. (1996). Nocturnal saturation improves by target-flow inspiratory muscle training in patients with COPD. *American Journal of Respiratory Critical Care Medicine, 153,* 260–265.

Hunt, S. M., McEwen, J., & McKenna, S. P. (1985). Measuring health status: A new tool for clinicians and epidemiologists. *Journal of the Royal College of General Practitioners, 35,* 185–188.

Jaeschke, R., Guyatt, G. H., Singer, J., Keller, J., & Newhouse, M. T. (1991). Mechanism of bronchodilator effect in chronic airflow limitation. *Canadian Medical Association Journal, 144,* 35–39.

Jaeschke, R., Guyatt, G. H., Willan, A., Cook, D., Harper, S., Morris, J., Ramsdale, H., Haddon, R., & Newhouse, M. (1994). Effect of increasing doses of beta agonists on spirometric parameters, exercise capacity, and quality of life in patients with chronic airflow limitation. *Thorax, 49,* 479–484.

Jones, D. J. M., Paul, E. A., Jones, P. W., & Wedzicha, J. A. (1995). Nasal pressure support ventilation plus oxygen compared with oxygen therapy alone in hypercapnic COPD. *American Journal of Respiratory and Critical Care Medicine, 152,* 538–544.

Jones, D. T., Thomson, R. J., & Sears, M. R. (1985). Physical exercise and resistive breathing training in severe chronic airways obstruction: Are they effective? *European Journal of Respiratory Diseases, 67,* 159–165.

Jones, P. W., Quirk, F. H., Baveystock, C. M., & Littlejohns, P. (1992). A self-complete measure of health status for chronic airflow limitation. *American Review of Respiratory Disease, 145,* 1321–1327.

Kaplan, R. M., & Bush, J. W. (1982). Health-related quality of life measurement for evaluation research and policy analysis. *Health Psychology, 1,* 61–80.

Katz, S., Ford, A. B., Moskowitz, R. W., Jackson, B. A., & Jaffe, M. W. (1963). Studies of illness in the aged. The index of ADL: A standardized measure or biological and psychosocial function. *Journal American Medical Association, 185,* 914–919.

Kim, M. J., Larson, J. L., Covey, M. A., Vitalo, C. A., Alex, C. G., & Patel, M. (1993). Inspiratory muscle training in patients with chronic obstructive pulmonary disease. *Nursing Research, 42,* 356–362.

Knowles, J. B., Fairbarn, M. S., Wiggs, B. J., Chan-Yan, C., & Pardy, R. L. (1988). Dietary supplementation and respiratory muscle performance in patients with COPD. *Chest, 93,* 977–983.

Knox, A. J., Morrison, J. F. J., & Muers, M. F. (1988). Reproducibility of walking test results in chronic obstructive airways disease. *Thorax, 43,* 388–392.

Lake, F. R., Henderson, K., Briffa, T., Openshaw, J., & Musk, A. W. (1990). Upper-limb and lower-limb exercise training in patients with chronic airflow obstruction. *Chest, 1990,* 1077–1082.

Lareau, S., Carrieri-Kohlman, V., Janson-Bjerklie, S., & Roos, P. (1994). Development and testing of the pulmonary functional status and dyspnea questionnaire (PFSDQ). *Heart & Lung, 23,* 242–250.

Lareau, S. C., Kohlman-Carrieri, V., Janson-Bjerklie, S., & Roos, P. J. (1986). Functional levels and dyspnea in patients with COPD [Abstract]. *American Review of Respiratory Disease, 133*, A163.

Larson, J. L., Covey, M. K., Berry, J., Wirtz, S., Alex, C. G., & Langbein, E. (1997). Inspiratory muscle training (IMT) and bicycle exercise training (EX) in patients with chronic obstructive pulmonary disease (COPD) [Abstract]. *American Journal of Respiratory and Critical Care Medicine, 155*, A497.

Larson, J. L., Covey, M. K., Vitalo, C. A., Alex, C. G., Patel, M., & Kim, M. J. (1993). Maximal inspiratory pressure: Learning effect and test-retest reliability in patients with chronic obstructive pulmonary disease. *Chest, 104*, 448–453.

Larson, J. L., Covey, M. K., Vitalo, C. A., Alex, C. G., Patel, M., & Kim, M. J. (1996). Reliability and validity of the 12-minute distance walk in patients with chronic obstructive pulmonary disease. *Nursing Research, 45*, 203–210.

Larson, J. L., Kim, M. J., Sharp, J. T., & Larson, D. A. (1988). Inspiratory muscle training with a pressure threshold breathing device in patients with chronic obstructive pulmonary disease. *American Review of Respiratory Disease, 138*, 689–696.

Leidy, N. (1994a). Using functional status to assess treatment outcomes. *Chest, 106*, 1645–1646.

Leidy, N. K. (1994b). Functional status and the forward progress of merry-go-rounds: Toward a coherent analytical framework. *Nursing Research, 43*, 196–202.

Leidy, N. K. (1995). Functional performance in people with chronic obstructive pulmonary disease. *IMAGE: Journal of Nursing Scholarship, 27*, 23–34.

Leidy, N. K., Abbott, R. D., & Fedenko, K. M. (1997). Sensitivity and reproducibility of the dual-mode actigraph under controlled levels of activity intensity. *Nursing Research, 46*, 5–11.

Leidy, N. K., & Haase, J. E. (1996) Functional performance in people with chronic obstructive pulmonary disease: A qualitative analysis. *Advances In Nursing Science, 18*(3), 77–89.

Leidy, N. K., & Traver, G. A. (1995). Psychophysiologic factors contributing to functional performance in people with COPD: Are there gender differences? *Research in Nursing & Health, 18*, 535–546.

Levine, S., Weiser, P., & Gillen, J. (1986). Evaluation of a ventilatory muscle endurance training program in the rehabilitation of patients with chronic obstructive pulmonary disease. *American Review of Respiratory Disease, 132*, 400–406.

Lewis, M. I., Belman, M. J., & Dorr-Uyemura, L. (1987). Nutritional supplementation in ambulatory patients with chronic obstructive pulmonary disease. *American Review of Respiratory Disease, 135*, 1062–1068.

Littlejohns, P., Baveystock, C. M., Parnell, H., & Jones, P. W. (1991). Randomised controlled trial of the effectiveness of a respiratory health worker in reducing impairment, disability, and handicap due to chronic airflow limitation. *Thorax, 46*, 559–564.

Mahler, D. A., Matthay, R. A., Snyder, P. E., Wells, C. K., & Loke, J. (1985). Sustained-release theophylline reduces dyspnea in nonreversible obstructive airway disease. *American Review of Respiratory Disease, 131*, 22–25.

Mahoney, F. I., & Barthel, D. W. (1965). Functional evaluation: The Barthel Index. *Maryland State Medical Journal, 14,* 61–65.

Martinez, F. J., Vogel, P. D., Dupont, D. N., Stanopoulos, I., Gray, A., & Beamis, J. F. (1993). Supported arm exercise vs unsupported arm exercise in the rehabilitation of patients with severe chronic airflow obstruction. *Chest, 103,* 1397–1402.

McDonald, C. F., Blyth, C. M., Lazarus, M. D., Marschner, I., & Barter, C. E. (1995). Exertional oxygen of limited benefit in patients with chronic obstructive pulmonary disease and mild hypoxemia. *American Journal of Respiratory Critical Care Medicine, 152,* 1616–1619.

McGavin, C. R., Gupta, S. P., Lloyd, E. L., & McHardy, G. J. R. (1977). Physical rehabilitation for the chronic bronchitic: results of a controlled trial of exercises in the home. *Thorax, 32,* 307–311.

McKay, S. E., Howie, C. A., Thomson, A. H., Whiting, B., & Addis, G. J. (1993). Value of theophylline treatment in patients handicapped by chronic obstructive lung disease. *Thorax, 48,* 227–232.

Mulloy, E., & McNicholas, W. T. (1993). Theophylline improves gas exchange during rest, exercise, and sleep in severe chronic obstructive pulmonary disease. *American Review of Respiratory Disease, 148,* 1030–1036.

Murciano, D., Aubier, M., Lecocguic, Y., & Pariente, R. (1984). Effects of theophylline on diaphragmatic strength and fatigue in patients with chronic obstructive pulmonary disease. *New England Journal of Medicine, 311,* 349–353.

Murciano, D., Auclair, M., Pariente, R., & Aubier, M. (1989). A randomized, controlled trial of theophylline in patients with severe chronic obstructive pulmonary disease. *New England Journal of Medicine, 320,* 1521–1525.

Newman, D., Tamir, J., Speedy, L., Newman, J. P., & Ben-Dov, I. (1994). Physiological and neuropsychological effects of theophylline in chronic obstructive pulmonary disease. *Israel Journal of Medical Sciences, 30,* 811–816.

Patessio, A., Carone, M., Ioli, F., & Donner, C. F. (1992). Ventilatory and metabolic changes as a result of exercise training in COPD patients. *Chest, 101*(S5), 274S–278S.

Preusser, B. A., Winningham, M. L., & Clanton, T. L. (1994). High- vs low-intensity inspiratory muscle interval training in patients with COPD. *Chest, 106,* 110–117.

Reardon, J., Awad, E., Normandin, E., Vale, F., Clark, B., & ZuWallack, R. L. (1994). The effect of comprehensive outpatient pulmonary rehabilitation on dyspnea. *Chest, 105,* 1046–1052.

Renston, J. P., DiMarco, A., & Supinski, G. S. (1994). Respiratory muscle rest using nasal BiPAP ventilation in patients with stable severe COPD. *Chest, 105,* 1053–1060.

Ries, A. L., Ellis, B., & Hawkins, R. W. (1988). Upper extremity exercise training in chronic obstructive pulmonary disease. *Chest, 93,* 688–692.

Ries, A. L., Kaplan, R. M., Limberg, T. M., & Prewitt, L. M. (1995). Effects of pulmonary rehabilitation on physiologic and psychosocial outcomes in patients with chronic obstructive pulmonary disease. *Annals of Internal Medicine, 122,* 823–832.

Ries, A. L., & Moser, K. M. (1986). Comparison of isocapnic hyperventilation and walking exercise training at home in pulmonary rehabilitation. *Chest, 90*, 285–289.

Rogers, R. M., Donahoe, M., & Costantino, J. (1992). Physiologic effects of oral supplemental feeding in malnourished patients with chronic obstructive pulmonary disease. *American Review of Respiratory Disease, 146*, 1511–1517.

Sassi-Dambron, D. E., Eakin, E. G., Ries, A. L., & Kaplan, R. M. (1995). Treatment of dyspnea in COPD: A controlled clinical trial of dyspnea management strategies. *Chest, 107*, 724–729.

Schols, A. M. W. J., Soeter, P. B., Mostert, R., Pluymers, R. J., & Wouters, E. F. M. (1995). Physiologic effects of nutritional support and anabolic steroids in patients with chronic obstructive pulmonary disease. *American Journal of Respiratory Critical Care Medicine, 152*, 1268–1274.

Shapiro, S. H., Ernst, P., Gray-Donald, K., Martin, J. G., Wood-Dauphinee, S., Beaupre, A., Spitzer, W. O., & Macklem, P. T. (1992). Effect of negative pressure ventilation in severe chronic obstructive pulmonary disease. *Lancet, 340*, 1425–1429.

Shapiro, S. H., Macklem, P. T., Gray-Donald, K., Martin, J. G., Ernst, P. P., Wood-Dauphinee, S., Hutchinson, T. A., & Spitzer, W. O. (1991). A randomized clinical trial of negative pressure ventilation in severe chronic obstructive pulmonary disease: Design and methods. *Journal of Clinical Epidemiology, 44*, 483–496.

Simpson, K., Killian, K., McCartney, N., Stubbing, D. G., & Jones, N. J. (1992). Randomised controlled trial of weightlifting exercise in patients with chronic airflow limitation. *Thorax, 47*, 70–75.

Singh, N. P., Despars, J. A., Stansbury, D. W., Avalos, K., & Light, R. W. (1993). Effects of buspirone on anxiety levels and exercise tolerance in patients with chronic airflow obstruction and mild anxiety. *Chest, 103*, 800–804.

Strijbos, J. H., Postma, D. S., van Altena, R., Gimeno, F., & Koeter, G. H. (1996). A comparison between an outpatient hospital-based pulmonary rehabilitation program and a home-care pulmonary rehabilitation program in patients with COPD. *Chest, 109*, 366–372.

Swerts, P. M. J., Kretzers, L. M. J., Terpstra-Linderman, E., Verstappen, F. T. J., & Wouters, E. F. M. (1990). Exercise reconditioning in the rehabilitation of patients with chronic obstructive pulmonary disease: A short- and long-term analysis. *Archives of Physical Medicine and Rehabilitation, 71*, 570–573.

Toevs, C. D., Kaplan, R. M., & Atkins, C. J. (1984). The costs and effects of behavioral programs in chronic obstructive pulmonary disease. *Medical Care, 22*, 1088–1100.

Toshima, M. T., Kaplan, R. M., & Ries, A. L. (1990). Experimental evaluation of rehabilitation in chronic obstructive pulmonary disease: Short-term effects on exercise endurance and health status. *Health Psychology, 9*, 237–252.

Tydeman, D. E., Chandler, A. R., Graveling, B. M., Culot, A., & Harrison, B. D. W. (1984). An investigation into the effects of exercise tolerance training on patients with chronic airways obstruction. *Physiotherapy, 70*, 261–264.

van Schayck, C. P., Dompeling, E., Rutten, M. P. M. H., Folgering, H., van den Boom, G., & van Weel, C. (1995). The influence of an inhaled steroid on quality of life in patients with asthma or COPD. *Chest, 107*, 1199–1205.

van Schayck, C. P., Rutten-van Molken, M. P. M. H., van Doorslaer, E. K. A., Folgering, H., & van Weel, C. (1992). Two-year bronchodilator treatment in patients with mild airflow obstruction. *Chest, 102*, 1384–1391.

Vergeret, J., Brambilla, C., & Mounier, L. (1989). Portable oxygen therapy: Use and benefit in hypoxaemic COPD patients on long-term oxygen therapy. *European Respiratory Journal, 2*, 20–25.

Wanke, T., Toifl, K., Merkle, M., Formanek, D., Lahrmann, H., & Zwick, H. (1994). Inspiratory muscle training in patients with Duchenne muscular dystrophy. *Chest, 105*, 475–482.

Ware, J. E., & Sherbourne, C. D. (1992). The MOS 36-Item Short-Form Health Survey (SF-36), Conceptual framework and item selection. *Medical Care, 30*, 473–483.

Weaver, T. E., & Narsavage, G. L. (1992). Physiological and psychological variables related to functional status in chronic obstructive pulmonary disease. *Nursing Research, 41*, 286–291.

Weiner, P., Azgad, Y., & Ganam, R. (1992). Inspiratory muscle training combined with general exercise reconditioning in patients with COPD. *Chest, 102*, 1351–1356.

Whittaker, J. S., Ryan, C. F., Buckley, P. A., & Road, J. D. (1990). Function in malnourished chronic obstructive pulmonary disease patients. *American Review of Respiratory Disease, 142*, 283–286.

Wijkstra, P., van der Mark, T. W., Kraan, J., van Altena, R., Koeter, G. H., & Postma, D. S. (1996). Long-term effects of home rehabilitation on physical performance in chronic obstructive pulmonary disease. *American Journal of Respiratory Critical Care Medicine, 153*, 1234–1241.

Wijkstra, P. J., Ten Vergert, E. M., van Altena, R., Otten, V., Kraan, J., Postma, D. S., & Koeter, G. H. (1995). Long term benefits of rehabilitation at home on quality of life and exercise tolerance in patients with chronic obstructive pulmonary disease. *Thorax, 50*, 824–828.

Younes, M. (1990). Load responses, dyspnea and respiratory failure. *Chest, 97*, 59S–68S.

Zibrak, J. D., Hill, N. S., Federman, E. C., Kwa, S. L., & O'Donnell, C. (1988). Evaluation of intermittent long-term negative-pressure ventilation in patients with severe chronic obstructive pulmonary disease. *American Review of Respiratory Disease, 138*, 1515–1518.

Chapter 11

Schizophrenia

JEANNE C. FOX AND CATHERINE F. KANE
UNIVERSITY OF VIRGINIA
SCHOOL OF NURSING
SOUTHEASTERN RURAL MENTAL HEALTH RESEARCH CENTER

ABSTRACT

Psychiatric nursing research has historically focused on psychosocial phenomena characteristic of personal experience or symptomatology associated with mental illness. The current climate of the mental health service system and basic science knowledge proliferation require nurse researchers to develop and evaluate interventions based on biological understanding of symptoms. This review examines psychiatric nursing and the broader psychiatric literature from 1990 to 1996 to provide a synthesis of the current research knowledge about important components of the field of schizophrenia research including causal processes, course and outcome, symptoms, treatment, relapse prevention, and consumer providers, followed by a discussion of directions for future research.

Keywords: Schizophrenia, Symptoms, Symptom Monitoring, Relapse and Relapse Prevention, Cognitive Behavioral Interventions, Skills Training, Psychotherapy, Family Interventions, Consumer Perspective

Historically, psychiatric nursing research has focused on psychosocial, intrapersonal, or interpersonal phenomena characteristic of personal experience or symptomatology associated with mental illness. Current dramatic changes in the health care delivery system and the mental health service systems dictate

287

a change in focus to developing and measuring the outcomes of interventions by psychiatric nurse researchers. In addition, basic science research has rapidly increased the understanding of the biological processes contributing to the cognitive, perceptual, and social interactive difficulties common in schizophrenia. Thus, system change and knowledge proliferation require the specialty of psychiatric nursing to provide conceptual and research-based linkages between examination of patients' experiences at the above designated levels and the biological processes contributing to these phenomena.

CONCEPTUAL FRAMEWORK

The stress-vulnerability-coping-competency model of major mental disorders explains the onset, course, and outcome of symptoms and social functioning as a complex interaction among biological, environmental, and behavioral factors (Liberman, 1982; Nuechterlein & Dawson, 1984) and is an enhancement of the well-known stress diathesis model of schizophrenia (Zubin & Spring, 1977). In this model, psychobiological vulnerability may result in psychotic symptoms when stressful life events exceed coping ability. Coping and competence can be attributes of the individual or of the social environment. Stressful life events that exceed the protective capacities of these factors can lead to symptomatic exacerbation. Even in the absence of a time-limited stressor, vulnerable individuals can succumb to ambient levels of challenge, tension, loss, or conflict if they lack the protections conferred by coping skills, social support, and/or appropriate biopsychosocial interventions. The model suggests the importance of improving and maintaining social and coping skills, developing and maintaining social supports, and encouraging treatment compliance.

METHODS

This review included research and review articles culled from a computerized literature search of *Index Medicus* and CINAHL (Cumulative Index of Nursing and Allied Health Literature) from 1990 to 1996. In addition the tables of contents of the following journals during the selected time frame were reviewed: *Archives in Psychiatric Nursing, Advances in Nursing Science, IMAGE: Journal of Nursing Scholarship, International Journal of Nursing Studies, Issues in Mental Health Nursing, Journal of Advanced Nursing, Journal of Psychosocial Nursing, Nursing Research, Perspectives in Psychiatric Nursing, Research in Nursing and Health*, and *Western Journal of Nursing*

Research. Of the over 1,500 references reviewed, fewer than 50 nursing articles were on schizophrenia. Articles on the topic of schizophrenia were assessed to determine their adequacy in meeting research standards in the following categories: purpose of the study, conceptual framework, study design, population description, sample criteria and size, instrumentation, data analysis, and conclusions. Following this assessment, it was determined that the nursing literature had few published reports that withstood this test of rigor in the topic area. In order to present a literature review that would reflect the vast literature in the field, identify areas of importance for research in general and nursing research specifically, and be of publishable length, the emphasis was on published reviews of the literature. Because of the rapid and extensive developments in psychopharmacological treatments for schizophrenia, we deleted such a focus from the review in deference to a separate review on this important topic. It should be noted that many reports of psychiatric nursing research do not exclusively include subjects with schizophrenia. Therefore, some studies related to the topical area are not included in this review. For a comprehensive review of the field of psychiatric nursing outcome research, readers are referred to Merwin and Mauck's (1995) thorough synopsis.

This review includes research from outside the discipline of nursing, which has greatly expanded knowledge about the interaction of biological and psychosocial processes contributing to the daily life of individuals with schizophrenia. A synthesis of the current research about the following important components of the field of schizophrenia research includes: causal processes, course and outcome, symptoms, treatment, relapse prevention, and consumer providers. This review is followed by a discussion of psychiatric nursing research on schizophrenia and recommended future directions.

CAUSAL PROCESSES

As Andreasen (1994) suggested, schizophrenia is a catastrophic, persistent, and complex illness that affects a broad range of cognitive and conceptual systems. The heterogeneity of the disorder significantly complicates the search for underlying causal processes. Four different types of biological mechanisms are believed to contribute to the etiology of the symptoms of schizophrenia. These include genetic/molecular causes, chemical anatomy, neural developmental, and neural circuitry. Research into each of these types of mechanisms has greatly increased general knowledge about biological correlates of this complex array of symptoms but simultaneously has produced competing and conflicting hypotheses about causal processes.

Twin and adoptive studies have confirmed the existence of genetic predisposition to schizophrenia that increases individual vulnerability for symptom expression. Family studies demonstrated an increased incidence of schizophrenia spectrum conditions in first-degree relatives of individuals with schizophrenia (Andreasen, 1994). Recently, the techniques of molecular genetics have been employed in numerous investigations in an attempt to identify a possible location of a specific genetic defect. To date this search has not resulted in conclusive evidence for the existence of a specific genetic disorder, but the field is relatively new and investigations continue with ever-advancing techniques.

The absence of complete concordance in monozygotic twins (concordance exists approximately 40% of the time) implicates the probable contribution of nongenetic factors to actual symptom expression (Andreasen, 1994). Which factors contribute significantly to symptom development and the mechanisms involved not well understood. Structural and functional brain abnormalities coupled with disturbed catecholamine processes have been the focus of numerous computed tomography scans (CT), magnetic resonance imaging (MRI), and postmortem and functional imaging studies.

Brain Anatomy

Reviews of CT literature (Andreasen, Swayze, et al., 1990; Chua & McKenna, 1995; Lewis, 1990; Raz & Raz, 1990; Van Horn & McManus, 1992) coupled with the work of Jones et al. (1994) demonstrated that lateral ventricular enlargement, although small, exists in schizophrenia. With the improvement of structural imaging through MRI, investigators have been able to examine the size of specific subcortical structures as well as cortical regions. Findings vary significantly, perhaps in part because of differences in control groups (age and gender) and in methodology. Lateral ventricular enlargement in schizophrenia was confirmed in studies (Andreasen, Erhardt et al., 1990; Bornstein, Schwartzkopf, Olson, & Nasrallah, 1992; Degreef et al., 1992; Gur & Pearlson, 1993; Kelsoe, Cadet, Pickar, & Weinberger, 1988; Suddath et al., 1989, 1990; Zipursky, Lim, Sullivan, Brown, & Pfefferbaum, 1992). As Chua and McKenna reported, however, other investigators did not confirm this finding (Harvey et al., 1993; Johnstone et al., 1989; Rossi et al., 1990, 1991; Shenton et al., 1992; Smith, Baumgartner, & Calderon, 1987; Young et al., 1991). According to Chua and McKenna, Suddath's study indicates that the overall pattern of MRI findings shows the only reportable difference in size (volume) of gray matter was in the left temporal lobe and specifically, in the hippocampus. In a sample of 15 monozygotic twins, hippocampal volume was smaller in schizophrenic twins in comparison with their matched monozygotic nonaffected twins in 14 of 15 cases on the left and 13 of 15 cases on the right. Chua and McKenna concluded that MRI findings strongly suggested that localized primarily subcortical and perhaps predominantly left-sided subcortical brain-substance abnormalities contributed to the disorder of schizophrenia.

Neuropathologic investigations have been reviewed by Bogerts (1993), Chua and McKenna (1995), Harrison (1995), Kirch and Weinberger (1986), Lantos (1988), Roberts (1991), and Shapiro (1993). As Roberts and Chua and McKenna suggested, investigations have primarily been conducted in the areas of overall brain size, basal ganglia size, limbic system structure, and histologic changes. Both lengths of schizophrenic patients' brains and fixed weights were significantly smaller than nonschizophrenic controls (Brown et al., 1986; Bruton et al., 1990; Chua & McKenna, 1995; Heckers, Heinsen, Heinsen, & Beckmann, 1991; Pakkenberg, 1987.)

Neuropathologic investigations of basal ganglia and limbic system structures have revealed mixed results with two studies demonstrating smaller internal segments of the globus palladius of the basal ganglia (Bogerts, David, Falkai, & Tapernon-Franz, 1990; Bogerts, Meertz, & Schonfeldt-Bausch, 1985) and three studies not replicating this finding (Brown et al., 1986; Heckers et al., 1991; Pakkenberg, 1990). Four of five studies reported reduced size of the parahippocampal gyrus, and in three of seven studies the hippocampus was found to be smaller in schizophrenic patients (Chua & McKenna, 1995).

Histologic investigations have focused on hippocampal cellular disarray as reported originally by Kovelman and Scheibel (1984) and Scheibel and Kovelman (1981). Altshuler, Conrad, Kovelman, and Scheibel (1987), however, reported no difference in cellular disarray between seven schizophrenic patients and six controls, and additional studies have failed to confirm this difference (Arnold, 1994; Benes, Sorensen, & Bird, 1991; Conrad, Abebe, Austin, Forsythe, & Scheibel, 1991; Christison, Casanova, Weinberger, Rawlings, & Kleinman, 1989). Reduced cell numbers in the hippocampus have also been reported (Falkai & Bogerts, 1986; Jeste & Lohr, 1989), but Benes and colleagues and Arnold found no significant differences in cell numbers in any hippocampal subregions (Chua & McKenna, 1995). Reduced cell numbers in a subregion of the para hippocampal gyrus were reported by Falkai, Bogerts, and Rozumek (1988) and Jakob and Beckmann (1986) but not confirmed by Arnold (1994). Reduced hippocampal cell size was reported by Benes et al. (1991) and Bogerts et al. (1985), whereas Arnold (1994) found smaller cell size in one of four cortical subregions of the hippocampus (Chua & McKenna, 1995). Thus, postmortem studies of schizophrenia do not yet conclusively support the notion of reduced brain size in schizophrenia, or the hypothesis of hippocampal cellular disarray.

Neural Development/Brain Circuitry

Investigators have proposed that the underlying causes for abnormalities in the brains of schizophrenics are neurodevelopmental in nature and may be caused by genetic programming defects or environmental injury that create a vulnerability, but remain dormant until some superimposed maturational process (i.e., pruning, sprouting, myelination, sex hormone changes during puberty on brain chemical systems) stimulates the diathesis to schizophrenia (Feinberg, 1982; Jernigan et al., 1991; Pettegrew et al., 1992; Stevens, 1992; Swayze, Andreasen, Alliger, Yuh, & Ehrhardt, 1992; Weinberger, 1987).

The chemical processes that have been most thoroughly studied include the dopamine and dopamine 2 receptors. These studies were based on the notion that an increase in a single neurotransmitter at a particular point in the series of events involved in chemical signaling in the brain led to the onset of illness and symptomatology (Carlsson, 1988). Recently, the advent of atypical neuroleptics, which have potent effects on other transmitter systems such as serotonin and D1 receptors, has stimulated investigations of other abnormalities including dysfunction of presynaptic autoreceptors through second messenger systems and the involvement of numerous neurotransmitter systems (Costall & Naylor, 1992; Niznik, Hubert, & Van, 1992; Simpson, Slater, Royston, & Deakin, 1992; Swerdlow & Geyer, 1993).

Functional brain studies of schizophrenia have included measures of cerebral blood flow, functional imaging, and functional imaging with task activation investigations. Chua and McKenna (1995) reported that in only 4 of 20 studies was there significant reduction in cerebral blood flow set/metabolism in schizophrenic patients, and one study (Paulman et al., 1990) actually reported significantly increased cerebral blood flow. Hypofrontality, although varying in definition across studies, has been reported in 10 of 27 studies. The inconclusiveness and conflicting findings related to hypo and hyperfrontality do not mask the probability that hypofrontality when measured in terms other than anterior:posterior ratio is related to deficit schizophrenia, negative symptoms, and possibly cognitive impairment.

Task-related hypofrontality has been investigated as a means of documenting deficit cerebral activity related to poor task performance among schizophrenics. In particular, schizophrenics' executive functioning task performance, which is associated with prefrontal cortex activation, frequently has been reported as impaired (Friston, Frith, Liddle, & Frackowiak, 1991; Goldberg, Weinberger, Berman, Pliskin, & Podd, 1987; McKenna, 1994; Shallice, Burgess, & Frith, 1991). Memory with functional image correlates of this activity involving the prefrontal cortex has recently emerged as a major area of impairment in schizophrenics (McKenna et al., 1990; Saykin et al., 1991; Shallice et al., 1991).

Weinberger, Berman, and Zec's 1986 investigation of executive functioning while resting and during performance blood flow, using the Wisconsin Card Sort Test with 20 schizophrenic and 25 age- and gender-matched controls, documented both difficulty with executive tasks among schizophrenic patients as well as smaller increase in blood flow to the prefrontal cortex during executive tasks. When the results were examined for differences in blood flow between control tasks and executive tasks, although differences between prefrontal blood flow between groups remained significant, overall analyses of variance across patients and controls became insignificant, however. Additional studies with variations in methodology and control groups have failed to confirm hypofrontality under resting conditions (Chua & McKenna, 1995). Recent investigations by Frith et al. (1995) were able to clearly separate specific components of tasks from the effects of speaking and using a semantic lexicon, which documented a tendency toward increased activation in the left superior temporal cortex, particularly in the most impaired patients (Chua & McKenna, 1995).

The most consistent brain abnormality is that of structural lateral ventricular enlargement, although this enlargement is small. Whether ventricular enlargement is primarily characteristic of male schizophrenics has not been resolved, and as Jones et al. (1994) suggested, this enlargement may be considered a risk factor or trait marker rather than be of direct causal relevance for schizophrenia (Chua & McKenna, 1995).

The questions related to hypofrontality remain and are extended by work of Dolan et al. (1993), Frith et al. (1995), Liddle et al. (1992), and Wolkin et al. (1992). Specifically, Dolan and colleagues demonstrated that both depressed and schizophrenic patients with poverty of speech had associated lower flow/metabolism in the left dorsolateral prefrontal cortex. As Chua and McKenna (1995) reported, however, the findings of Frith et al. (1995) suggested no evidence of task-activated hypofrontality, but instead a decoupling of normal reciprocal patterns of activity in the frontal and temporal lobe. Thus Chua and McKenna concluded that instead of simple reductions in regional brain activity, schizophrenia may be characterized by complicated alterations in normal patterns of reciprocal activity between anatomically related areas of the cerebral cortex.

Currently, neurodevelopmental rather than neurodegenerative explanations for structural characteristics of the brains of schizophrenics prevail (Harrison, 1995). Structural brain abnormalities, although small, are present at or before the onset of symptoms and are relatively nonprogressive thereafter (Marsh, Suddath, Higgins, & Weinberger, 1994). Malnutrition, birth complications, maternal influenza, a high frequency of physical anomalies among schizophrenics, and abnormal dermatoglyphics (both associated with intrauterine maldevelopment as well as the presence of neuromotor and behavioral abnormalities in young preschizophrenic children) have all been cited to support a neurodevelopmental explanatory model for this complex illness.

Though no nursing research was found in this area, biological mechanism research for schizophrenia has continued to explicate the neurobiologic processes underlying the symptoms, behavior, and coping strategies of individuals experiencing schizophrenia. These findings target possible bases for nursing-intervention studies. Unfortunately, the extant research is far from conclusive. Understanding causal mechanisms is further hampered by lack of knowledge regarding the intricate functioning of the brain in whole and in part. Prenatal and early developmental prevention efforts are suggested by the findings. It is probable that intervention research and biological-mechanism research in the near future will proceed symbiotically, one potentially illuminating the other. As Andreasen (1994) suggested, the ever-expanding technology and opportunity to integrate findings from the molecular level through membranes, cells, circuits, and systems will continue to provide a rich challenge to investigators exploring the causality and complexity of schizophrenia.

COURSE AND OUTCOME

A number of reviews of the literature on course of schizophrenia have been conducted in recent years (Eaton, Bilker, et al., 1992; Eaton, Mortensen, et al., 1992; Edgerton & Cohen, 1994; Harding, 1988; Harding, Zubin, & Strauss, 1992; McGlashan, 1988; Ram, Bromet, Eaton, Pato, & Schwartz, 1992). This chapter summarizes the findings of these reviews and highlights recent controversies and correlates of schizophrenia related to its course. McGlashan reviewed 10 North American outcome studies of at least 10 years duration with acceptable design criteria. Overall, these studies indicate that schizophrenia frequently has a chronic course with an outcome usually worse than other major mental illnesses. Schizophrenia has an increased risk for suicide, physical illnesses, and mortality. The evidence indicates that the course is not necessarily progressive, appearing to plateau after 5 to 10 years of apparent illness. The outcome of schizophrenia is heterogenous; no clear picture has emerged regarding predictors of long-term outcome probably because of lack of uniformity in the methods used in longitudinal studies.

One of the most extensive follow-up studies was conducted by Harding and colleagues on a cohort of patients with schizophrenia from the Vermont State Hospital (Harding, Brooks, Ashikaga, Strauss, & Breier, 1987a, 1987b).

Conducting a rediagnosis from each patient's hospital record, 82 individuals were identified with an average age of 61 years and interviewed 20–25 years after their entry into a rehabilitation project initiated by the hospital. Outcome varied widely but one half to two thirds of the sample had achieved considerable improvement or recovered. This finding contrasts with other longitudinal studies of shorter duration that found either little or no change in function at follow-up (Gardos, Cole, & LaBrie, 1982; McGlashan, 1984a, 1984b). The Vermont group differed from other studies in ways that could be linked to better outcome: (a) they resided in a rural setting, (b) they responded to pharmacotherapy, (c) they had a considerably later age of onset, and (d) they were involved in a psychiatric rehabilitation program involving work placements postdischarge. Subsequently, Harding and colleagues have completed a follow-up study with persons from a Maine state psychiatric facility where no psychiatric rehabilitation program was in place (DeSisto, Harding, McCormick, Ashikaga, & Brooks, 1987a, 1987b). A comparison of these two cohorts showed better function for the Vermont group at follow-up.

More recent studies conducted in the United States (Breier, Schreiber, Dyer, & Pickar, 1991; Carpenter & Strauss, 1991) indicated that initial prognostic indicators and treatment response were important predictors of outcome. In an analysis of the data from the International Pilot Study of Schizophrenia's Washington cohort, 40 schizophrenic subjects were observed 11 years after index admission (Carpenter & Strauss, 1991). Prognostic data at initial evaluation included ratings from the Prognostic Scale (J. S. Strauss & Carpenter, 1974) and from a modified Phillips (1953) Scale. Five items on the Prognostic Scale were significantly associated with future outcome. Patients with more frequent social contacts and more stable heterosexual relationships showed a better 11-year outcome in terms of frequency of social contacts, employment status, symptom severity, and overall outcome. Shorter hospitalizations were associated with higher frequency of social contacts and more stable employment at follow-up. The presence and severity of either thought disorder, delusions, or hallucinations at initial assessment were significantly related to symptom severity at follow-up. Breier et al. (1991) followed 58 patients with schizophrenia (mean [M] age = 26, standard deviation [SD] = 7). Follow-up assessments were conducted 2–12 years post discharge from the National Institute of Mental Health (NIMH) Intramural Program. Results indicated substantial functional impairment and symptom severity with only 20% of the sample exhibiting good outcome. Levels of positive and negative symptoms evaluated when patients were receiving optimal neuroleptic treatment during the index hospitalization significantly predicted outcome levels of symptoms, functioning, and time spent hospitalized in the follow-up period. The two studies reflected the manifest illness period of chronic schizophrenia as opposed to the later period of the illness course found in the Harding studies.

Difficulties with this body of research plague most other longitudinal efforts. The studies were actually conducted retrospectively rather than prospectively. Representation is compromised because of an inability to locate all members of the cohort. Variation in levels of biological and social interventions are not well accounted for. Because human subject protection dictates that treatment cannot be withheld in such cases, the true course of untreated schizophrenia may never be known. Planned, extended longitudinal follow-up in intervention studies would go a long way to explicating variations in illness outcome, however.

MORBIDITY AND MORTALITY

Two reviews of the literature regarding schizophrenia and medical illness confirm that morbidity and mortality rates for persons with schizophrenia are higher than for the nondiagnosed population (Adler & Griffith, 1991; Holmberg & Kane, 1995). Epidemiological studies of schizophrenia morbidity and mortality are extensive. Studies of morbidity indicate that physical illnesses are underdiagnosed in schizophrenia. Findings indicated that the higher death risk was not associated with the illness itself nor neuroleptic treatment, except through physical conditions that were contributing, coincidental, or iatrogenic to schizophrenia. Though the morbidity risk for males with schizophrenia has been considered higher than for females, evidence from a German epidemiological study designed to minimize methodological flaws found no significant gender differences (Hambrecht, Reicher-Rossler, Fatkenheuer, Louza, & Hafner, 1994).

The incidence of suicide among persons with schizophrenia is comparable to that found in affective disorder. With a suicide rate of 10% to 13%, suicide is the number one cause of premature death among persons with schizophrenia. Caldwell and Gottesman (1990) reviewed the literature on this disturbing topic. Their review determined that depression, especially the symptom of self-reported or perceived hopelessness, is an important factor to consider in assessing suicide risk in this population. According to Caldwell and Gottesman, the most salient and well-documented risk factors are being young, Caucasian, male, experiencing a chronic pattern of acute remissions and exacerbations, perception of the deteriorative effects of schizophrenia, realistic nondelusional assessment of the future, fear of further mental deterioration, extreme treatment dependence, and loss of faith in treatment. Apparently, the strongest predictor of suicide is a past history of suicide attempts, which is similar to the general population.

There is no published nursing research literature in this important area to date. Little published research exists generally, which explicates the clinical indicators of morbidity and mortality in schizophrenia. Research attention to this area is critically needed.

Symptoms

Positive and negative.   The characterization of the symptom phenomenology of schizophrenia is relevant to determining the subsequent course of the illness and treatment regimens appropriate to the presenting symptom clusters. By the end of the 19th century, Hughlings-Jackson (1894/1931) recommended that the positive symptoms, hallucinations, and delusions be kept separate from negative symptoms of anhedonia and a motivation in conceptualizing psychoses. Kraepelin (1896) and Bleuler (1911/1950) both viewed negative symptoms as fundamental to a diagnosis of schizophrenia, until Schneider (1950/1959) introduced the concept of "first-rank symptoms," which were all positive symptoms. In the 1980s Crow (1980) and Andreasen and Olsen (1982) argued for the importance of considering negative symptoms in etiology, course, and treatment response. For a period of time the dichotomous model of positive and negative symptoms held sway, but recently a variety of studies (Andreasen, Arndt, Miller, Flaum, & Nopoulos, 1995; Andreasen et al., 1994; M. E. Strauss, 1993; von Knorring & Lindstrom, 1995) indicated a multifactorial model of schizophrenic symptoms.

Although negative symptoms have generally been an internally consistent construct, positive symptoms were internally heterogeneous (M. E. Strauss, 1993). The measurement instrument used for the analysis of symptom configurations seemed to determine the number of factors identified. Andreasen developed the Scale for the Assessment of Negative Symptoms (SANS) and the Scale for the Assessment of Positive Symptoms (SAPS) (Andreasen & Olsen, 1982). The current form of the SANS and SAPS assesses a total of 49 individual signs and symptoms, grouped in like categories to create the original listing of five negative symptoms and five positive symptoms for which global ratings could be assigned. Negative symptoms are alogia, affective blunting, avolition, anhedonia, and attentional impairment. Positive symptoms are hallucinations, delusions, positive formal thought disorder, bizarre behavior, and inappropriate affect. In a recent report, Andreasen et al. (1995) reviewed the results of five studies conducted at the Iowa Clinical Research Center in which factor analyses were employed to determine the underlying factor structure. Combining three separate samples of similar subjects ($N = 209$), the analyses supported the presence of three factors. Factor one was a negative factor, with high loadings on avolition, anhedonia, affective blunting, alogia, and attentional deficit. Factor two was a disorganization factor, with high loadings on positive thought disorder and bizarre behavior. Factor three was a psychoticism factor, with loadings on delusions and hallucinations. In another sample ($N = 90$) not included in the previous studies (Miller, Arndt, & Andreasen, 1993), results of a preliminary principal-components analysis with varimax rotation indicated the presence of three factors that accounted for 64% of the total variance. The most recent study (Andreasen et al., 1995) examined a sample of 243 patients including the 90 subjects from the Miller et al. study and again found validation for the three-factor structure.

Another symptom measure was developed by Kay, Fiszbein, and Opler (1987) and named the Positive and Negative Syndrome Scale (PANSS) for schizophrenia. The scale included 30 items, 18 items for the Brief Psychiatric Rating Scale (BPRS) (Overall & Gorham, 1962) and 12 items from the Psychopathology Rating Scale (PRS) (Singh & Kay, 1975). Later, Kay (1991) introduced the Structured Clinical Interview for the PANSS (SCI-PANSS). Kay and Sevy (1990) conducted a principal-component analysis on PANSS ratings from 240 chronic schizophrenic patients. Seven factors emerged and four (positive, negative, excited, and depressed) were retained and included in a four-factor pyramidal model. In principal-component analysis of the PANSS by von Knorring and Lindstrom (1995) a five-factor model emerged adding a cognitive dimension to the Kay and Sevy model. Lindenmayer, Bernstein-Hyman, and Grochowski (1994) found a similar five-factor model as did Bell, Lysacker, Beam-Goulet, Milstein, and Lindenmayer (1994).

The multifactorial models of schizophrenia have great potential for determining the neurochemical and neurostructural causes of schizophrenia. Such efforts can further result in the development of more specific antipsychotic medications to target an individual's predominant symptoms. The potential for the further development of specific nonpharmaceutical interventions can also be predicted.

Symptom monitoring.   Amador and colleagues presented an extensive and integrative review of the literature on insight and awareness in schizophrenia (Amador, Strauss, Yale, & Gorman, 1991). These authors concluded that poor insight is a fundamental attribute of schizophrenia unrelated to various sociocultural or demographic characteristics. More recent studies indicated that insight and severity of illness were independent of each other, and though poorly understood, evidence for a variety of neuroanatomical causes of poor illness insight had relevance in schizophrenia. They posited that the concept of insight into illness appears to consist of at least four distinct dimensions: (a) awareness of the signs, symptoms, and consequences of the illness; (b) general attributions about illness and specific attributions about symptoms and their consequences; (c) self-concept formation; and (d) psychological defensiveness. They noted that the distinction between neurogenic and psychogenic contributions to poor awareness must be examined and required different therapies. In general, further work on unawareness of illness in schizophrenia will need to address its multidimensional nature and use more reliable and valid measures to better understand the phenomenon.

Regarding awareness of impending relapse in schizophrenia, O'Connor (1991) reviewed the literature on the stress–vulnerability model of schizophrenic relapse proposed by Goldstein (1987). Studies regarding prodromal symptoms of relapse are marred by difficulties in determining actual symptoms of relapse from prodromal symptoms. Not all early signs result in relapse, and not all relapses are preceded by detected early signs. Evidence indicates that the majority of psychotic relapses in schizophrenia are preceded by prodromal symptom increases of at least 2 weeks and can be as long as 8 weeks. The earliest signs are often anxiety or depression resulting in sleep disturbance, agitation, anger, hostility, somatic concerns, preoccupation, social withdrawal, and amotivation. When increased symptomatology is closely monitored and treated appropriately, a high rate of restabilization is observed.

Hamera and colleagues recently examined the process of self-regulation and symptom monitoring in schizophrenia. Using the Self-Regulation Interview for Schizophrenia (McCandless-Glimcher et al., 1986), target symptoms indicative of the relapse prodrome were identified in a community-living sample of persons with schizophrenia (Hamera, Peterson, Handley, Plumlee, & Frank-Ragan, 1991). Forty-one percent of the subjects' target symptoms were anxiety related, 28% were related to depression, and 31% to psychosis. Seventy-five percent of the interviewees reported that their marker symptoms always occurred with decompensation, and 60% said that when the symptom was not present, they did not get worse. However, 60% of the subjects said that their marker occurred weekly or more often. Forty-nine of the 51 subjects reported taking actions ($M = 3$) to regulate the symptom. The most frequent action was to add new activities or focus on existing ones. Other activities included cognitive strategies such as "self-talk" and reducing stimuli by resting and social withdrawal. Persons with psychotic indicators had significantly lower functioning than subjects reporting anxiety or depression as markers.

In an additional analysis of these data, Hamera, Peterson, Young, and Schaumloffel (1992) observed that subjects reported anxiety-based markers more frequently than depression or psychotic indicators. Psychotic and depressive markers were rated as significantly more troublesome than anxiety-based indicators. The 1-year follow-up of 28 original subjects resulted in the finding that half of the subjects reported using the same indicator or an indicator from the same category. There was no pattern identified in the switch from one marker to another. Hamera proposed a symptom self-regulation model, adapted from Leventhal, Norenz, and Strauss' (1982) model of illness representation and Carver and Scheier's (1981) control theory. The symptom self-regulation model describes the process of managing relapse as a negative feedback loop, where individuals note discrepancies over time between their present state and a standard of reference that is their desired state. Specific discrepancies are associated with their illness status and actions are taken to reduce the discrepancy between their standard of reference and their current state. The data provided support for this model. Subjects easily identified indicators of illness that were disturbing and represented the need for action when they were present. Baker's (1995) qualitative study of the ability of persons with schizophrenia to detect early signs lends support to Hamera's model. Baker's interviews indicated that the level of disturbance caused by prodromal symptoms motivate individuals to take action to relieve the distress. Baker's study further explicated the developmental process of individuals with schizophrenia becoming aware of the need to monitor their distress and take action when needed.

Symptom monitoring provides one avenue for a person with schizophrenia to exert control over the illness. The insight necessary for such action may not be reliable or require interpretation by clinicians or significant others, however. Issues remain regarding how best to conceptualize and measure symptom awareness, as well as how to promote symptom awareness in a way that ensures functional client response. Symptom monitoring is a research area that integrates the course of schizophrenia, personal awareness, and intervention development and is a promising area for nursing research.

RELAPSE/RELAPSE PREVENTION

Zubin, Steinhauer, and Condray (1992) reviewed the issue of vulnerability to relapse in schizophrenia. Examining seven studies of relapse in first-episode schizophrenia conducted since 1978, they derived four major hypotheses supported by the findings: (a) vulnerability to relapse can be investigated by comparing relapsers with nonrelapsers using accepted measures of clinical change; (b) life stress is associated with relapse, possibly as a prodromal event preceding full relapse, leading to stress-producing responses from the environment that serve as circular feedback for the development of a full-blown episode; (c) prediction of relapse as an internal disturbance of homeostasis can be examined in medication withdrawal trials that may mimic natural relapse;

and (d) investigating patients who relapse despite depot neuroleptic treatment should reveal relapse because of the loss of the protective value of therapeutic intervention.

Hirsch and colleagues examined schizophrenic relapse in a controlled treatment withdrawal trial (Hirsch et al., 1996). Chronic schizophrenic patients ($N = 71$) were followed for 4 months, half were treated with effective doses of neuroleptic medication, and half were withdrawn from medication. Multivariate analyses demonstrated that life events made significant cumulative contribution over time to the risk of relapse and that medication withdrawal made an independent contribution. Patients on regular medication had 80% less risk of relapse than those who had been withdrawn by choice or under controlled conditions. This study supported the hypothesis that life events contributed to risk of relapse but did not confirm the life events trigger model of relapse. Another recent study examined the "revolving-door" phenomenon in persons with schizophrenia ($N = 135$) who were frequently readmitted (Haywood et al., 1995). Substance abuse and medication noncompliance were the major predictors of readmission frequency.

Hogarty (1993) concluded that new treatments are promising in reducing relapse rates. He noted that the control of such factors as noncompliance, the dose of neuroleptic, the level of stimulation in the patient's therapeutic and home environments, extrapyramidal side effects, attention and arousal deficits, and life stress can reduce the rate of relapse in most patients. Hogarty concludes that a relapse rate of 65%–70% in the first year following hospital discharge can be reduced to 40% by neuroleptic medications, and by a further 20% with the addition of psychosocial therapy.

Compliance is defined as adherence to a prescribed and appropriate treatment (Bebbington, 1995). Noncompliance with prescribed neuroleptics may occur in up to 50% of persons with schizophrenia. Bebbington's review of the literature found support for alcohol abuse being the main predictor of nonadherence to a medication regimen. Bebbington interpreted research findings in terms of the health belief model (Becker, 1979; Becker & Maiman, 1975) and identified several techniques for increasing compliance. These techniques included providing information about the illness and the therapeutic benefits of medication and use of the therapeutic relationship to encourage and prompt compliance to establish adaptive views of the illness and medication.

Another factor associated with noncompliance is the side effects of neuroleptic medication (Whitworth & Fleischhacker, 1995). Disturbing side effects of medication range from neurological extrapyramidal side effects (acute and tardive dystonia, acute akathisia, parkinsonism, and tardive dyskinesia) to physical side effects such as anticholinergia; antiadrenergia; dermatologic, hematologic, and ophthalmologic effects; sexual dysfunction; and weight gain.

In general, adverse effects can often be treated by dose reduction or switching to an antipsychotic of a different class. Whitworth and Fleischhacker recommended that future research focus on the side effects that most interfere with activities of daily life and impact the self-esteem of the person with schizophrenia.

In order to reduce noncompliance and the risk of development of tardive dyskinesia, studies evaluating the effect of reducing dosage after stabilization in long-term treatment of schizophrenia have been conducted (Schooler, 1991). Schooler reviewed the research on two methods of dosage reduction: continuous low dose and intermittent or targeted medication. Both methods required attentive patient monitoring and treating relapse by increasing medication dosage. Schooler found support for the contention that both strategies are feasible for many persons with schizophrenia, but were related to higher rate of relapse than maintaining an established moderate dose. Relapse rates in the studies reviewed were inversely related to dosage, but low-dose medication had the advantage of reduced adverse side effects and improved subjective well-being. Targeted medication was found to result in lower administered dose overall, but did not benefit tardive dyskinesia or social functioning. These two forms of medication administration are being compared in the NIMH Treatment Strategies in Schizophrenia Study (Schooler, 1993).

Depot administration of neuroleptic medications has been found to have advantages over oral administration leading to lower rates of relapse (Gerlach, 1994). These advantages include increased compliance, lack of absorption problems, stable plasma drug concentrations, regular contact with clinicians, and adjustment of medication to lowest effective dose. Disadvantages include delayed disappearance of potentially irreversible and unpleasant side effects and, for many patients, a feeling of being controlled (Gerlach, 1995). However, Gerlach (1995) concluded that administered in the proper way, with suitable information to the patient and relatives, depot neuroleptics improve the quality of antipsychotic treatment, reduce relapse frequency, stabilize the therapeutic effect, and diminish the level of side effects.

Clearly, the most reliable and effective mode of preventing relapse is adherence to an appropriate medication regimen. The research indicates that life stress, substance abuse, and medication side effects contribute to relapse in treatment-responsive individuals. Noncompliance is associated with side effects. The development of improved psychosocial and pharmacological interventions that can prevent relapse is essential to improving the lives of those afflicted with schizophrenia and of particular relevance to psychiatric nursing research.

PSYCHOSOCIAL INTERVENTIONS

A thorough examination of the vast literature addressing the various aspects of psychosocial interventions available for schizophrenia is beyond the scope of this review. Four areas of continuing development, controversy, promise, and interest to psychiatric nursing will be briefly summarized and discussed: cognitive behavioral therapy, social skills training, psychotherapy, and family interventions.

Cognitive Behavioral Interventions

Corrigan and Storzbach (1993) have reviewed behavioral interventions in treating schizophrenic symptoms. These interventions are frequently based on operant conditioning and reinforcement strategies and on training in coping skills. Reinforcement strategies are apparently useful in decreasing the rate of confused speech, delusional talk, and other bizarre behaviors, but they have little effect on the patient's subjective distress associated with the symptoms. Behavioral strategies for coping with psychotic symptoms include cognitive reframing, nonconfrontational methods that explore alternative explanations for delusions, and humming to interfere with auditory hallucinations. Corrigan and Storzbach concluded that operant and skills-based approaches to decreasing psychotic symptoms had significant effects on the manifestation of hallucinations, delusions, and conceptual disorganization. These approaches also provided promising heuristics for guiding future research and directing treatment development (Corrigan & Storzbach, 1993). An entire issue of *Schizophrenia Bulletin (18)* was devoted to examining cognitive treatments with a wide range of support and criticism.

Findings regarding cognitive training and social skills training have been reported by Fox and Kane (1996). Briefly, Brenner's Integrated Psychological Therapy (IPT) is an extensive cognitive intervention applied to schizophrenia. IPT consists of five subprograms (cognitive differentiation, social perception, verbal communication, social skills, and interpersonal problem solving) designed to progressively improve the cognitive dysfunction and social deficits of schizophrenia. Intervention studies have demonstrated that IPT is effective in affecting elementary cognitive processes evident in the first few weeks of treatment, but findings are mixed with regard to IPT's effect on more complex cognitive skills (Brenner, Hodel, Roder, & Corrigan, 1992). In a recent review of the literature concerning cognitive training, Hodel and Brenner (1994) noted the continuing criticism of cognitive interventions and concluded that continued development of cognitive approaches to treatment hold promise for reducing schizophrenic symptoms and deficits.

Skills Training

Skills training is an extensive psychiatric rehabilitation program developed specifically for schizophrenia that is based on social learning concepts. Skills training focuses on improving individual functioning in social learning situations by fostering sustained attention, problem solving, and goal setting. Education modules on a variety of social skills topics incorporate learning activities to enhance cognitive and behavioral performance. Social skills training has emerged as an important clinical technology with a large body of literature to document its efficacy (Liberman, 1992; Liberman & Kopelowicz, 1995; Liberman, Mueser, Wallace, Jacobs, & Eckman, 1986).

Psychotherapy

An NIMH collaborative study compared the relative benefit of exploratory, insight-oriented psychotherapy (EIO) to reality-adaptive supportive psychotherapy (RAS) in a nonchronic sample of persons with schizophrenia (Gunderson et al., 1984; Stanton et al., 1984). EIO was given 3 hours weekly for 2 years, and RAS was given 1 hour per week for 2 years. This study demonstrated a better outcome for persons in the RAS group in terms of recidivism and role performance in spite of the fact that EIO patients had three times as much therapy. This seminal study provided the basis for future studies discriminating psychoanalytic from supportive psychotherapy (Conte, 1994). Supportive psychotherapy involves strengthening the therapeutic alliance, environmental interventions, education, advice and suggestion, encouragement and praise, limit setting and prohibitions, and undermining maladaptive defenses while strengthening adaptive defenses with emphasis on strengths and talents (Rockland, 1993). The utility of supportive interventions in combination with pharmacological treatment has significant promise (Coursey, 1989).

Clearly, the whole field of psychosocial interventions in schizophrenia research needs further depth, specificity, and rigor. Each area addressed here has promise for psychiatric nursing research, and though psychiatric nurses are engaged in delivering these types of interventions, the paucity of published research by psychiatric nurses in this area is alarming. One hopes that in the next decade we will see an increase in published results of psychiatric nursing interventions in schizophrenia.

FAMILY INTERVENTIONS

Over the last 20 years, the perspective on the family of the person with schizophrenia has evolved from considering the family as a causal factor in the illness to seeing the family as an ally in the treatment of the illness (Kane, 1994). Family psychoeducational programs were designed to help the family develop skills to cope with the challenges of schizophrenic symptoms and prevent relapse. Goldstein (1995) referred to family-intervention studies conducted in the 1980s as first-generation studies of family psychoeducational programs. These controlled studies primarily compared interventions intended to modify family interactional processes believed to exacerbate symptoms. These studies were formulated around the concept of family-expressed emotion, which was related to increased rates of relapse and are reviewed elsewhere (Kane, 1994; Lam, 1991). Though family psychoeducational programs fairly consistently were found to reduce relapse over and above rates obtained through regular antipsychotic medication, change in levels of family-expressed emotion was seldom documented.

Second-generation family-intervention studies conducted in the 1990s propose to refine our understanding of the applicability of these programs to a broader selection of client conditions, determine the programmatic essentials, and determine effectiveness in varying situations. Randolph et al. (1994) studied a Behavioral Family Management intervention compared to treatment as usual only at a Veterans Administration hospital in Los Angeles ($N = 41$). Clients and families were treated and followed for 16 months with relapse rates at 1 year of 14.3% and 55%, respectively. High expressed emotion was not affected in either condition.

Cole, Lehman, and colleagues (Cole, Kane, Zastowny, Grolnick, & Lehman, 1993; Zastowny, Lehman, Cole, & Kane, 1992) compared a Behavioral Family Management (Falloon, Boyd, & McGill, 1984) to a Supportive Family Counseling Model (Bernheim & Lehman, 1985), each intervention continuing for 16 months ($N = 30$) in individual sessions with families. During the intervention, patient functional status improved in both interventions, and relapse rates were similar. Family outcomes were similar with no differential impact on expressed emotion.

In Finland, the Turku Psychiatric Clinic (Lehtinen, 1994) examined the effects of a new family intervention aimed at giving the psychosis meaning linked to the family's present life situation, interactional patterns, and history, based on the techniques of the Milan group (Selvini, Boscolo, Cecchini, & Prata, 1978; Selvini-Palazzoli, Boscolo, Cecchini, & Prata, 1980). Outcome comparisons were made of patients on disability pension at 5-year follow-up to patients who had received the family intervention. There were significantly fewer schizophrenics on disability pension in the family-intervention group than in the old program. Continuity of clinicians in treatment was identified as an important component of successful long-term outcome. The methods in this study were not as strong as in other studies, and the effects of medication were not evaluated. This program is of interest, however, because it demonstrated the in vivo evolution of a family-focused intervention in a clinical setting, and suggested that family involvement in patient treatment, where continuity is maintained over long periods, has positive outcomes.

McFarlane (1994) has examined the relative efficacy of multiple family groups when compared to single-family interventions in treating schizophrenia. Predicated on the perspective that families coping with schizophrenia are isolated and stigmatized, a psychoeducational multifamily group (PEMFG) was hypothesized to be more effective in expanding family social networks, consequently developing problem-solving abilities and reducing relapse. In one study (McFarlane, Lukens, Link, & Dushay, 1995), schizophrenic patients ($N = 41$) were randomly assigned to three treatment conditions: PEMFG, psychodynamically oriented multiple family therapy, or psychoeducational single-family treatment (PESFG). PEMFG was associated with lower relapse rates at 12 and 24 months than PESFG, and both were lower than the psychodynamic therapy. Four-year relapse rates indicated that PEMFG and the psychodynamic group were superior to the single-family intervention. In New York a multisite test of PEMFG versus PESFG (McFarlane, Link, Dushay, & Marchal, 1995) was conducted over a 2-year period. For cases completing the treatment protocol (80%) PEMFG had significantly lower relapse rates than PESFG. In both groups employment and medication adherence increased. PEMFG uses one half the staff time needed for PEMSG.

The above studies were rigorous and methodologically sound, and suggested that there was no added advantage to behavioral family-management programs over quality supportive family interventions, nor possibly over intensive high-quality individual interventions. These studies were of long-term family interventions. An inclusive review of short-term compared to long-term family interventions has been written by Kane (1994). A substantive review of the effects of family programs and adherence to treatment regimens has been written by Tarrier (1991).

CONSUMER PROVIDER

Because of efforts of persons with mental illness, as well as lay mental health advocacy groups, NIMH and Community Mental Health Services (CMHS), a surge of involvement in consumer-advocacy initiatives has occurred in the United States. The most intriguing result of these efforts is the development of consumer-provider positions in community psychiatric service agencies. In recent years the variety and extent of consumer-delivered mental health services have grown (Solomon & Draine, 1994). Mental health consumers operate drop-in centers and companion programs, and work as case managers and job coaches (Attkisson et al., 1992; Mowbray, Chamberlain, Jennings, & Reed, 1988; Sherman & Porter, 1991). Only recently have empirical evaluations of these new forms of service delivery been conducted.

Solomon and Draine (1994) tested the hypothesis that because consumer case managers and clients shared common experiences, clients would be more satisfied with services provided by a consumer team of case managers than a nonconsumer case management team. Clients with serious and persistent mental illness ($N = 91$), randomly assigned to consumer and nonconsumer case management teams, were interviewed after 1 year of service. The consumer team was comprised entirely of consumer case managers. Both teams provided services in an assertive community treatment model based on work done by Stein and Test (1980) and Bond, Miller, Krumweid, and Ward (1988). Case managers delivered care in vivo rather than in their offices. Case managers had their own caseloads and functioned relatively independently in serving their own clients. Case management included an array of housing, rehabilitation, treatment, social services, and activities necessary for or desired by clients. Case managers performed brokering, assistance, and support functions as opposed to clinical management and treatment. The data revealed that clients were less satisfied with service from the consumer team than from the nonconsumer team. Further analysis revealed that assignment alone to consumer or nonconsumer teams was not the overriding factor associated with dissatisfaction. Personal characteristics of the case managers were the only significant predictors of satisfaction. Clients who perceived their case manager as positively possessing these characteristics were more satisfied with service. Solomon and Draine stressed the importance of emotional engagement in helping persons with severe mental illness (SMI). They noted that the hiring and training process for new case managers should be aimed at recruiting case managers with positive personal characteristics and developing these characteristics through skill-building training. In a companion report to this study Solomon and Draine (1996) noted that consumer managers (individuals with SMI who are stabilized and working as case managers) were concerned about how they were accepted by other mental health professionals. The consumer-case-manager team maintained less collateral contact with other professionals and more interpersonal contact with clients than the nonconsumer-case-manager team. Consumer case managers did not report any greater signs of stress, diminished self-esteem, or burnout than the nonconsumer case managers.

Lyons, Cook, Ruth, Karver, and Slagg (1996) investigated a model of consumer service delivery in a mobile assessment program designed to assist homeless people with severe psychiatric disorders. Consumer providers were considered well suited to this form of service delivery, in which staff members worked directly with clients in nontraditional locations. A naturalistic study was devised to identify the similarities and differences in the nature and amount of services delivered by consumer as opposed to nonconsumer staff. Staff of the mobile assessment service were interviewed and followed for a 2-year period using empirical service data. Findings indicate few differences between the consumer and nonconsumer staff. Two significant differences were noted: consumer staff engaged in more mobile outreach than did nonconsumer staff, and consumer staff dyads were less likely to be dispatched to an emergency. Given the greater level of street outreach by consumer staff, they were possibly less available in the office for emergency dispatches.

Mowbray et al. (1996) used focus group interviews with consumer providers who were employed as case manager extenders to vocational specialists to determine the roles and benefits of these positions. Their findings indicated that implementation of the peer-support specialists (consumer providers) role was much more complex and difficult than had been imagined. Suggestions for consideration in developing similar programs included the need to develop a progressive human resource system that requires the establishment of a mission and a culture conducive to consumer-role innovation, the availability of mentoring and consistent supervision, and the establishment of opportunities for education and advancement of consumer providers.

LINKAGES TO PSYCHIATRIC NURSING RESEARCH

The previous review of research in schizophrenia provides a generous grounding for psychiatric nursing research. As Fox (1992) suggests, the specialty of psychiatric nursing has access to knowledge necessary to develop models that link information about neurostructural, neurochemical, and neurofunctional deficits underlying psychiatric disorders with treatment and environmental strategies and the daily life of individuals experiencing psychiatric illnesses. Quality intervention development requires successful adaptation and linkage of biological knowledge to social intervention and caring. Promising areas of research for psychiatric nursing directly related to this review and a practice focus on daily adaptation and coping include (a) information-processing deficits and the experience with psychosocial stressors common to individuals experiencing schizophrenia, and (b) the development of psychoeducational and other environmental interventions to promote targeted compensation for specific deficits (Fox & Kane, 1996).

A theoretical structure that provides a framework for linking basic research knowledge about perceptual, cognitive, and information-processing deficits with psychiatric nursing practice is needed. Ciompi's (1989) proposed model of the linkage of biological and psychosocial systems in schizophrenia provides such a framework and protects against splitting into biological or psychosocial reductionism. Ciompi's model of the long-term evolution of schizophrenia highlights the interaction of vulnerability, stressors, biological reactivity, social responsiveness, and the complexity of the interactions of complex systems (Fox & Kane, 1996). This model describes the course of schizophrenia in three phases. The first phase or the premorbid phase exists from conception until the first episode of psychosis and reflects a period when a combination of unfavorable biological and psychosocial conditions interact to increase susceptibility. The second or psychotic decompensation phase frequently occurs in adolescence, reflecting increasing overtaxation and final psychotic decompensation of the overly vulnerable information-processing system. In this phase increasingly destructive interactions among vulnerability, inadequate reality-reinforcing environmental conditions, and other variable situational influences contribute to the process of switching from a functional reality-based interpretation of stimuli and appropriate responses to stressors to a psychotic interpretation and response. The third phase is open and variable with chronic states of residual deficits or remissions.

Examples of psychiatric nursing research questions derived from such a model include but are not limited to (a) What factors protect vulnerable individuals from the deteriorating cognitive processes associated with onset of psychotic symptoms? (b) What prodromal symptoms or symptom patterns can be recognized early and what interventions are appropriate for altering the course of prodromal symptoms? (c) What interventions in what format are most effective during different phases of illness? (d) What interventions are additive to psychopharmacologic treatment? (e) What perceptual-cognitive dysfunctions contribute to paranoid ideation? (f) Which interventions can successfully interrupt the cascading disintegration of information processing associated with psychosis? and (g) What interventions can assist families and significant others to assess the vulnerability of patients and effectively modify the environment to deescalate the interaction of unfavorable biological and environmental conditions to decrease the likelihood that psychoses will develop?

Most nursing research in schizophrenia reported in the literature is focused on either an examination of the experience of illness from the individual client's or family's perspectives or on some specific intervention rather than on causality or biological processes, as described in this review. Although the link between this research and nursing research may not be obvious, a second theoretical perspective that highlights the importance of this link is that of Brenner (1989). This author emphasized that client-impaired processes frequently operate at the interface of biological abnormalities and external stressors and significantly affect micro social and macro social functioning. The interactions of neural systems such as dopamine with cognitive and emotional processes of behavioral control in conjunction with external stressors create the dysfunction or deficits observed in all stages of information processing commonly experienced by individuals suffering from schizophrenia. Disturbances in attention, perception, conceptualization, memory, and recall are reflected in the characteristic difficulties of discriminating between relevant and irrelevant stimuli, maintaining focused attention, and relating previous experience to ongoing processes.

These disturbances, although rarely characterized in biological terms in the nursing research literature, are the focus of much nursing descriptive and intervention research. Even more specifically, Brenner (1989) articulated the two cycles that must be interrupted to effectively treat schizophrenia. The first cycle involves linkage of perceptual and conceptual processes and their integration. The second cycle involves the positive feedback loops that exist between cognitive dysfunctions and psychosocial stressors. This second cycle is most often the focus of nursing research in schizophrenia.

A review of nursing research related to schizophrenia published during the past few years reveals a predominant pattern of qualitative investigations examining patients' experiences, symptom monitoring, and family-caretaker characteristics and experiences. In the preceding review, investigations of the life course of schizophrenia (Harding, 1988; Harding et al., 1987a, 1987b, 1992) and investigations of symptoms (Hamera et al., 1991, 1992; O'Connor, 1991) were all examples of studies conducted by psychiatric nurses. Additionally, qualitative descriptive studies of small nonrandom samples by Howard (1994), Eakes (1995), Main, Gerace, and Camilleri (1993), and Najarian (1995) about family members' experiences, Chavetz's (1996) study of patients' perceptions of their life experience with schizophrenia, and Baker's (1995) investigation of client ability to detect signs of relapse reflect significant attention to a family–client topical area for research. This focus is consistent with previous psychiatric nursing research and relies heavily on qualitative methods. Although this focus will no doubt provide insight and perhaps aid in the clarification of research questions, there is a need to provide conceptual and research-based bridges between the extant knowledge base and intervention development.

SUMMARY AND CONCLUSIONS

The extensive and prolific research literature on schizophrenia published in the recent past reflects increased interest in this field. Despite both the increase in research effort and the quality of investigations reported, many unanswered questions exist. Schizophrenia and effective care of individuals suffering this disabling mental disorder remain fertile areas for research programs and careers for nurses and members of related disciplines.

Although the topics and need for additional research in this field are unbounded, examples include investigations of causal attributes and processes, clinical indicators of morbidity and mortality, methodological approaches to examining different levels of processes and phenomena accompanying schizophrenia and course of illness (i.e., neurodevelopmental circuitry or biochemical disturbances in conjunction with cognitive symptoms). Of equal importance are investigations of cultural contributions to the course of schizophrenia in cross-cultural studies employing methodologic consistency across cultures. There is a continuing need for increasing specification and refinement of multifactorial models of the disorder and its course; individual awareness or unawareness of symptoms and illness; and innovative models for combining targeted cognitive interventions with community supportive interventions such as psychosocial rehabilitation, outreach, family support, and consumer-provider interventions.

From a clinical research perspective there is a particular need to test effectiveness of alternative models of intervention targeting different dimensions of the disabling symptoms and course of the disorder. Through research and practice the specialty of psychiatric nursing has consistently demonstrated a sensitivity and concern for clients' perceptions, daily coping, and adaptation. This concern includes attention to physical, psychological, and social care needs, and the interaction of these needs. There remains a critical need for the specialty to prepare investigators who can determine the interventions that most effectively accommodate or diminish the effects of underlying perceptual, cognitive, and informational-processing deficits of individuals with schizophrenia. Research on interventions that specifically enhance daily coping, adaptation, general health status, and quality of life despite these deficits is a potentially powerful arena for psychiatric nursing research contributions.

REFERENCES

Adler, L. E., & Griffith, J. M. (1991). Concurrent medical illness in the schizophrenic patient: Epidemiology, diagnosis and management. *Schizophrenia Research, 4,* 91–107.

Altshuler, L. L., Conrad, A., Kovelman, J. A., & Scheibel, A. (1987). Hippocampal pyramidal cell orientation in schizophrenia: A controlled neurohistologic study of the Yakovlev Collection. *Archives of General Psychiatry, 44,* 1094–1098.

Amador, X. F., Strauss, D. H., Yale, S. A., & Gorman, J. M. (1991). Awareness of illness in schizophrenia. *Schizophrenia Bulletin, 17,* 113–132.

Andreasen, N. C. (1994). The mechanisms of schizophrenia. *Current Opinion in Neurobiology, 4,* 245–251.

Andreasen, N. C., Arndt, S., Miller, D., Flaum, M., & Nopoulos, P. (1995). Correlational studies of the Scale for the Assessment of Negative Symptoms and the Scale for the Assessment of Positive Symptoms: An overview and update. *Psychopathology, 28,* 7–17.

Andreasen, N. C., Ehrhardt, J. C., Swayze, V. W., Alliger, R. J., Yuh, W. T., Cohen, G., & Ziebell, S. (1990). Magnetic resonance imaging of the brain in schizophrenia. *Archives of General Psychiatry, 47,* 35–44.

Andreasen, N. C., Nopoulos, P., Schultz, S., Miller, D., Gupta, S., Swayze, V., & Flaum, M. (1994). Positive and negative symptoms of schizophrenia: Past, present, and future. *Acta Psychiatrica Scandinavica, 90*(suppl. 384), 51–59.

Andreasen, N. C., & Olsen, S. (1982). Negative v. positive schizophrenia: Definition and validation. *Archives of General Psychiatry, 39,* 789–794.

Andreasen, N. C., Swayze, V. W., Flaum, M., Yates, W. R., Arndt, S., & McChesney, C. (1990). Ventricular enlargement in schizophrenia evaluated with computed tomographic scanning: Effects of gender, age, and stage of illness. *Archives of General Psychiatry, 47,* 1008–1015.

Arnold, S. E. (1994). Investigations of neuronal morphology and the neuronal cytoskeleton in the hippocampal region in schizophrenia. *Neuropsychopharmacology, 10,* 634S.

Attkisson, C., Cook, J., Karno, M., Lehman, A., McGlashan, T. H., Meltaer, H. Y., O'Connor, M., Richardson, D., Rosenblatt, A., Wells, K., Williams, J., & Hohmann, A. (1992). Clinical services research. *Schizophrenia Bulletin, 18,* 561–626.

Baker, C. (1995). The development of the self-care ability to detect early signs of relapse among individuals who have schizophrenia. *Archives of Psychiatric Nursing, 9,* 261–268.

Bebbington, P. E. (1995). The content and context of compliance. *International Clinical Psychopharmacology, 9*(suppl. 5), 41–50.

Becker, M. H. (1979). Understanding patient compliance: The contribution of attitudes and other psychosocial factors. In S. J. Cohen (Ed.), *New directions in patient compliance* (pp. 1–31). Lexington, MA: D. C. Heath.

Becker, M. H., & Maiman, L. A. (1975). Sociobehavioral determinants of compliance with health and medical care recommendations. *Medical Care, 13,* 10–24.

Bell, M. D., Lysacker, P. H., Beam-Goulet, J. L., Milstein, R. M., & Lindenmayer, J. P. (1994). Five-component model of schizophrenia: Assessing the factorial invariance of the Positive and Negative Syndrome Scale. *Psychiatry Research, 52,* 295–303.

Benes, F. M., Sorensen, I., & Bird, E. D. (1991). Reduced neuronal size in posterior hippocampus of schizophrenic patients. *Schizophrenia Bulletin, 17,* 597–608.

Bernheim, K. F., & Lehman, A. F. (1985). *Working with families of the mentally ill.* New York: Norton.

Bleuler, E. (1911/1950). *Dementia Praecox or the group of schizophrenias.* New York: International Universities Press.

Bogerts, B. (1993). Recent advances in the neuropathology of schizophrenia. *Schizophrenia Bulletin, 19,* 431–445.

Bogerts, B., David, S., Falkai, P., & Tapernon-Franz, U. (1990, September). *Quantitative evaluation of astrocyte densities in schizophrenia* [Abstract]. Presented at the 17th Congress of Collegium Internationale Neuro-Psychopharmacologicum, Kyoto, Japan.

Bogerts, B., Meertz, E., & Schonfeldt-Bausch, R. (1985). Basal ganglia and limbic system pathology in schizophrenia. *Archives of General Psychiatry, 42,* 784–791.

Bond, G. R., Miller, L. D., Krumweid, R. D., & Ward, R. S. (1988). Assertive case management in three CMHC's: A controlled study. *Hospital and Community Psychiatry, 39,* 411–418.

Bornstein, R. A., Schwartzkopf, S. B., Olson, S. C., & Nasrallah, H. A. (1992). Third-ventricle enlargement and neuropsychological deficit in schizophrenia. *Biological Psychiatry, 31,* 954–961.

Breier, A., Schreiber, J. L., Dyer, J., & Pickar, D. (1991). National Institute of Mental Health Longitudinal Study of chronic schizophrenia. *Archives of General Psychiatry, 48,* 239–246.

Brenner, H. D. (1989). The treatment of basic psychological dysfunctions from a systematic point of view. *British Journal of Psychiatry, 155*(suppl. 5), 74–83.

Brenner, H. D., Hodel, B., Roder, V., & Corrigan, P. (1992). Treatment of cognitive dysfunctions and behavioral deficits in schizophrenia. *Schizophrenia Bulletin, 18,* 21–26.

Brown, R., Colter, N., Corsellis, J. A. N., Crow, T. J., Frith, C. D., Jagoe, R., Johnstone, E. C., & Marsh, L. (1986). Postmortem evidence of structural brain changes in schizophrenia: Differences in brain weight, temporal horn area, and parahippocampal gyrus compared with affective disorder. *Archives of General Psychiatry, 43,* 36–42.

Bruton, C. J., Crow, T. J., Frith, C. D., Johnstone, E. C., Owens, D. G., & Roberts, G. W. (1990). Schizophrenia and the brain: A prospective clinico-neuropathological study. *Psychological Medicine, 20,* 285–304.

Caldwell, C. B., & Gottesman, I. I. (1990). Schizophrenics kill themselves too: A review of risk factors for suicide. *Schizophrenia Bulletin, 16,* 571–589.

Carlsson, A. (1988). The current status of the dopamine hypothesis of schizophrenia. *Neuropsychopharmacology, 1,* 179–186.

Carpenter, W. T., & Strauss, J. A. (1991). The prediction of outcome in schizophrenia IV: Eleven-year follow-up of the Washington IPSS Cohort. *Journal of Nervous and Mental Disease, 179,* 517–525.

Carver, C. S., & Scheier, M. F. (1981). *Attention and self-regulation: A control-theory approach to human behavior.* New York: Springer-Verlag.

Chavetz, L. (1996). The experience of severe mental illness: A life history approach. *Archives of Psychiatric Nursing, 10*(1), 24–31.

Christison, G. W., Casanova, M. F., Weinberger, D. R., Rawlings, R., & Kleinman, J. E. (1989). A quantitative investigation of hippocampal pyramidal cell size, shape, and variability of orientation in schizophrenia. *Archives of General Psychiatry, 46,* 1027–1032.

Chua, S. E., & McKenna, P. J. (1995). Schizophrenia—a brain disease: A critical review of structural and functional cerebral abnormality in the disorder. *British Journal of Psychiatry, 166,* 563–582.

Ciompi, L. (1989). The dynamics of complex biological-psychosocial systems: Four fundamental psycho-biological mediators in the long-term evolution of schizophrenia. *British Journal of Psychiatry, 155*(suppl. 5), 15–21.

Cole, R., Kane, C. F., Zastowny, T., Grolnick, W., & Lehman, A. (1993). Expressed emotion communication and problem solving in the families of chronic schizophrenic young adults. In R. E. Cole & D. Reiss (Eds.), *How do families cope with chronic illness* (pp. 141–172). Hillsdale, NJ: Lawrence Erlbaum.

Conrad, A. J., Abebe, T., Austin, R., Forsythe, S., & Scheibel, A. B. (1991). Hippocampal pyramidal cell disarray in schizophrenia as a bilateral phenomenon. *Archives of General Psychiatry, 48,* 413–417.

Conte, H. R. (1994). Review of research in supportive psychotherapy: An update. *American Journal of Psychotherapy, 48,* 494–504.

Corrigan, P. W., & Storzbach, D. M. (1993). The ecological validity of cognitive rehabilitation for schizophrenia. *Journal of Cognitive Rehabilitation, 11,* 14–21.

Costall, B., & Naylor, R. J. (1992). The psychopharmacology of 5-HT3 receptors. *Pharmacological Toxicology, 71,* 401–415.

Coursey, R. D. (1989). Psychotherapy with persons suffering from schizophrenia: The need for a new agenda. *Schizophrenia Bulletin, 15,* 349–353.

Crow, T. J. (1980). Positive and negative schizophrenia symptoms and the role of dopamine. *British Journal of Psychiatry, 137,* 383–386.

Degreef, G., Ashtari, M., Bogerts, B., Bilder, R. M., Jody, D. N., Alvir, J. M., & Lieberman, J. A. (1992). Volumes of ventricular system subdivisions measured from magnetic resonance images in first-episode schizophrenic patients. *Archives of General Psychiatry, 49,* 531–537.

DeSisto, M. J., Harding, C. M., McCormick, R. V., Ashikaga, T., & Brooks, G. W. (1987a). The Maine-Vermont three decade studies of serious mental illness: Matches comparison of cross-sectional outcome. *American Journal of Psychiatry, 141,* 718–726.

DeSisto, M. J., Harding, C. M., McCormick, R. V., Ashikaga, T., & Brooks, G. W. (1987b). The Maine-Vermont three decade studies of serious mental illness: Longitudinal course comparisons. *British Journal of Psychiatry, 167,* 338–342.

Dolan, R. J., Bench, C. J., Liddle, P. F., Friston, K. J., Frith, C. D., Grasby, P. M., & Frackowiak, R. S. (1993). Dorsolateral prefrontal cortex dysfunction in the major psychoses; symptom or disease specificity? *Journal of Neurology, Neurosurgery, and Psychiatry, 56,* 1290–1294.

Eakes, G. G. (1995). Chronic sorrow: The lived experience of parents of chronically mentally ill individuals. *Archives of Psychiatric Nursing, 9,* 77–84.

Eaton, W. W., Bilker, W., Haro, J. M., Herrman, H., Mortensen, P. B., Freeman, H., & Burgess, P. (1992). Long-term course of hospitalization for schizophrenia: Part II. Change with passage of time. *Schizophrenia Bulletin, 18,* 229–255.

Eaton, W. W., Mortensen, P. B., Herrman, H., Freeman, H., Bilker, W., Burgess, P., & Wooff, K. (1992). Long-term course of hospitalization for schizophrenia: I. Risk for rehospitalization. *Schizophrenia Bulletin, 18,* 217–228.

Edgerton, R. B., & Cohen, A. (1994). Culture and schizophrenia: The DOSMD Challenge. *British Journal of Psychiatry, 164,* 222–231.

Falkai, P., & Bogerts, B. (1986). Cell loss in the hippocampus of schizophrenics. *European Archives of Psychiatry and Neurological Sciences, 236,* 154–161.

Falkai, P., Bogerts, B., & Rozumek, M. (1988). Quantitative study of gliosis in schizophrenia and Huntington's chorea. *Biological Psychiatry, 24,* 515–520.

Falloon, I. R. H., Boyd, J. L., & McGill, C. (1984). *Family care of schizophrenia.* New York: Guilford.

Feinberg, I. (1982). Schizophrenia: Caused by a fault in programmed synaptic elimination during adolescence? *Journal of Psychiatric Research, 17,* 319–334.

Fox, J. C. (1992). Psychiatric nursing: Directions for the future. In L. Aiken & C. Fagin (Eds.), *Charting nursing's future* (pp. 216–234). Philadelphia: J. B. Lippincott.

Fox, J. C., & Kane, C. F. (1996). Information processing deficits in schizophrenia. In A. B. McBride & J. K. Austin (Eds.), *Psychiatric mental health nursing: Integrating the behavioral and biological sciences* (pp. 321–347). Philadelphia: W. B. Saunders.

Friston, K. J., Frith, C. D., Liddle, P. F., & Frackowiak, R. S. (1991). Investigating a network model of word generation with positron emission tomography. *Proceedings of the Royal Society of London B, 244,* 101–106.

Frith, C. D., Friston, K. J., Herold, S., Silbersweig, D., Fletcher, P., Cahill, C., Dolan, R. J., Frackowiak, R. S., & Liddle, P. F. (1995). Regional brain activity in chronic schizophrenic patients during the performance of a verbal fluency task: Evidence for a failure of inhibition in left superior temporal cortex. *British Journal of Psychiatry, 167,* 343–349.

Gardos, G., Cole, J. O., & LaBrie, R. A. (1982). A twelve-year follow-up study of chronic schizophrenics. *Hospital and Community Psychiatry, 33,* 983–984.

Gerlach, J. (1994). Oral versus depot administration of neuroleptics in relapse prevention. *Acta Psychiatrica Scandinavica, 89*(suppl. 382), 28–32.

Gerlach, J. (1995). Depot neuroleptics in relapse prevention: Advantages and disadvantages. *International Clinical Psychopharmacology, 9*(suppl. 5), 17–20.

Goldberg, T. E., Weinberger, D. R., Berman, K. F., Pliskin, N. H., & Podd, M. H. (1987). Further evidence for dementia of prefrontal type in schizophrenia? A controlled study of teaching the Wisconsin Card Sorting Test. *Archives of General Psychiatry, 44,* 1008–1014.

Goldstein, M. J. (1987). Psychosocial issues. *Schizophrenia Bulletin, 13,* 157–171.

Goldstein, M. J. (1995). Psychoeducation and relapse prevention. *International Clinical Psychopharmacology, 9*(suppl. 5), 59–69.

Gunderson, J. G., Frank, A. F., Katz, H. M., Vannicelli, M. L., Frosch, J. P., & Knapp, P. H. (1984). Effects of psychotherapy in schizophrenia: II. Comparative outcome of two forms of treatment. *Schizophrenia Bulletin, 10,* 564–598.

Gur, R. E., & Pearlson, G. D. (1993). Neuroimaging in schizophrenia research. *Schizophrenia Bulletin, 19,* 337–353.

Hambrecht, M., Reicher-Rossler, A., Fatkenheuer, B., Louza, M. R., & Hafner, H. (1994). Higher morbidity risk for schizophrenia in males: Fact or fiction? *Comprehensive Psychiatry, 35,* 39–49.

Hamera, E. K., Peterson, K. A., Handley, S. M., Plumlee, A. A., & Frank-Ragan, E. (1991). Patient self-regulation and functioning in schizophrenia. *Hospital and Community Psychiatry, 42,* 630–631.

Hamera, E. K., Peterson, K. A., Young, L. M., & Schaumloffel, M. M. (1992). Symptoms monitoring in schizophrenia: Potential for enhancing self-care. *Archives of Psychiatric Nursing, 6,* 324–330.

Harding, C. (1988). Course types in schizophrenia: An analysis of European and American studies. *Schizophrenia Bulletin, 14,* 633–643.

Harding, C. M., Brooks, G. W., Ashikaga, T., Strauss, J. S., & Breier, A. (1987a). The Vermont Longitudinal Study of persons with severe mental illness: II. Long-term outcome of subjects who retrospectively met DSM-III criteria for schizophrenia. *American Journal of Psychiatry, 144,* 718–726.

Harding, C. M., Brooks, G. W., Ashikaga, T., Strauss, J. S., & Breier, A. (1987b). The Vermont Longitudinal Study of persons with severe mental illness: I. Methodology, study sample, and overall status 32 years later. *American Journal of Psychiatry, 144,* 718–726.

Harding, C. M., Zubin, J., & Strauss, J. S. (1992). Chronicity in schizophrenia: Revisited. *British Journal of Psychiatry, 161,* 27–37.

Harrison, P. J. (1995). On the neuropathology of schizophrenia and its dementia: Neurodevelopmental, neurodegenerative, or both? *Neurodegeneration, 4,* 1–12.

Harvey, I., Ron, M. A., Du Boulay, G., Wicks, D., Lewis, S. W., & Murray, R. M. (1993). Reduction of cortical volume in schizophrenia on magnetic resonance imaging. *Psychological Medicine, 23,* 591–604.

Haywood, T. W., Kravitz, H. M., Grossman, L. S., Cavanaugh, J. L., Davis, J. M., & Lewis, D. A. (1995). Predicting the "revolving door" phenomenon among patients with schizophrenic, schizoaffective and affective disorders. *American Journal of Psychiatry, 152,* 856–861.

Heckers, S., Heinsen, H., Heinsen, Y. C., & Beckmann, H. (1991). Cortex, white matter, and basal ganglia in schizophrenia: A volumetric postmortem study. *Biological Psychiatry, 29,* 556–566.

Hirsch, S., Bowen, J., Emami, J., Cramer, P., Jolley, A., Haw, C., & Dickinson, M. (1996). A one year prospective study of the effect of life events and medication in the etiology of schizophrenic relapse. *British Journal of Psychiatry, 168,* 49–56.

Hodel, B., & Brenner, H. D. (1994). Cognitive therapy with schizophrenic patients: Conceptual basis, present state, future directions. *Acta Psychiatrica Scandinavica, 90*(suppl. 384), 108–115.

Hogarty, G. E. (1993). Prevention of relapse in chronic schizophrenic patients. *Journal of Clinical Psychiatry, 54*(Suppl.), 18–23.

Holmberg, S. K., & Kane, C. F. (1995). Severe psychiatric disorder and physical health risk. *Clinical Nurse Specialist, 9,* 287–292, 298.

Howard, P. B. (1994). Lifelong maternal caregiving for children with schizophrenia. *Archives of Psychiatric Nursing, 8,* 107–114.

Hughlings-Jackson, J. (1894/1931). The factors of insanities. *Medical press and circular.* In J. Taylor (Ed.), *Selected writings.* London: Hodder and Stoughton.

Jakob, H., & Beckmann, H. (1986). Prenatal developmental disturbances in the limbic allocortex in schizophrenics. *Journal of Neural Transmission, 65,* 303–326.

Jernigan, T. L., Zisook, S., Heaton, R. K., Moranville, J. T., Hesselink, J. R., & Braff, D. L. (1991). Magnetic resonance imaging abnormalities in lenticular nuclei and cerebral cortex in schizophrenia. *Archives of General Psychiatry, 48,* 881–890.

Jeste, D. V., & Lohr, J. B. (1989). Hippocampal pathologic findings in schizophrenia. *Archives of General Psychiatry, 46,* 1019–1024.

Johnstone, E. C., Owens, D. G. C., Crow, T. J., Frith, C. D., Alexandropolis, K., Bydder, G., & Cotler, N. (1989). Temporal lobe structure as determined by nuclear magnetic resonance in schizophrenia and bipolar affective disorder. *Journal of Neurology, Neurosurgery and Psychiatry, 52,* 736–741.

Jones, P. B., Harvey, I., Lewis, S. W., Toone, B. K., Van, O. J., Williams, M., & Murray, R. M. (1994). Cerebral ventricle dimensions as risk factors for schizophrenia and affective psychosis: An epidemiological approach to analysis. *Psychological Medicine, 24,* 995–1011.

Kane, C. F. (1994). Psychoeducational programs for families of the mentally ill: From blaming to caring. In E. Kahana, D. E. Biegel, & M. Wykle (Eds.), *Family caregiving across the lifespan* (pp. 219–239). Beverly Hills: Sage.

Kay, S. R. (1991). Positive and negative syndromes in schizophrenia. Assessment and research. In *Clinical and experimental research. Monograph Series of the Department of Psychiatry, Albert Einstein College of Medicine of Yeshiva University.* New York: Brunner/Mazel.

Kay, S. R., Fiszbein, A., & Opler, L. A. (1987). The positive and negative syndrome scale (PANSS) for schizophrenia. *Schizophrenia Bulletin, 13,* 261–276.

Kay, S. R., & Sevy, S. (1990). Pyramidal model of schizophrenia. *Schizophrenia Bulletin, 16,* 537–545.

Kelsoe, J. R, Jr., Cadet, J. L., Pickar, D., & Weinberger, D. R. (1988). Quantitative neuroanatomy in schizophrenia: A controlled magnetic resonance imaging study. *Archives of General Psychiatry, 45,* 533–541.

Kirch, D. G., & Weinberger, D. R. (1986). Anatomical neuropathology in schizophrenia: Post-mortem findings. In H. A. Nasrallah & D. R. Weinberger (Eds.), *Handbook of schizophrenia: The neurology of schizophrenia* (Vol. 1, pp. 325–348). Amsterdam: Elsevier.

Kovelman, J. A., & Scheibel, A. B. (1984). A neurohistological correlate of schizophrenia. *Biological Psychiatry, 19,* 1601–1621.

Kraepelin, E. (1896). *Lehrbuch der Psychiatrie.* Leipzig: J. A. Barth.

Lam, D. H. (1991). Psychosocial family intervention in schizophrenia: A review of empirical studies. *Psychological Medicine, 21,* 423–441.

Lantos, P. (1988). The neuropathology of schizophrenia: A critical review of recent work. In P. Bebbington & P. McGuffin (Eds.), *Schizophrenia: The major issues* (pp. 73–89). Oxford: Heinemann/Mental Health Foundation.

Lehtinen, K. (1994). Need-adapted treatment of schizophrenia: Family interventions. *British Journal of Psychiatry, 164*, 89–96.

Leventhal, H., Norenz, D., & Strauss, A. (1982). Self-regulation and the mechanism for symptom appraisal. In D. Mechanic (Ed.), *Psychological epidemiology* (pp. 56–86). New York: Academic Press.

Lewis, S. W. (1990). Computerized tomography in schizophrenia 15 years on. *British Journal of Psychiatry, 157*(suppl. 9), 16–24.

Liberman, R. P. (1982). What is schizophrenia? *Schizophrenia Bulletin, 8*, 435–437.

Liberman, R. P. (1992). *Handbook of psychiatric rehabilitation.* New York: MacMillan.

Liberman, R. P., & Kopelowicz, A. (1995). Basic elements in biobehavioral treatment and rehabilitation of schizophrenia. *International Clinical Psychopharmacology, 9*(suppl. 5), 51–58.

Liberman, R. P., Mueser, K. M., Wallace, C. J., Jacobs, H. E., & Eckman, T. (1986) Training skills in the psychiatrically disabled: Learning coping and competence. *Schizophrenia Bulletin, 12*, 631–647.

Liddle, P. F., Friston, K. J., Frith, C. D., Hirsch, S. R., Jones, T., & Frackowiak, R. S. (1992). Patterns of cerebral blood flow in schizophrenia. *British Journal of Psychiatry, 160*, 179–186.

Lindenmayer, J. P., Bernstein-Hyman, R., & Grochowski, S. (1994). Five factor model of schizophrenia: Initial validation. *Journal of Nervous and Mental Disease, 182*, 631–638.

Lyons, J. S., Cook, J. A., Ruth, A. R., Karver, M., & Slagg, N. B. (1996). Service delivery using consumer staff in a mobile crisis assessment program. *Community Mental Health Journal, 32*, 33–40.

Main, M. C., Gerace, L. M., & Camilleri, D. (1993). Information sharing concerning schizophrenia in a family member: Adult siblings' perspective. *Archives of Psychiatric Nursing, 7*, 147–153.

Marsh, L., Suddath, R. L., Higgins, N., & Weinberger, D. R. (1994). Medial temporal lobe structures in schizophrenia: Relationship of size to duration of illness. *Schizophrenia Research, 11*, 225–238.

McCandless-Glimcher, L., McKnight, S., Hamera, E., Smith, B. L., Peterson, K. A., & Plumlee, A. A. (1986). Use of symptoms by schizophrenics to monitor and regulate their illness. *Hospital and Community Psychiatry, 37*, 929–933.

McFarlane, W. R. (1994). Multiple-family groups and psychoeducation in the treatment of schizophrenia. *New Directions in Mental Health Services, 62*, 13–22.

McFarlane, W. R., Link, B., Dushay, R., & Marchal, J. (1995). Psychoeducational multiple family groups: Four-year relapse outcome in schizophrenia. *Family Process, 34*, 127–144.

McFarlane, W. R., Lukens, E., Link, B., & Dushay, R. (1995). Multiple-family groups and psychoeducation in the treatment of schizophrenia. *Archives of General Psychiatry, 52*, 679–687.

McGlashan, T. H. (1984a). Testing four diagnostic systems for schizophrenia. *Archives of General Psychiatry, 41*, 141–144.

McGlashan, T. H. (1984b). The Chestnut Lodge follow-up study: I. Follow-up methodology and study sample. *Archives of General Psychiatry, 41*, 573–585.

McGlashan, T. H. (1988). A selective review of Recent North American long-term follow-up studies of schizophrenia. *Schizophrenia Bulletin, 14,* 515–542.

McKenna, P. J. (1994). *Schizophrenia and related syndromes.* Oxford: Oxford University Press.

McKenna, P. J., Tamlyn, D., Lund, C. E., Mortimer, A. M., Hammond, S., & Baddeley, A. D. (1990). Amnesic syndrome in schizophrenia. *Psychological Medicine, 20,* 967–972.

Merwin, R., & Mauck, A. (1995). Psychiatric nursing outcome research: The state of the science. *Archives of Psychiatric Nursing, 9,* 311–331.

Miller, D., Arndt, S., & Andreasen, N. C. (1993). Alogia, attentional impairment, and inappropriate affect: Their status in the dimensions of schizophrenia. *Comprehensive Psychiatry, 34,* 221–226.

Mowbray, C. T., Chamberlain, P., Jennings, M., & Reed, C. (1988). Consumer-run mental health services: Results from five demonstration projects. *Community Mental Health Journal, 24,* 151–156.

Mowbray, C. T., Moxley, D. P., Trasher, S., Bybee, D., McCrohan, N., Harris, S., & Clover, G. (1996). Consumers as community support providers: Issues created by role innovation. *Community Mental Health Journal, 32,* 47–67.

Najarian, S. P. (1995). Family experience with positive client response to clozapine. *Archives of Psychiatric Nursing, 9,* 3–10.

Niznik, H. B., Hubert, H. M., & Van, T. (1992). Dopamine receptor genes: New tools for molecular psychiatry. *Journal of Psychiatry and Neuroscience, 17,* 158–180.

Nuechterlein, K., & Dawson, M. (1984). A heuristic vulnerability/stress model of schizophrenic episodes. *Schizophrenia Bulletin, 10,* 300–312.

O'Connor, F. W. (1991). Symptom monitoring for relapse prevention in schizophrenia. *Archives of Psychiatric Nursing, 5,* 193–201.

Overall, J. E., & Gorham, D. R. (1962). Brief Psychiatric Rating Scale. *Psychological Reports, 10,* 799–912.

Pakkenberg, B. (1987). Post-mortem study of chronic schizophrenic brains. *British Journal of Psychiatry, 151,* 744–752.

Pakkenberg, B. (1990). Pronounced reduction of total neuron number in mediodorsal thalamic nucleus and nucleus accumbens in schizophrenics. *Archives of General Psychiatry, 47,* 1023–1028.

Paulman, R. G., Devous, M. D., Gregory, R. R., Herman, J. H., Jennings, L., Bonte, F. J., Nasrallah, H. A., & Raese, J. D. (1990). Hypofrontality and cognitive impairment in schizophrenia: Dynamic single-photon tomography and neuropsychological assessment of schizophrenic brain function. *Biological Psychiatry, 27,* 377–399.

Pettegrew, J. W., Keshavan, M. S., Panchalingam, K., Strychor, S., Kaplan, D. B., Tretta, M. G., & Allen, M. (1991). Alterations in brain high-energy phosphate and membrane phospholipid metabolism in first-episode, drug-naive schizophrenics: A pilot study of the dorsal prefrontal cortex by in vivo Phosphorus 31 nuclear magnetic resonance spectroscopy. *Archives of General Psychiatry, 48,* 563–568.

Pettegrew, J. W., Strychor, S., McKeag, D. S., Keshavan, M., Tretta, G., & Allen, M. (1992). Membrane alterations in schizophrenia [Abstract]. *Biological Psychiatry, 27*(suppl.), 113A.

Phillips, L. (1953). Case history data and prognosis in schizophrenia. *Journal of Nervous and Mental Disease, 117,* 515–525.

Ram, R., Bromet, E. J., Eaton, W. W., Pato, C., & Schwartz, J. E. (1992). The natural course of schizophrenia: A review of first-admission studies. *Schizophrenia Bulletin, 18,* 185–207.

Randolph, E. T., Eth, S., Glynn, S. M., Paz, G. G., Leong, G. B., Shaner, A. L., Strachen, A., VanVort, W., Escobar, J., & Liberman, R. P. (1994). Behavioural family management in schizophrenia: Outcome of a clinic based intervention. *British Journal of Psychiatry, 164,* 501–506.

Raz, S., & Raz, N. (1990). Structural brain abnormalities in the major psychoses: A quantitative review of the evidence from computerized imaging. *Psychological Bulletin, 108,* 93–108.

Roberts, G. W. (1991). Schizophrenia: A neuropathological perspective. *British Journal of Psychiatry, 158,* 8–17.

Rockland, L. H. (1993). A review of supportive psychotherapy, 1986–1992. *Hospital and Community Psychiatry, 44,* 1053–1060.

Rossi, A., Stratta, P., D'Albenzio, L., Tartaro, A., Schiazza, G., diMichele, V., Bolino, F., & Casacchia, M. (1990). Reduced temporal lobe areas in schizophrenia: Preliminary evidences from a controlled multiplanar magnetic resonance imaging study. *Biological Psychiatry, 27,* 61–68.

Rossi, A., Stratta, P., Dimichele, V., Galluci, M., Splendiani, A., Decataldo, S., & Cassacchia, M. (1991). Temporal lobe structure by magnetic resonance in bipolar affective disorders and schizophrenia. *Journal of Affective Disorders, 21,* 19–22.

Saykin, A. J., Gur, R. C., Gur, R. E., Mozley, P. D., Mozley, L. H., Resnick, S. M., Kester, D. B., & Stafiniak, P. (1991). Neuropsychological function in schizophrenia: Selective impairment in memory and learning. *Archives of General Psychiatry, 48,* 618–624.

Scheibel, A. B., & Kovelman, J. A. (1981). Disorientation of the hippocampal pyramidal cell and its processes in the schizophrenic patient. *Biological Psychiatry, 16,* 101–102.

Schneider, K. (1950/1959). *Clinical psychopathology.* New York: Grune and Stratton.

Schooler, N. (1991). Maintenance medication for schizophrenia: Strategies for dose reduction. *Schizophrenia Bulletin, 17,* 311–324.

Schooler, N. (1993). Reducing dosage in maintenance treatment of schizophrenia: Review and Prognosis. *British Journal of Psychiatry, 163*(suppl. 22), 58–65.

Selvini, M. P., Boscolo, L., Cecchini, G., & Prata, G. (1978). *Paradox and counterparadox.* New York: Jason Aronson.

Selvini-Palazzoli, M., Boscolo, L., Cecchini, G., & Prata, G. (1980). Hypothesizing-circularity-neutrality: Three guidelines for the conductor of the session. *Family Process, 19,* 3–12.

Shallice, T., Burgess, P. W., & Frith, C. D. (1991). Can the neuropsychological case-study approach be applied to schizophrenia. *Psychological Medicine, 21,* 661–673.

Shapiro, R. M. (1993). Regional neuropathology in schizophrenia: Where are we? Where are we going. *Schizophrenia Research, 10,* 187–239.

Shenton, M. E., Kikinis, R., Jolesz, F. A., Pollak, S. D., LeMay, M., Wible, C. G., Hokama, H., Martin, J., Metcalf, D., & Coleman, M. (1992). Abnormalities of the left temporal lobe and thought disorder in schizophrenia: A quantitative magnetic resonance imaging study. *New England Journal of Medicine, 327,* 604–612.

Sherman, P. S., & Porter, R. (1991). Mental health consumers as case management aides. *Hospital and Community Psychiatry, 42,* 494–498.

Simpson, M. D. C., Slater, P., Royston, C., & Deakin, J. F. W. (1992). Regionally selective deficits in uptake sites for glutamate and gamma-aminobutyric acid in the basal ganglia in schizophrenia. *Psychiatry Research, 42,* 273–282.

Singh, M. M., & Kay, S. R. (1975). A comparative study of haloperidol and chlorpromazine in terms of clinical effects and therapeutic reversal with benzotropine in schizophrenia. *Psychopharmacology, 43,* 103–113.

Smith, R. C., Baumgartner, R., & Calderon, M. (1987). Magnetic resonance imaging studies of the brains of schizophrenic patients. *Psychiatry Research, 20,* 33–46.

Solomon, P., & Draine, J. (1994). Satisfaction with mental health treatment in a randomized trial of consumer case management. *Journal of Nervous and Mental Disease, 182,* 179–184.

Solomon, P., & Draine, J. (1996). Perspectives concerning consumers as case managers. *Community Mental Health Journal, 32,* 41–46.

Stanton, A. H., Gunderson, J. G., Knapp, P. H., Frank, A. F., Vannicelli, M. L., Schnitzer, R., & Rosenthal, R. (1984). Effects of psychotherapy in schizophrenia: I. Design and implementation of a controlled study. *Schizophrenia Bulletin, 10,* 520–563.

Stein, L. I., & Test, M. A. (1980). Alternative to mental hospital treatment: I. conceptual model, treatment program, and clinical evaluation. *Archives of General Psychiatry, 37,* 392–397.

Stevens, J. R. (1992). Abnormal reinnervation as a basis for schizophrenia: A hypothesis. *Archives of General Psychiatry, 49,* 238–243.

Strauss, J. S., & Carpenter, W. T. (1974). Prediction of outcome in schizophrenia: II. Relationships between predictor and outcome variables. *Archives of General Psychiatry, 31,* 37–42.

Strauss, M. E. (1993). Relations of symptoms to cognitive deficits in schizophrenia. *Schizophrenia Bulletin, 19,* 215–231.

Suddath, R. L., Casanova, M. F., Goldberg, T. E., Daniel, D. G., Kelsoe, J. R., Jr., & Weinberger, D. R. (1989). Temporal lobe pathology in schizophrenia: A quantitative magnetic resonance imaging study. *American Journal of Psychiatry, 146,* 464–472.

Suddath, R. L., Christison, G. W., Torrey, E. F., Casanova, M. F., & Weinberger, D. R. (1990). Anatomical abnormalities in the brains of monozygotic twins discordant for schizophrenia. *New England Journal of Medicine, 322,* 789–794.

Swayze, V. W., II, Andreasen, N. C., Alliger, R. J., Yuh, W. T. C., & Ehrhardt, J. C. (1992). Subcortical and temporal structures in affective disorder and schizophrenia: A magnetic resonance study. *Biological Psychiatry, 31,* 221–240.

Swerdlow, N. R., & Geyer, M. A. (1993). Clozapine and haloperidol in an animal model of sensorimotor gating deficits in schizophrenia. *Pharmacology and the Biochemistry of Behavior, 44,* 741–744.

Tarrier, N. (1991). Some aspects of family interventions in schizophrenia: I. Adherence to intervention programs. *British Journal of Psychiatry, 159,* 475–480.

Van Horn, J. D., & McManus, I. C. (1992). Ventricular enlargement in schizophrenia: A meta-analysis of studies of the ventricle: Brain ratio (VBR). *British Journal of Psychiatry, 160,* 687–697.

von Knorring, L., & Lindstrom, E. (1995). Principle components and further possibilities with the PANSS. *Acta Psychiatrica Scandinavica, 91*(suppl. 388), 5–10.

Weinberger, D. R. (1987). Implications of normal brain development for the pathogenesis of schizophrenia. *Archives of General Psychiatry, 44,* 660–669.

Weinberger, D. R., Berman, K. F., & Zec, R. F. (1986). Physiologic dysfunction of dorsolateral prefrontal cortex in schizophrenia: I. Regional cerebral blood flow evidence. *Archives of General Psychiatry, 43,* 114–124.

Whitworth, A. B., & Fleischhacker, W. W. (1995). Adverse effects of antipsychotic drugs. *International Clinical Psychopharmacology, 9*(suppl. 5), 21–27.

Wolkin, A., Sanfilipo, M., Wolf, A. P., Angrist, B., Brodie, J. D., & Rotrosen, J. (1992). Negative symptoms and hypofrontality in chronic schizophrenia. *Archives of General Psychiatry, 49,* 959–965.

Young, A. H., Blackwood, D. H. R., Roxborough, H., McQueen, J. K., Martin, M. J., & Kean, D. (1991). A magnetic resonance imaging study of schizophrenia. *British Journal of Psychiatry, 158,* 158–164.

Zastowny, T. R., Lehman, A. F., Cole, R. E., & Kane, C. F. (1992). Family management of schizophrenia: A comparison of behavioral and supportive family treatment. *Psychiatric Quarterly, 63,* 159–186.

Zipursky, R. B., Lim, K. O., Sullivan, E. V., Brown, B. W., & Pfefferbaum, A. (1992). Widespread cerebral gray matter volume deficits in schizophrenia. *Archives of General Psychiatry, 49,* 195–205.

Zubin, J., & Spring, B. (1977). Vulnerability—A new view of schizophrenia. *Journal of Abnormal Psychology, 86,* 103–126.

Zubin, J., Steinhauer, S. T., & Condray, R. (1992). Vulnerability to relapse in schizophrenia. *British Journal of Psychiatry, 161*(suppl. 18), 13–18.

Index

suicidal behavior and, 91, 93
DeSisto, J. J., 295
Desmond, S. M., 147
Diabetes mellitus; *see also* Childhood diabetes, behavioral research on
diet and, 4
DiClemente, F. J., 127
Diener, M., 227, 228
Diet; *see also* Childhood nutrition;
    School-age child health care
death by disease and, 4
Dietary Intervention Study in Children
    (DISC I), 11
Dietrich, D. R., 85
Dietz, W. H., 13, 15, 125
DiIorio, C., 127
DISC I (Dietary Intervention Study in
    Children), 11
Dishman, R. K., 146
Divorce
    adolescent antisocial behavior and,
        86
    conduct disorder and, 96
    psychosocial health of children and,
        50, 85
Docherty, D., 152
Dolan, R. J., 293
Domel, S. B., 8, 22
D'Onofrio, C. N., 43
Dopamine, schizophrenia and, 292
Dorius, G. L., 123
Downey, A. M., 154
Drotar, D., 71, 77
Dryfoos, J. G., 96, 104–105, 222
Dubbert, P., 17
DuBois, D. L., 89
Duerst, B., 130
Duffy, J., 229
Duffy, M. E., 181
Dullinger, D., 258–260
Durham, M. L., 190
Dyspnea Questionnaire, 256

E
Eakes, G. G., 310
Ealing Teen Mums' Club, 231

East, P., 226–227, 232
Eating disorders
    cultural factors and, 20–21
    depression comorbidity with, 91
    of diabetic children, 71
    prevention of and programs for, 105
    risk factors of, 97–98
Eaton, M. L., 258–259, 294
Eaton, W. W., 294
Eccles, J. S., 146, 149
Economic malnutrition, of children,
    23–25
Edgerton, R. B., 294
Edmundson, E., 159, 163
Educational Resource Informational Center (ERIC), 140
Efthimiou, J., 273–274
Ehrhardt, A., 131
EIO (Exploratory, insight-oriented psychotherapy), for schizophrenia,
    304
Elderly health promotion
    abstract regarding, 173
    behaviors vs. outcomes, longitudinal
        studies of, 176–177
    age difference studies and,
        177–179
    clinical preventive services study
        of, 184
    correlate identification studies of,
        182–183
    descriptive studies of, 177
    gender difference study of, 183
    gender and socioeconomic factors
        study of, 183–184
    health-seeking behavior study of,
        180
    internal locus of control studies
        and, 179–182
    interpersonal relationship and physical activity study of, 182
    rural female study of, 183
    rural vs. urban study of, 181
    self-care management studies of,
        180–181

Contents of Previous Volumes

VOLUME II

ORDER FORM

Save 10% on Volume 17 with this coupon.

___Check here to order the ANNUAL REVIEW OF NURSING RESEARCH, Volume 17, 1999 at a 10% discount. You will receive an invoice requesting prepayment.

Save 10% on all future volumes with a continuation order.

___Check here to place your continuation order for the ANNUAL REVIEW OF NURSING RESEARCH. You will receive a prepayment invoice with a 10% discount upon publication of each new volume, beginning with Volume 17, 1999. You may pay for prompt shipment or cancel with no obligation.

Name _____

Institution _____

Address _____

City/State/Zip _____

Examination copies for possible adoption are available to instructors "on approval" only. Write on institutional letterhead, noting course, level, present text, and expected enrollment (include $3.50 for postage and handling). Prices slightly higher overseas. Prices subject to change.

Mail this coupon to:
SPRINGER PUBLISHING COMPANY
536 Broadway, New York, N.Y. 10012

S *Springer Publishing Company*

Developing Research in Nursing and Health
Quantitative and Qualitative Methods

Carol Noll Hoskins, PhD, RN, FAAN

"It is a clear and unencumbered 'snapshot' of essential information that can serve as a study guide for graduate students, a handy reference for researchers and faculty, and an 'instructor's manual' for teaching research. I would certainly use this guide...."
—**Harriet R. Feldman**, *PhD, RN, FAAN*
Dean and Professor, Pace University Lienhard School of Nursing

This handy volume is an excellent adjunct to traditional research texts and courses, and a boon to educators and researchers challenged to "know all" about the processes of research. Some of the important general features include:

• an outline format designed to highlight key information
• clarification of confusing and difficult information
• exemplars used throughout each chapter and in the appendices

This valuable guide stands out from traditional texts by offering a succinct overview of key sources of nursing and related literature; differentiation of the theoretical framework of quantitative and qualitative studies; a guide to abstracting research studies; clear presentation of the types, rules, and procedures of sampling; and a conceptual appproach to organizing descriptive and inferential statistics and qualitative data analysis.

Contents: Research in Nursing • The Research Question — Hypotheses • The Literature Review, Definition of Terms, and Theoretical Framework • Research Designs • Sampling in Qualitative Designs—-Basic Issues and Concepts • Data Analysis and Interpretation—-Qualitative Designs • Principles of Measurement • Development of Quantitative Measures

1998   130pp   0-8261-1185-8   softcover

536 Broadway, New York, NY 10012-3955 • (212) 431-4370 • Fax (212) 941-7842